THE UPSIDE TO EVERYTHING, EVEN BREAST CANCER

Theresa Drescher

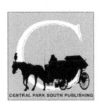

The Upside to Everything, Even Breast Cancer

Published by Central Park South Publishing, 2021
www.centralparksouthpublishing.com

Cover Art Direction: X Baczewska
Cover Designer: Val Gyorgy
Interior Designer: Victor Marcos
Author Photo: Franklin Thompson
Cover Photo: Tomekbudujedomek/Getty Images

ISBN:
978-1-956452-90-7 (Hardback)
978-1-956452-00-6 (Paperback)
978-1-956452-01-3 (E-book)

Dedication

To my mother, Margaret Alice Drescher, *who never met a cancer patient she would not help.*

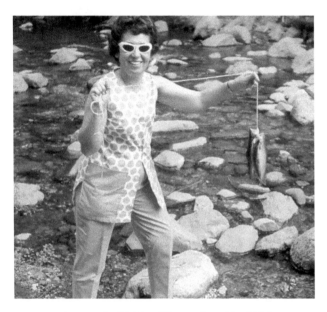

August 8, 1918 – November 19, 1990

Table of Contents

THE UPSIDE TO EVERYTHING, EVEN BREAST CANCER

Prologue

My relationship with cancer began when I was nine years old. I did not have cancer, but that was when the disease became all I thought about.

My family has been inundated with it: breast, kidney, pancreatic, lung, brain, liver or blood cancer has affected one or more individuals on both sides of my family, both genders, at all ages for generations.

Even though my family gathered and prayed, went to church and lit candles for those diagnosed, no one ever talked about the disease. Everyone knew who had what kind and how each one was doing, but that's where it ended. Probably, no one knew enough about their cancer diagnosis to give anything more than basic information anyway. In the 1950s, '60s and '70s, people did not question doctors about their disease or how they planned to address the illness. Much of medicine was a complete mystery to the public. Doctors were gods. Their word was sacrosanct, and decisions were final. I would hear someone was sick with it and then not hear anything about them again until they were either better or dead. It was more often the latter, at which time my parents would dress up and go to a funeral. The end.

The lack of conversation about anyone's cancer instilled a deep dread in me. I did not know if you could catch cancer like a cold or the flu, get it by touching someone who had it, or if it came from something you ate or drank. What if it really was God's punishment for bad behavior, as the nuns told me? Their explanation for cancer made me fearful, and I second-guessed all my actions. It also made me dissect the behavior of everyone in my family. This way, when one of them was diagnosed, I would know how she got the disease and would avoid doing whatever I thought her bad behavior was. This was before the internet, so my only sources of information were the dictionary and the Encyclopedia Britannica. The one thing I understood from reading them was that cancer kills you.

My parents met and married when they both were in the Army in San Francisco during World War II. After the war was over, they focused on starting a family. It took eleven years for my mother to get pregnant with me. Once she did, she left the service and became a stay-at-home mom. Two years later my sister was born. My father, a career military man, continued to serve through the Korean and Vietnam Wars before he retired as a master sergeant.

We settled into life on the base as much as a military family can. My dad spent a lot of time building things in his workshop, buying camping equipment, reading or bowling with the Army league. My mom was very social, arranging cookouts, cocktail parties and kids' activities with the other military wives. I was a Brownie in the Girl Scouts, and my mom was the leader of our troop. We also belonged to the community center where we swam and played with other children. We could have been the poster people for the all-American family living the dream.

When my dad received his orders to go to Vietnam, my parents felt it would be easier for my mom if we lived in an apartment in the nearby town of Yuma City, about thirty miles away, while he was gone. There were more services there, and she would not have to manage the upkeep of a house by herself. So, we packed up all our belongings, left our friends behind and moved.

I was nine, my sister, Bonnie, was seven, and we had recently started the fall semester at our new grade school, Blessed Sacrament. My dad had been gone a few weeks. On a Monday morning, my mom drove us to school as usual, but as she was dropping us off, she told us she had a doctor's appointment that afternoon and a neighbor in our apartment complex was going to pick us up. We were to stay with the neighbor until my mom came to get us. This was odd because we barely knew our neighbors, but our mom assured us everything was fine. That afternoon, when the neighbor picked us up she told us our mom was sick, so we were going to stay with her and her kids that evening. She would not elaborate on what was wrong with my mom or where she was.

That night Bonnie and I slept on their couch end to end, with our feet touching in the middle. I lay there and stared at the reflection of the water from the complex's pool on the walls and ceiling. I could not imagine what was so wrong with my mother that she could not be home with us. Or why she did not call us. She could not be fine if she just left us like this. I knew she would never do that. I thought about my little sister at the other end of the couch and worried if I would have to take care of her.

The next afternoon, when the neighbor picked us up, she told us our mom was very sick and would not be home for a while. She also told us she did not have enough room for us to continue staying with her, so she had a new plan. She would take us to school in the morning and pick us up in the afternoon and we could have dinner with her family in the evening, but we were to stay up in our apartment alone. She told us we were big girls now and was confident we could take care of ourselves. With no word from my mom or dad and no one to call or a familiar face to turn to, Bonnie and I had no other option but to go back to our apartment, so we left and went home.

Two weeks went by like that. Then one afternoon, while we were watching TV after school, my dad walked in the front door with one of his military buddies. We did not know he was coming home from Vietnam, so we were surprised—and wildly happy—to see him. He told us our mom was in the hospital and he had already been to see her. He said he would take us to visit her tomorrow. He did not go into any detail as to what was wrong with her or how sick she was.

The next day, when we got to the hospital they told my dad that Bonnie and I were too young to go into the patients' rooms. We had to stay out in the waiting room. My sister and I sat in chairs by the door that led to the patients' rooms, and my dad left to get my mom. A short while later with a nurse's help, he brought her out in a wheelchair to the waiting room to see us.

She was hunched over, wrapped in blankets, shivering and in tremendous pain. We were told she was very sick, and we could not touch, kiss or get too close to her, so we just stood and stared. As I later learned, she had had a radical mastectomy for breast cancer. She was 47 years old. Her surgery was so extensive that her skin and muscle from her chest, under her arm and part of her back had been removed. The surgeon had grafted skin from the front of both her thighs on to her chest and around her body to replace all that was taken in the surgery.

My mom behaved as if nothing was wrong. She smiled and assured us things were going to be fine. She would be home soon. She was able to visit with us for only five minutes, and when that time was up, she blew us kisses and my dad and the nurse took her back to her room. Stunned, I watched them go. Bonnie and I sat quietly and waited for him to come back. I knew my mom was not coming home anytime soon.

My dad came out about twenty minutes later with a grim look on his face, and in silence, we walked to the car. He took us to a toy store and told us to get whatever we wanted. Bonnie and I wandered around aimlessly in the small, hot, creaky toy store without saying a word. Finally, we said there was nothing we wanted. My dad picked out a couple of toys for us, and we left. No one said a word the entire thirty-minute drive home.

That was the last day we saw my mom for about six months. She was able to have surgery at the hospital in Yuma City, but there were no facilities where she could have chemotherapy or radiation treatments. My dad made arrangements for her to have them in Phoenix, more than three hours away, and she went there directly from the hospital. I questioned him about what was going on, but he would not discuss it. I heard she had cancer by eavesdropping on his conversation with others.

Our aunts and uncles had their own families to contend with and could not come to Yuma to take care of us. After taking care of my mom, my dad met the neighbors and set up a tag team of care to make sure

Bonnie and I ate, went to school and had clean clothes. He bought us a puppy. Then one morning, he took us to school, and that afternoon, when we came home, he was gone. Without a word, he had returned to the war. The Army had given him two weeks stateside to take care of his family.

Bonnie and I stayed alone in our apartment and took care of ourselves in the following months. In the morning, we would get ready and I would walk the puppy then go to the neighbors' to be taken to school. After school, they would bring us home and we would have dinner with them or another neighbor who lived in the apartment below us. Sometimes we would watch TV after we ate before we'd go home to do our homework, take a bath and go to bed. Other times we just ate dinner then went back to our apartment and watched TV, dressed up our Barbie dolls or played records and danced. We had turned Kleenex boxes and paper towel rolls into guitars and danced around the apartment like we were in a band. If The Beatles or The Monkeys were on TV, we would play our Kleenex guitars and sing along with them.

The Vietnam War dominated the news every day with images of flag-draped coffins coming off airplanes, antiwar protests and footage from the front lines. During the dinner hour, people were glued to the TV watching the war, and we knew that was where our dad was. My mom called regularly and would ask us about school and how we were doing, but she was too sick and weak to talk for very long. She would always act upbeat, but I could hear the strain in her voice. A few times, my dad called from Vietnam, and those too were short conversations. He would send us different Vietnamese porcelain dolls dressed in traditional outfits and ask if we got them. I questioned them both about cancer during those phone calls, but neither would engage. They told me, "Let it go. It is nothing for you to worry about."

Late one afternoon, as Bonnie and I were watching TV after school, without warning my mom came walking through the front door with the help of a friend. We were shocked and thrilled to see her. She behaved as if everything was normal again and she was just home now. We were shaken by how frail she looked and by how dark her skin was from the radiation. True to form, though, my mom promised us she was fine and was home to stay. She quickly picked up the routine the three of us had before she left and went on like nothing happened. A month or so later, my father came home from Vietnam, and we were a family again. He received his next assignment, and we packed up the apartment and moved to Fort Bliss, Texas, and never again spoke about what happened that year.

From then on, every time my mom went to the doctor, I lived in fear she would not come home. I asked to go to her appointments with her, but my parents always insisted I go to school. When we got the news my mom's mother was diagnosed with breast cancer and my dad's sister with brain cancer, my first response was relief that it was not my parents—then guilt that I had those feelings, followed by paranoia about bad karma.

As I got into my teens, cancer started getting more attention. The president declared a war on cancer; awareness campaigns were showing up on television and in magazines; and money was being spent on research and a cure. Breast cancer was front and center. All this attention on it triggered my fears. I changed the channel when a public announcement came on TV. I avoided any movies in which someone was diagnosed with cancer. As soon as magazines arrived, I went through them and ripped out any advertisements, awareness campaigns or stories about breast cancer. Later I could flip through them leisurely without the fear of running across anything to do with the disease.

My mother's first recurrence happened when I was twenty-three. I knew something was wrong because she got sick and began throwing up. Then I saw a wig on the dresser in my parents' bedroom. When I questioned them about it, they told me they were taking care of it, she was fine. Despite my objections, they continued to behave as if nothing was wrong.

My mom survived that round, after which she began volunteering to support other women, driving them to get their treatments. When I asked about what she was doing, she would give me only tidbits of information.

Her proximity to others with cancer made me very uncomfortable, and I constantly worried about her health. I could not understand why she wanted to be around people with that awful, gross disease all the time.

Fourteen years after my father came home from Vietnam I found out he was sick on Christmas Eve from a cousin who assumed I knew about his diagnosis. I confronted my parents, and they said, "We were going to tell you when the time was right."

"When was that?" I cried. "At his funeral?" Five weeks later, my dad was dead from lung cancer from exposure to Agent Orange while in Vietnam. He was sixty-one years old.

Twenty-six years—and three recurrences—after my mother's initial diagnosis, on a Monday morning before Thanksgiving, she died of a pulmonary embolism while undergoing chemotherapy for the fourth time. She was seventy-three.

When I was twenty-four, I was able to start getting annual mammograms because of my family history. I thought if I was diligent about getting tested every year, I was being responsible and that in itself was prevention. I was very restless in the months and weeks that led up to the tests and then lived in fear as I waited for the results. If everything was OK, I got a letter in the mail letting me know the results and a reminder to make an appointment in another year. If something suspicious appeared, I got a call to schedule an appointment for another mammogram and then I'd have to wait for the letter or phone call again. I have dense and cystic breasts and often got called to come back for more images. This whole process could take weeks, during which time I would barely sleep, eat or think of anything but breast cancer and how I was going to handle getting that diagnosis.

Once I got clean results, I would feel incredible relief for a couple of months before the dread of going through it again would creep up on me. I would not do a self-exam for fear of feeling something new. I left that up to my gynecologist to do. I reasoned that I saw her once a year and not much could happen in that one year.

Any kind of pain anywhere in my body made me anxious. If I had a backache or a headache for any length of time, I would become convinced it was cancer. I would not go to a doctor, though, for fear of her telling me I was right. I knew there was no logic to this thinking, but cancer convoluted everything and warped my ability to be rational.

My lifestyle choices and behavior did nothing to help my anxiety, but I loathed the idea of changing any of them. I believed everything would be okay because I was thin and healthy, or at least nothing was wrong with me. I never watched what I ate or went anywhere near a gym. I was lazy when it came to food: If it was not in the deli down the block or on a takeout menu, I did not bother. As years passed, my lifestyle did not evolve or improve. I smoked two packs of Marlboro Reds a day, drank black coffee all morning and Cokes all afternoon and had popcorn or cheese sticks for dinner.

My career was in product development, so I traveled to trade shows and factories around the world and was on and off planes and in different time zones all the time and never got much sleep. Every once in a while, I would decide I needed to address my stress and got a massage in the hotel followed by cocktails with co-workers. Little about my life was healthy. I was torn and guilt-ridden about being so irresponsible for someone with a strong family history of cancer.

Thirty-four years after my mom's initial diagnosis, at the end of my second day of a two-week business trip to Asia, I was taking off my clothes to shower when I saw a stain in the right cup of my bra. At first, I was confused by it because I knew I had brought clean clothing on the trip. Then it hit me what it could be.

It felt as if someone had kicked me in the stomach, and I bent over to catch my breath. I broke out in a cold sweat and I had to sit on the edge of the bathtub with my head between my legs to keep from fainting. I sat there taking deep breaths and shaking for a long time until I could get up and splash water on my face. I washed the bra, then tossed and turned anxiously all night. I did not call my husband, Michael, because talking about it would have confirmed that something was wrong.

The next evening when I took off my bra, the stain was there again, but this time, it was bigger, and I could tell it was blood. I was hugely disappointed. I sat on the floor of the bathroom feeling defeated and called Michael.

It was about seven p.m. on a Sunday evening, and I was in Hong Kong. There was nothing I could do until the clock hit 9 a.m. in New York City two hours later. As soon as my gynecologist's office opened, I was on the phone with her and explained to her what had happened. She told me I needed to see a breast cancer surgeon quickly and recommended someone. There was no way I was going to be able to focus on anything related to the factories or product over the next two weeks, so I changed my plans and flew home in the morning.

I met the surgeon on Wednesday morning, and she determined I was bleeding from a milk gland in my nipple and scheduled me for a surgical biopsy that Friday morning. The findings were lobular carcinoma in situ, or LCIS, in my right breast. It is when abnormal cells develop in the lobules of the breast. It is sometimes referred to as stage "zero" cancer, or a pre-cancerous condition, but it is not considered cancer and does not require treatment.

Being diagnosed with LCIS does indicate that you have an increased risk of developing breast cancer. I had two choices: do nothing and be watched very carefully by adding more diagnostic tests to my routine such as an ultrasound and an MRI, or start taking the drug tamoxifen, a hormone therapy drug used to treat early and advanced stage breast cancer. I did research on tamoxifen and its side effects, such as menopausal symptoms, an increased risk for blood clots and endometrial cancer, and decided watching myself very carefully was the better option for me.

This scare made me take a more active role in my breast health, albeit uneasily. The following year, my surgeon told me about a new study comparing the results of mammograms, ultrasounds and MRIs on high-risk patients and suggested I participate. The study needed women with a family history of breast cancer, who had had a scare themselves and whose breasts were currently disease-free. The plan was to follow the women over years comparing the results of all three tests. The whole situation made me feel very uncomfortable, and I did not want to do it. I felt deep shame at the thought of not taking advantage of the advanced diagnostic imaging, though, so I volunteered.

The mammogram was scheduled on a Thursday, the ultrasound on Friday and the MRI on Monday. On Friday afternoon, I receive a call that my MRI scheduled for Monday had been canceled because something suspicious showed up in my left breast on the mammogram. I was no longer a candidate for the study. I called the radiation department at the hospital and asked the person there to please reconsider and proceed with the MRI, but he did not budge. I was frantic and called my surgeon's office for help. I wanted my doctor to have every possible image of the questionable spots. I managed to convince everyone that if an MRI is as effective as it is supposed to be, then they should want to see how these spots would appear on all three types of screening. They finally relented, and I had the additional screening.

Getting bad news any day of the week is stressful, but on a Friday afternoon, it is a special kind of hell and makes for a very long weekend. We had social activities planned all weekend, and I moved through them in a fog. That Friday night, John F. Kennedy Jr., his wife and his sister-in-law were flying to Nantucket, when their plane went missing over the ocean. It was all anyone talked about all weekend, and, sad as it was, for me it became a welcome distraction. I explained my subdued behavior as a lack of sleep and the oppressive humidity, but I just felt anxious and nauseous all weekend.

After the MRI late Monday morning, a nurse told me to get dressed but not to leave. The radiologist scheduled me for a core biopsy later that day. I sat in the waiting room for about two hours, then a nurse came and took me to a small room with a couple of chairs and said she would be back. I'd had the surgical biopsy the year before, but I had no idea what a core biopsy was or what was involved.

a few people I knew to get referrals for breast surgeons for a second opinion. I chose two based on the experience others had had with them and, by that afternoon, had set up appointments for a second and third opinion over the next two days.

I was instructed to bring copies of my pathology reports, slides, and films with me to the appointments. I thought *Okay, no problem.* I was unaware there were procedures for getting copies of medical records. I could get the written reports from my surgeon the next day, but images and slides needed to come from the radiology department. That department required that I go there, make the request in writing, show ID and fill out a release form. This could be done between the hours of 9:00 a.m. and 11:00 a.m. Monday through Friday. I then had to return five days later between the hours of 1:00 p.m. and 3:00 p.m. to pick up everything.

I had not anticipated all these extra steps to get my records. I had to call and reschedule the appointments set up for the next two days with the additional surgeons to the following week. I had taken everything on with extreme urgency, and this time delay wreaked havoc on my emotions. Now that I was diagnosed, I believed I was in a race against time.

Within twenty-four hours of my diagnosis, I had done everything I had to do. I ordered test results, set up appointments for doctors, scheduled pre-op tests and had a date for the surgery. Now I just had to wait seven days for the first appointment to see another surgeon. It was hell. I do not wait well for anything, but I soon found out that is what you do with cancer. You wait...for everything, all the time.

As that week dragged by, I picked up and put down magazines and newspapers without understanding a thing I read and flipped through TV channels but could not stop on one for more than a few moments. I felt if I was not doing something related to my cancer all the time, I was not taking the disease seriously. But I did not know what to do.

One month before my diagnosis, I had left my corporate job and started my own product design and development business. My diagnosis stopped me cold in my tracks. I had no idea what was going to happen next. I could not fathom how I was going to start a new company now. I remembered my mother's experience with breast cancer when she was incapable of doing much for almost a year after her first diagnosis. I was also terrified that potential clients were going to find out about my cancer and not hire me, thinking I would not be reliable. I tried to focus on building the business but ended up only staring into space. I had moved from motivational fear to shutdown fear.

I finally had the appointment with the second surgeon, a highly respected breast surgeon at New York Presbyterian Hospital. Michael and I got off the elevator on the cancer floor, and I abruptly stopped, staggered by what I saw. My doctor's office was in the ambulatory surgery center of Beth Israel Medical Center, located a few blocks away from the main hospital. The cancer doctors there had individual offices and waiting rooms assigned by their specialty. This hospital had all the cancer doctors located in the main building on the same floor, and they shared a common waiting room. It was the biggest waiting room I had ever been in, and it was filled with patients with all kinds of cancer.

Michael stood beside me and said, "Just breathe." Then he put his arm around my waist and walked me to the front desk. A receptionist asked me my name and the time of my appointment. Once she found me on the schedule, she started assembling the forms I needed to fill out. "I need your insurance card and ID," she said as she handed me the forms. "Fill these out and bring them back to me."

Michael and I found two seats together and sat down. I began filling out the forms. I held back tears when I wrote down breast cancer as the reason for my visit. When I returned the forms the receptionist said, "You are going to have a wait; you are a last-minute drop-in." Most cancer doctors have very full schedules, and it can take weeks or months to get an appointment with them. Many are willing to give a second opinion to a patient on short notice, but you may have a wait.

For the next three hours, Michael and I watched people in different stages of cancer come and go. Some looked fine; others were hunched over or slumped in their chair, or in a wheelchair, gaunt and very sick. Several people had young children with them who ran around while their parents watched television, read magazines or talked with each other. I was grateful I had the appointment, but I was agitated by the wait and terrified at the sight of such sick patients. The longer we waited the closer I got to my first public meltdown. The comfort of Michael's arm around me was the only thing that saved me from bursting into sobs.

The surgeon was patient, informative and thoughtful in his manner. His approach was calm and direct. He looked at my mammogram and pathology report and slides and agreed that a lumpectomy followed by treatment was the best option for me. By now, I was over the initial shock of my diagnosis and had questions.

"How can a lumpectomy get rid of my cancer?" I asked. "Do calcifications come from eating too much dairy? How can the cancer show up in my left breast when I had LCIS in my right? Wouldn't it show it in the same breast?"

He described how a lumpectomy could get all my cancer and I would not have to lose my whole breast. He also said it was a common procedure for early breast cancer. He explained that calcifications have nothing to do with eating or drinking dairy and that it was not unusual for cancer to show up in the opposite breast than the one that had LCIS.

When he saw my surgeon's name on top of one of the documents, he said, "You are in excellent hands. She is a great surgeon and considered the artisan of breasts. She does an amazing job preserving them." When I told him she recommended I get the second opinion, he replied, "She is very confident in her work. That's great."

After learning more about my diagnosis, and hearing his thoughts about my surgeon, I felt better about my prognosis.

The third surgeon was also associated with a large New York City hospital, but I saw him at his private office. He read the reports and looked at the images and in a blasé and dismissive manner said, "You just have garden-variety cancer."

I am not sure if his intent was to make me feel better or if he was disappointed because my cancer was not exotic, but it made me feel insignificant, and I immediately hated him. He also agreed with the other surgeons on my diagnosis, treatment and prognosis.

When we left, I fumed about the flippant way he said it was "garden-variety cancer." As we stood on the sidewalk in front of his office, I turned to Michael and said, "It's still cancer, though, right?" I wanted to march back into the arrogant doctor's office and say, "Fuck you! Want to trade places?" That would not be the only time I felt incredibly lucky to have a doctor I trusted and felt comfortable with to help me through my cancer.

Not every community will have multiple doctors; there may be only one doctor who specializes in your cancer, or you cannot switch to another one for insurance or location reasons. It is not ideal if you do not have a big pool of doctors to choose from and you do not like the one you have, but not all is lost. You have a team of physician assistants, nurse practitioners, nurses and caregivers around you. They can support you, answer your questions and help you with your concerns if your doctor is not able or willing.

How many doctors will you have?

Everyone's cancer is different, and how many doctors you need varies. Minimally you will have the following:

- Surgical oncologist: physician who performs breast surgery
- Radiology oncologist: manages radiation treatments (if you have radiation treatments)
- Medical oncologist: manages chemotherapy and medications
- Plastic surgeon: breast reconstruction (should you choose this procedure)

Your surgeon will be the one to determine the best surgical option for you. The oncologist and radiologist are the ones who will give you your treatment choices for chemotherapy, radiation and medication.

The breast surgeon specializes in breast cancer. Oncologists and radiologists work with patients who have various types of cancer. A plastic surgeon may specialize in breasts but will also be able to reconstruct or enhance other areas of the body.

The following professionals are available to support you and your doctor:

- Nurse practitioner: works with the doctor, performs physical examinations, diagnoses and treats illnesses, orders and analyzes lab work and other diagnostic tests, prescribes medications and can serve as a patient's regular health-care provider
- Physician's assistant: works with the doctor and performs physical examinations, recommended tests, helps with surgery, manages treatments and side effects and counsels people about cancer

- Hospitalist: doctors whose primary professional focus is the general medical care of hospitalized patients

The following medical professionals can also be a part of a cancer team. You may not require their services but should be aware that they exist.

- Oncology nurse: monitors the patient's physical condition, prescribes medication, administers chemotherapy and other treatments
- Pain management doctor or physiatrist: usually an anesthesiologist who has been certified or trained on the relief and/or management of pain

The following health-care professionals may be added to your team if your health warrants it:

- Physical therapist: a health-care professional who administers treatment for a disease or an injury with massage, exercises, heat and other modalities to reduce pain and increase mobility
- Registered dietitian: a dietitian specially trained to provide medical nutritional therapy to patients in hospitals and long-term care facilities

Additionally, the professionals below are available to help you manage your situation:

- Patient navigator: nurse, social worker or lay health worker who helps the patient "navigate" the health-care system. The navigator coordinates patient care, connects patients with resources, explains their treatment options, makes appointments, and provides advice and support
- Social worker: a professional who provides help and support services to the economically, physically, mentally and socially disadvantaged

Why second (and third) opinions?

Below are questions I have been asked when I have suggested a woman get a second opinion.

"Why? I already go to the best surgeon in my area."

"He was my friend's doctor when she had breast cancer. He did a great job. I trust him. Why would I see someone else?"

"She was voted one of the best breast cancer doctors by *New York* magazine. How do you find better than that?"

Getting a second opinion is not about the doctor; it is about *you*. You should be getting as much useful information and as clear an understanding as possible about your disease and all your options. The more you know, the better prepared you will be, and the more confident you will feel when making decisions.

Seeking a second opinion was the most valuable advice my breast surgeon could have given me. It did not occur to me to get a second opinion from another surgeon, and I do not know that I would have readily gotten one if she had not recommended it. I liked her, I knew she would be my doctor and I also thought, *Why*? It was only after I met the other doctors and heard their take on my diagnosis, prognosis, treatment options and outcome that I truly began to understand my situation.

When my surgeon recommended a lumpectomy, I was skeptical at first. I did not understand enough about my cancer or the procedure to feel confident that removing only part of my breast, not all of it, would successfully remove my cancer. I thought you had to lose your whole breast for that to happen. After speaking to other doctors, I understood a lumpectomy was a common and very successful procedure for early-stage breast cancer and the right one for me.

Also, by the time I saw the second and third surgeons, I was prepared to listen and able to hear what I was being told. Every doctor agreed with my surgeon's plan, but I heard it differently each time. They emphasized distinct aspects of the surgery or treatment and told it in their own way. Finally, I had a better understanding of what I was up against and what was going to happen. Once I knew that, I could figure out what to ask, and that changed everything for me.

The more information I got, the easier it was to formulate questions for my surgeon that both educated me and calmed my fears. It gave me back some control. My questions helped my surgeon understand my concerns and take steps to alleviate or reduce my anxiety about the things that mattered to me. She explained my chest would not look like my mother's did after her radical mastectomy. She confirmed I could still be intimate with my husband and told me I would be able to work and resume most of my normal activities. That reduced my depression and made me feel less helpless.

Once, when I recommended that a woman get a second opinion when she was uncertain how to proceed with treatment, she said, "I did that. I asked my radiologist for a recommendation for an oncologist for a second opinion. He told me I didn't need one. I was already with a good oncologist and didn't need to go to someone else for another opinion."

Her current oncologist was a part of the radiologist's practice, and he refused to give the woman a referral to another one. She was intimidated and frightened by his response, so she dropped it. She was afraid he would not continue to treat her if she consulted someone else about her diagnosis. That was not his choice to make; it was hers. It is your right to get an independent second opinion. It is important to understand everything that is happening to you. A doctor should not resist your getting a second opinion, and you want her to be interested in the report when you do.

To get a true second opinion, see a doctor who is not associated with your surgeon's practice. Ask doctors or people outside her circle for referrals to another surgeon. Most likely anyone on your team is going to refer you to another person who is on their team or someone who follows their same line of thinking or works in their hospital. You want an independent second opinion.

If you live in an area where you have few choices to get a true second opinion, you still have options. There are online services offered by well-regarded large urban hospitals such as the Dana-Farber Cancer Institute in Boston and the Cleveland Clinic where a patient can get a second opinion from renowned specialists without traveling to the facilities.

Tip

To get a true second opinion, see a doctor who is not associated with your surgeon's practice.

The patient sends their medical records to the hospital and specialist(s) review them and provide a written report with their opinion. Before you contact an online service, check with your insurance company to find out if you will be reimbursed for the expense. Online second opinion services do not take insurance. (See Badass Cancer Resources, Second Opinions, page 256.)

Seeking a second, or third, opinion on your diagnosis, prognosis and protocol is a smart way to educate yourself so you can make informed decisions. There comes a point, however, where you need to take the information you have and move forward. I have spoken to women who have gone for five and six opinions about their prognosis or treatment options. The information was the same each time, but the process prolonged their having to make a decision. The purpose of getting another opinion is to help you become knowledgeable about your diagnosis and choices so you feel confident about your next steps, not slow your progress.

You are not hurting anyone's feelings by seeking a second opinion. Doctors understand why you do it. Many expect it and do it themselves. Just be gracious when you see other doctors and thank them for their time.

Doctor-patient relationship

A doctor-patient relationship forms when a doctor provides a person with medical care. What that statement does not convey is how personal it should be. Your doctor is not going to know you like a close friend, but there is more than your diagnosis that she should know.

It is important to establish an open and honest connection with her from the beginning. Talk to her; tell her about yourself, the best way to communicate with you and how much information you will want from her. Some people want every detail about their diagnosis, treatment and

> **Tip**
>
> *You are not hurting anyone's feelings by seeking a second opinion. Doctors understand why you do it. Many expect it and do it themselves.*

medications, and others want broad strokes. Discuss if you want her to make all the decisions about your health care or if you want to be given the options and be the final word, or a mix of both.

Communicate, participate, engage and create a partnership with her. The better she knows you, the easier it will be for her to help you with questions, guide you on decisions, and determine if there are changes in both your physical and mental health.

It is not always easy to know what to ask, especially in the beginning as you are trying to figure out what is going on. A good place to begin is with family and friends. Once you start telling them about your cancer, people are going to ask you questions. Write down anything that you do not know about. This will help you formulate questions to ask your doctor. The more information you gather, the more you will know what to ask.

Once your doctor knows your concerns, she will have a starting place to help dispel incorrect information, confirm things that are accurate and help fill in the blanks on what you do not know. Do not feel hesitant or embarrassed about asking questions. You really have no idea what your doctor is thinking, and she truly has heard it all before.

Many times, women do not want to bother their doctor with too many questions. They are afraid she will get annoyed and not give them the best care or drop them as a patient. When I suggest a woman call her doctor to ask a question, I often hear the following:

"He has a very busy practice. I do not want to bug him."

"I'm sure I can find the information somewhere. I do not need to bother her for it."

"I already called her once after my appointment. I'm afraid if I call again, she will get annoyed with me."

I understand. The mere thought of losing your cancer doctor can push panic buttons you did not even know you had. No one wants to mess

Tip

A doctor will not dismiss you for asking too many questions about your health care. It benefits her when you know about your diagnosis and protocol.

up anywhere or do anything that will possibly diminish their chances of getting the best care.

A doctor can dismiss a patient in her care for several reasons such as a patient refusing to follow treatment recommendations, failing to keep appointments, behaving in such a way that could harm staff and other patients or failing to pay. A doctor will not dismiss you for asking too many questions about your health care. It benefits her when you know about your diagnosis and protocol. It is easier for her to engage and partner with you if she knows when you do not understand what she is saying or what she means.

Let her know how to best communicate with you. I preferred to be told the importance of information on a scale of one to ten. One was nothing to worry about, and ten meant it was a big deal. I also found my doctors and health-care workers understood me better when I communicated using that scale regarding how I was feeling.

One way to make sure you have the correct information is to repeat back to the doctor what you heard her say. After she explains something to you, say to her, "If I understand you correctly, you said…" and tell her what you heard. It clarifies quickly if you are both on the same page. Stop her and ask for an explanation when she says something you do not understand. Do not wait until the end of the appointment.

Another way is to bring someone with you to appointments to hear what is said and take notes. That person can act as a second set of eyes and ears for you. Prior to asking someone to accompany you, check with your doctor or the hospital regarding Covid protocols.

I have spoken with women who were upset they were not given more information but when asked for details realized they had been told more. It just was not what they wanted to hear. It is completely understandable to not want to hear some of the things being told to you. It can be frightening and painful information, but selective hearing or tuning out some of what is said does not change anything and can be detrimental to your well-being.

When you feel overwhelmed with information, it is helpful to break it down, so it is manageable instead of attempting to tackle it all at once. It will help you clarify and absorb the material more quickly if you can deal with each aspect of it individually.

A simple place to start: Write down topics of information—for example, diagnosis, medication, treatment, tests. Under each topic, write down what you understand about it and what you do not know and the next steps. Go through each point and note where you need further explanations and whom you need to contact to get it. For example, under treatment: *radiation start date, March 1. Tattoo markings? What are they? Where do I get them done? Contact radiation oncologists' office for details.* You will soon understand your next steps and be able to effectively handle what is in front of you.

Give your doctor time to discuss things with you. Review your notes and questions before your appointment, and be prepared. Voice your questions early in the appointment or when she says something you do not understand. Do not wait until the end, as you are getting ready to leave. She will not be able to give you the time and attention you deserve if you wait until your appointment is over. She can spend more time addressing your concerns if you bring them up at the beginning of your appointment or as they come up.

What not *to do*

Put down your phone when in an appointment. Better yet, turn it off. It will not help you to be distracted by your phone during a conversation with your doctor about your cancer. You do not know what she is going to say, and you could miss vital information if otherwise engaged on your phone. In addition, it is

Tip

Voice your questions early in the appointment or when your doctor says something you do not understand. Do not wait until the end, as you are getting ready to leave. She will not be able to give you the time and attention you deserve if you wait until your appointment is over.

disrespectful to the person trying to save your life to not give her your full attention.

It is not a good idea to walk into your doctor's office pushing research and treatments that you read about online. Doctors appreciate an informed patient but not one who tries to tell them what to do. No matter how much you know about your cancer, she knows infinitely more and has experience dealing with it. If you have questions about information you find, however, you should ask her. It is always good to have a conversation about advances in medicine, new approaches to treatment and whether something is appropriate for you.

What your doctor needs to know about you

Tell your doctor what is important to you and the quality of life you want now and in the future. This includes your plans and desires. A bilateral mastectomy rules out breast-feeding. Your fertility may be affected by different treatments. If you are young and want to have children, this may matter to you. Discuss your plans to have or grow your family and what options are available for preserving your fertility before and during cancer treatment. Talk with her about protecting your hormonal health after treatment. Conserving as much of your breast as possible may be very important to you. These are extremely emotional and weighty issues your doctor needs to know from you *before* you have surgery or start treatment. Be honest and open about your fears.

- Tell her about your life and what you are afraid of losing.
- Discuss your plans and desires for the future.
- Tell her what you are worried about.
- Let her know if you have a support system.

Your doctor's success will be measured against your expectations, and unless you tell her what those are, how can she get you close to your desired outcome? Maintaining as much of your life as possible helps minimize the depression that often accompanies cancer. Communicate with your doctor so she can support you.

Traditional versus alternative versus integrative medicine

There are different practices of medicine. Traditional medicine is the most recommended when treating cancer, but it is good to know all the practices. You may want to incorporate more than one into your health-care plan.

The different protocols break down as follows:

- Traditional medicine: Practiced by your surgeon, radiologist, oncologist, gynecologist, primary care physician, etc. It is evidence-based medicine.
- Alternative medicine: Includes acupuncture, acupressure, massage therapy, yoga and t'ai chi as well as hypnotherapy, spiritual healing, art and music therapy, meditation, guided imagery and visualization. It also includes nutritional counseling and general well-being.
- Integrative medicine: A combination of the two. Integrative medicine is when alternative medicine is used in conjunction with traditional medicine to incorporate the entire body and enhance healing.

After my surgery, I started looking at alternative medicine as a way to support my overall health. Over time, I added acupuncture, massage therapy and yoga into my traditional medicine protocol. Also, I learned about nutrition and began to eat healthy food instead of whatever was fastest and most convenient. I felt better mentally, emotionally and physically, and my mood improved.

You will find people willing to offer you remedies and recipes for alternative ways to handle cancer and its side effects. Always research anything before you try it. Whatever you choose to do regarding integrative or alternative medicine, over-the-counter supplements and herbs, keep all your health-care providers informed. Some alternative protocols may have an impact on various traditional medicines. (See Badass Cancer Resources, Complementary and Integrative Health, page 246.)

Myth

If I am not offered all the tests, procedures and treatments available, I am not getting the best cancer care.

Truth

Not every test, treatment or procedure is right for every person. You and your doctor should discuss which ones will increase your chance of recovery and help you maintain the best quality of life and which could increase your risk of side effects and lead to unnecessary costs.

—CANCER.NET

The important people on your journey

It has been said the most powerful people in a company are the assistants, secretaries and support staff. They hold the key to everyone and everything you need. It is no different in the medical world.

Doctors are a critical component in your care, but they have the smallest role in taking care of you. It is the physician assistants, nurses, technicians, receptionists and administrative personnel—the ones working with you one-on-one every day—who play the biggest part.

If your doctor does not have the patience or is not willing to take the time to answer all your questions, reach out to the other members on your team. Her support staff can provide you information if she is not available, explain things you do not understand or get you what you need. Ask her nurse to sit with you, or make an appointment to see her assistant to address your concerns. She will know as much as your doctor about your health care and will have access to your records. If something comes up they cannot answer, they will contact your doctor and get back to you. They can become your advocate, as well as a compassionate ear, to get you through the tough times or direct you to others who can help.

It benefits you to view all the health-care workers as individuals on your team there to help you and not just as people behind the counter, desk or machine or as someone there to serve you. It is hard, and it hurts to have cancer, and understandably you can get very angry and want to lash out. But you need these people, and they all want the best outcome for you. Nobody wants to work with someone who does not cooperate, yells or refuses to listen, especially when her only objective is to help save your life. It makes everything so much harder than it needs to be. Treat each staff person with the respect you want in return.

You have the right to, and should, speak up if you are not getting what you want or need. It is important that you use your voice as you deal with breast cancer. This is about how you do it. Your number-one job is to take care of yourself; sometimes that means helping others by being engaged and courteous. If you are grateful in your own way for everyone on your team, you will be the benefactor.

CHAPTER 3

Next Steps

The first order of business after you hear your diagnosis is to find out the specifics about your cancer before you start making decisions. This may be obvious, but most people say, "I didn't hear a thing after she said, 'You have cancer.'"

Most of the women I've spoken with were completely dumbfounded and caught off guard on getting their diagnosis. Even the ones who anticipated the news were surprised when they heard it. Many of them heard it over the phone entirely out of context with what they were doing. They were standing in line at the grocery store, taking the kids to school, on vacation, in their office or home alone. All of them were too shocked to ask more than a few—if any—questions or know where to begin.

If you received your diagnosis over the phone, the first move is to request an appointment with your doctor to discuss the specifics. If you receive a letter in the mail from her, open it and read it right away. If you do not want to open it when you are alone, ask a family member or friend to be with you.

Everything starts and advances based on your diagnosis, so understanding it is essential. Once you receive the news, the next step is to understand what it means.

Tip

Your cancer doctor just recently met you. She does not know how you think or how much or how little you know or what matters to you unless you tell her. Many doctors do not say much or tell you anything unless you ask them. It is up to you to speak up and ask questions about your diagnosis, or she will assume you have what you need and keep moving forward.

Every patient, along with her wants, needs and desires, is as different and unique as her diagnosis. Your doctor has an obligation to explain everything to you. But your cancer doctor just recently met you. She does not know how you think or how much or how little you know or what matters to you unless you tell her. Many doctors do not say much or tell you anything unless you ask them. It is up to you to speak up and ask questions about your diagnosis, or she will assume you have what you need and keep moving forward.

When discussing your diagnosis, it is important that your doctor communicates with you using terms you understand rather than complicated medical jargon. It will not help if you do not comprehend what she is telling you. She does not expect you to understand everything she is saying, but she will not know how much you are processing unless you tell her. Speak up about anything you do not understand. Simply say to her, "I don't know what that means," "I don't understand what you are saying," "Please, explain that again" or "Please, slow down. I can't keep up with everything you are telling me."

My doctor was always thorough in her explanations, but many times I stayed muddled in my understanding. One time, I asked her to draw me a picture, so I could *see* what she was telling me. As soon as I saw her sketch, everything became clear. From that point on, I asked all my doctors to draw me a picture of anything I did not understand.

Do not be afraid or embarrassed to ask your doctor to repeat what she said, draw pictures or communicate in a specific way that allows you to fully comprehend what she is saying. Cancer is not a world you are familiar with, and the information is too important not to know. She will

- Inpatient: A person is admitted to the hospital, usually for more than one night.
- Observational: A person is usually admitted to the hospital for observation while it is determined if she needs to be an inpatient. Always ask how your visit is being classified. Insurance does not always pay for observational.

Discuss with your doctor if she expects your surgery to be outpatient or if you will be admitted.

The timeline from diagnosis to surgery to treatment can move very quickly. There is never a good time to try to figure out all that is happening, but it is especially difficult when you are still shell-shocked from getting the diagnosis. It is okay to take your time, ask the questions and make sure you have what you need before you move forward. Ask your doctor how much time you have to make a decision before moving ahead with each step. Then take advantage of the time to become informed about your options. Work with her to slow down the schedule of events until you are comfortable with your choices. She most likely will not let you put off your next steps for a few months, but she will give you another week or two to gather information and ask more questions.

Be patient and understanding with yourself. Maneuvering in the world of cancer is complicated. No one expects you to know what to do or how to do it. Ask questions, and lean on your doctor and her team for guidance. They are there to help you.

CHAPTER 4

Now What?

After all those years of worrying when I would be told I had cancer, I never considered what would happen beyond the diagnosis. I read the brochures, handouts, booklets, and cards that told me what to do about my cancer, but I did not know what I was supposed to do with myself. I had no idea that expecting to have cancer would feel so completely different from actually having it.

I did not think about the turmoil my life would undergo. Michael and I had just celebrated our third wedding anniversary, and I felt horrible about what my cancer diagnosis meant to him. He continued to assure me we would get through this together, but I thought, *Oh, you poor man, you have no idea*. He did not grow up around the disease and experience the hell it can bring to everyone. How could I make him live that? Will he hate me soon into it? Want to leave? Feel horribly guilty about doing so or angry because his guilt would not let him? Should I leave him, so he does not have to make that decision? How do I shield him from what is about to happen?

I did not want to address these feelings and could not sit with my thoughts or wait for things to unfold, so I did what I do best: charged forward. The singular focus on my left breast caused me to scramble, backtrack or start over on numerous things all at the same time. I had information faxed to a wrong number and claims sent to the wrong address, and I double-booked appointments. This spinning of my wheels only fueled my frustration. I asked questions but wasn't listening to the answers. I was too intimidated by the disease to do anything constructive anyway. I took notes on random pieces of paper and often reviewed them, but they were incomplete or made no sense. And there were many that I simply misplaced.

Myth
Small-breasted women have less chance of getting breast cancer.

Truth
There is no connection between the size of your breasts and your risk of getting breast cancer.

—HEALTH.COM

My take-charge attitude made people believe I had it all under control, so they did not step in to help me and I did not ask for it—or want it. Asking for help or a favor of any kind made me feel weak, bothersome and vulnerable. Like everything else in my life, I thought I could do it all by myself and that the pieces would just fall into place as long as I kept forging ahead. That kind of thinking is not a plan; it is just a mess. I was making matters worse for myself.

Moving for the sake of doing something does not accomplish anything. I would have done better if I had slowed down, figured out what I needed and put strategies in place to stabilize my life mentally and emotionally before charging ahead. It would have put me on more solid ground and at a much better advantage to handle all that came at me. I was already doing everything I could to take care of my disease. I needed to do something positive for my life.

Calming the chaos

I function better with familiarity and routine, and both were gone. Clarity, integrity and dependability are the three things that make my world right. I did not question anyone's integrity. I believed they were all acting in the best interest of my health. But clarity and dependability were harder to find. I had a difficult time understanding the vocabulary of cancer, and there was no consistency to my routine. The unexpected happened all the time, different people came and went, and every day felt unfamiliar and scary. It was grueling to operate with such uncertainty.

Finally exhausted with my unfocused method, I figured out the one thing I had control over: how I handled myself as a person with cancer. I did not know what that was, though. Just telling myself to relax was not working. I needed to *do* something to calm down, and I craved some predictability.

I was good at business and enjoyed it. I understood how to move things forward and excelled in time and crisis management and problem solving. So I decided to treat my cancer like a job with tasks, projects and meetings.

Once I began to use my business skills of organization, communication and negotiating to manage my cancer, I was able to deal with things less emotionally. My life became more familiar to me. I understood how to be productive in that environment, and it gave me a sense of stability.

I got a notebook to keep everything in. It kept me organized and became my cancer bible. I wrote my to-do list, notes, questions, information, suggestions, phone numbers and appointments. I also tucked copies of my test results in it. I took it with me to every appointment and had it at hand for every conversation regarding my cancer. It helped me recall important information, remember things to do and prepare and prioritize questions for the next time I spoke with someone. My notebook also became a safe place to write down all my fears and frustrations as I sat in waiting rooms, sometimes for hours.

The goal is to be informed and make fewer decisions in emotionally charged moments. Working your cancer through a system, a method, a procedure, a routine or an art that you know and are comfortable with can help you manage the situation with some familiarity. Once I approached my cancer like a job, I was less frenzied and overwhelmed all the time. I could manage my cancer in a way that I understood.

I met an art teacher who described how she designated an area in her kitchen as her cancer spot to keep her organized and on task. She put up a bulletin board where she pinned information, to-do lists, questions and appointment times. She invited her family to add notes and anything they wanted her to discuss with her doctor. This made it easy to keep her family informed about her schedule and progress—and to keep them involved.

"I used colored craft paper to identify areas to pin questions they wanted me to ask and post magazine articles. It looked like those boards you see on cop shows, with pictures and arrows and question marks," she laughed. "Before an appointment, I gathered all the notes, articles and questions posted and went through them, then discussed them with my doctor."

She also included a countdown calendar on the board to mark off the days she had left of treatment. Her kids pinned healthy recipes, motivational quotes, funny pictures, and useful information and tips on the board.

"It helped everyone stay engaged in my process, and it kept me organized and on track with my schedule. I would have my cup of coffee in front of the board every morning and review my to-do list and any new information posted. I felt in charge and prepared."

Some cancer treatments can take many months or longer to get through. A helpful way to chart your progress and stay motivated is to create a countdown calendar to mark the days left of chemotherapy or radiation. It can give you a sense of achievement as you reach your goal of completion.

It can be a traditional calendar where you simply cross off each day, or it can be elaborate with pictures, benchmarks and rewards. Pinterest has a large selection of creative and inspirational chemotherapy and radiation countdown calendars to help you with ideas. In the search bar of a search engine—for example, Google or Yahoo!—type in *Pinterest*. In the search bar of Pinterest type in *chemo calendar countdown* or *cancer calendar countdown,* and images of calendars people have created will appear.

After you begin treatment, the mental state of panic and confusion you felt when first diagnosed will lessen. You will have a schedule to follow, and your days will become more predictable. A routine will take shape, and you will be able to make plans and keep them. The anticipation, fear and dread of the unknown will begin to lessen as your life becomes familiar again.

Once you receive your diagnosis, the medical world takes over and keeps moving forward—which is what it is designed to do and you want it to do. You can get swept away in it very quickly or paddle the boat yourself. Either way, you will travel this road. It is how you do it that can make a difference in your life. Give yourself all the tools you need to manage it in a way that is productive and understandable for you.

Where to begin

Before you can make informed decisions about your health or your next steps, there are several questions you should answer first. They will help you to outline what you already know or have in place and what you still need to do. You will gain a better understanding of what you need to focus on.

- Do I understand my diagnosis?
- Do I understand the distinction between the different medical protocols?
- How much do I know about my health insurance?
- Whom do I want to know or not know about my diagnosis?
- Where can I get information on cancer helplines?
- Do I know my rights as a patient? My responsibilities?

As you review and prioritize your list, make a note on the follow-up action you need to take beside each item. It will become clear what your next steps for taking care of yourself should be. Once you understand what you have and what you need, you can plan accordingly and secure what is missing or head off any issues before they become a problem.

The easier you make gathering information from your doctor, hospital and insurance company, the more likely you are to get what you need. A simple method to save yourself time and frustration is to write down all your questions before you start calling people. Be clear about what you want from each call before you make it: to set up an appointment; to get test results, information, a second opinion, a

> **Tip**
>
> *Once you receive your diagnosis, the medical world takes over and keeps moving forward—which is what it is designed to do and you want it to do. You can get swept away in it very quickly or paddle the boat yourself. Either way, you will travel this road. It is how you do it that can make a difference in your life.*

referral, etc. You will take better notes, hear what is said and accomplished more. It will also help you stay focused and on task.

Stabilizing your life

All cancers need to be dealt with quickly. But there are things you can take care of first that will help you better comprehend your situation fully, so you can manage it to your benefit.

The first thing to understand about this disease is that most cancers grow very slowly. In most instances, it takes six to ten years for cancer to develop to a detectable stage. Regardless of the stage of your cancer, your doctor will tell you if you need to take any urgent steps when she gives you your diagnosis.

Keep in mind, not every decision needs to be made in the moment. Ask your doctor what your timeline is to determine your next steps. It will give you some time to think through your choices and steady your personal and work life early. Restoring some order in your life will allow you to focus on the disease.

A place to start putting things in order is to write down everything you need to support your cancer.

- A doctor you trust
- A support team of family and friends you can rely on
- Health insurance
- Child, elder or pet care
- Transportation
- Coverage at work

Writing down thoughts helps clarify them. It will give you a starting point on what you need to do next. Once I had everything down, I found I had and knew more than I thought in some areas and less in others. It will do the same for you too. Make sure to leave room or make columns beside each point so you can add notes such as "the next steps."

Next, prioritize your list. A simple way to do that is to use the MoSCoW Method that Dai Clegg, a specialist in data modeling, developed. It is a straightforward method that business managers use to help people understand the importance they put on each task they are required to do. Using it will help you get and stay organized and reduce your stress as you work your way through your to-do list.

The method works by dividing your list into four categories: must have, should have, nice to have, and will not have (at this time). Must have is anything critical to the success of your situation. Should have is anything that is important but not immediate. And nice to have is just that—nice, but it can come later, or you can live without it. Will not have is anything that is not going to be of benefit to you, requires too much time or energy with little or no payback, or really does not matter right now. Categorizing your priorities will help you focus on exactly what you need to do next.

Once you know the level of urgency to give each task, pace yourself as you work down your list. It is exhausting to try to do everything all at once, and, as I can attest, the result is not always effective or efficient. Accept that plans and priorities are going to change frequently. Decide whether each new task goes in the must have, should have, nice to have or will not have column. Doing this will help you stay focused and spend your energy wisely.

A way to manage all you have to do is to take your list of priorities and create a one-goal-a-day plan, such as call insurance about an outstanding claim, get an updated referral for an oncologist or research clinical trials. The objective is to complete one task a day, every day, to address your illness. By the end of the week, you will have taken seven productive measures to help yourself manage your situation; by the end of two weeks, you will have accomplished fourteen.

The purpose is to divide your tasks so you can accomplish tasks without feeling overwhelmed. Taking baby steps every day can make the road in front of you more manageable. A plan to steady your home and work life will give you the most options, help you stay engaged in your health care and help you feel as if you have some control back in your life.

Doing research

As you do research, stay focused on understanding your diagnosis, treatment options and next steps. Look for information that will help you, not theories that will distract you. It is easy to get ahead of yourself and start looking up chemotherapy side effects and survival rates. One website becomes another and another, and the next thing you know, you are way off-course, reading unhelpful details that fill you with fear.

When first diagnosed, I did a lot of research in the library and on the internet, but it was unfocused and therefore unproductive. I let my mood determine what I looked for. If I was in an optimistic mood, I would look for information that gave me good news, and if I was in a pessimistic place, I would find reports and articles to confirm my doomed fate. This scattershot approach did not accomplish much more than to fuel my fears.

When doing research, you want facts on your type of cancer and your options to treat it, not predictions on life expectancy. Research is helpful, but there is an endless amount of information available, both correct and incorrect. You are going to find evidence that proves anything you want to know, good or bad. It is better for your mental health if you limit the amount of time you spend on research and set boundaries for where you look for information.

The Badass Cancer Resources guide in the back of this book has more than 140 national and international resources to help you focus on information that will benefit you and limit the time you spend on sites that are not helpful in your research. I reviewed each site with an understanding of what kind of information a cancer patient wants so as to not waste your time. (See Badass Cancer Resources, page 241.)

The best approach for getting any information is to go to the source: your doctor. I did not go to my surgeon when I needed information

> *Tip*
>
> *It is better for your mental health if you limit the amount of time you spend on research and set boundaries for where you look for information.*

at first. I let my pride get in the way and thought I could find what I needed myself. I also felt that, given my family history, I should have known more than I did. By admitting I knew so little, I felt selfish and that I had somehow failed myself and my family. So I floundered in the dark, which only fueled my anxiety until I finally picked up the phone and called my doctor.

If your doctor is not available or does not get you the information you need, remember that you have a team to support you. Reach out to them; they are there to help you.

Why you should know your family history

Sharing your family's medical history with your doctor is crucial. Many women over the years have told me they found out that a grandmother had breast cancer, an aunt died of ovarian cancer or a grandfather had colon cancer only after they had been diagnosed with breast cancer themselves. That information would have been very helpful for their doctors to know.

All I knew about my family history was that my mom had breast cancer and my dad died of lung cancer. As to any of my relatives, I just knew they had cancer. It did not occur to me to ask the details such as what age they were diagnosed, or what kind, stage or treatment anyone had. Even if I had thought about it, my fear of getting a cancer diagnosis would have prevented me from asking. By the time I got cancer and understood how helpful that information is to a doctor, everyone had passed away.

I did not know until years after my experience that during my mother's autopsy, they found cancer cells in her ovaries. Because of that, a breast cancer diagnosis increased my risk of developing ovarian cancer. Providing my doctors with that information would have made them look at me more closely, run additional tests or recommend different treatment options.

Tip

It is important to understand your family's medical history and share it with your doctor. It gives her a bigger picture of your health and how to better take care of you.

Find out what type of cancer family members have been diagnosed with and what age they were diagnosed. Doctors look at the disease differently if someone was diagnosed at thirty-five than if they were diagnosed at seventy-five.

Some people are uncomfortable talking about cancer or their family's medical history. Some cultures frown upon talking about it, and there are others who simply do not know such discussions are critical.

Whatever the reason, know that it is important to understand your family's medical history and to share it with your doctor. It gives her a bigger picture of your health, where you may be at risk and how to better take care of you. She may suggest you do more frequent follow-ups or request different tests to rule out something. Whether it is cancer, heart disease, diabetes or something else, make a point to find out details and tell all your doctors.

Building your team

You will have a team made up of all the people who are going to help you through your diagnosis. As soon as you choose a doctor, her nurses, staff, hospital administrators and lab technicians will follow as a part of your team. When you bring family and friends in to help, you begin to fill it out.

You will not have a say in the people your doctor includes, but you have complete control over which family and friends are on your team. As you maneuver through cancer, you need the people you *know* will show up, not just the ones you *want* to show up. It is key that you pick the right person for the task, any task, when you ask for their help and support. The people you ask for help should be reliable and responsible.

You also want them to be good at what you are asking of them. It does not make sense to ask someone to help you with something they are not good at, or know little about or are not capable of doing. You would not ask a friend who is allergic or does not like animals to walk your dog or take care of your cat. No one wins in that situation.

It is important that you are reasonable in your requests and consider each person's capabilities before you ask. You may not have the perfect candidate for every task, but it is not helpful to put people in a position in which they will fail, feel obligated or otherwise be uncomfortable around you. They may start to avoid you' so they do not have to tell you no all the time. Hurt feelings develop, and this is a time when friendships can fall apart. Just be fair and ask the right people for each task. It will reduce the stress in everyone's life if loved ones are supporting you in a way in which they are comfortable and competent. This will give you a better chance of getting what you want and need.

Lean on your team and ask for their help, but remember, you are obligated to do only what you feel is right for you. Supporting you does not give someone a say in your care. You will find there will be loved ones, as well as complete strangers, who will tell you what you should do or what they would do in your situation. They will freely tell you what they have read, heard or seen or what you should eat, wear or have. Some of this advice will be helpful, and some will not. Take what you want and discard the rest. Something to say to anyone pushing their opinion on how you should handle cancer: "Thank you for your advice on my cancer. I am considering treating it in a different way. I have to go with what I believe is best for me. I am sure you understand."

There is no right or wrong, good or bad, smart or dumb way to do cancer. There is only the way that is right for you.

When I was first diagnosed, I looked to how my parents managed their diagnosis for guidance. They did not discuss or share information; no one broke down and cried, showed anger or frustration or asked for help, at least not in front of me. They went on with life as if nothing out of the ordinary was happening. I figured if I just kept going and behaved as if nothing was wrong, it proved how resilient I was too. It did not. It just made me tired.

Tip

If you have to talk yourself into or out of an idea, then you are not following your gut instinct.

Every crack in my veneer caused me to judge myself harshly against their behavior, then obsess about how I could do better. No matter what I did, I did not feel it measured up to how well they handled their disease. Until I stopped comparing myself with my parents, and others who appeared to know how to handle cancer, I did not feel brave, strong or confident in my ability to confront the disease.

There is only one journey you should be concerned about: yours. Follow your gut instinct, and make the choices that feel right for you. It can be difficult to sort out your own thoughts and follow your intuition with the confusing information, contradicting opinions and well-meaning voices telling you what to do. Here is a helpful tip: If you have to talk yourself into or out of an idea, then you are not following your gut instinct.

Cancer is a difficult experience. Some days will be easy, and others will feel just awful. Do not fight it or work to make every day okay. Some days will not be fine no matter what you do. There will be times when you are feeling good about things and that you have it together; other times, when it will seem as if the world is falling apart around you and you are just over it. There may be moments when you do not even recognize your thoughts or behavior. That is neither good nor bad; it just is. Acknowledge those feelings, then let them go. They are part of having cancer. Keep your eye on the big picture: managing your cancer and regaining your health.

CHAPTER 5

Appointments, Tests and Procedures

When first diagnosed with cancer you will find your days are quickly filled with various appointments, tests and procedures. The paperwork, what to bring or follow-up on can be overwhelming. The good news is the information required for most appointments is basically the same. But each doctor's office might word the requests differently. A way to reduce the stress around appointments is to prepare for them in advance.

The easiest way to keep track of all details is to write them down in your notebook, or electronic device, and have them with you at every appointment. You will be surprised how easily you forget basic information—even things you have known for years—when you're under stress. The dates of previous surgeries, details of my family's medical history or simply how many milligrams of a medication or which supplements I took every day continually tripped me up on forms until I wrote down everything. Having the information in my notebook made filling out the forms easy and tension-free.

It is essential that all your information, health and otherwise, be correct and consistent with all your doctors, the hospital, medical labs and the insurance company. Missing or incorrect data can cause insurance headaches and appointment hassles and take up a lot of time.

Tip

Being prepared enhances the likelihood of having productive interaction with everyone. Before you pick up the phone or go to a doctor's appointment, have all your information available at your fingertips.

Information and paperwork to prepare

Being prepared enhances the likelihood of having productive interactions with everyone. Before you pick up the phone or go to a doctor's appointment, have all your information available at your fingertips. You will be better able to concentrate on the call or appointment if you are not riffling through paper or are otherwise distracted.

Below are the specifics you will need to know or have on hand when making an appointment.

- Reason for the appointment: follow-up, images, blood tests, scans, second opinion, treatment, etc.
- Referring physician's information; name, address, phone number, fax number
- Insurance information: company name, phone number, policy ID/group number, policy holder's name and relationship, if you are not the primary individual on the policy
- If your insurance company requires medical referrals
- Pharmacy information: name, phone number, and address

Below is what you will need to have on hand when you go to the appointment.

- Valid picture ID: driver's license, passport, state ID, etc.
- Insurance card
- Referral for appointment (if not electronically submitted by your referring physician)
- Information on primary care physician: name, address, phone number, fax number
- Surgeon's information: name, address, phone number, fax number
- Name, phone number and relation of someone to contact in case of emergency
- List of medications you are taking—reason for taking, dosage, number of times taken per day, what time of day
- Allergies to medication and your reaction; for example, hives, difficulty breathing

- Information on any surgeries and overnight hospital stays—dates and reasons
- Personal medical history—cancer, heart disease, kidney disease, etc., as well as measles, chicken pox, malaria, etc.
- Family history of illness—cancer, tuberculosis, diabetes, heart disease, etc.; age of diagnosis; their relation to you—mother, father, sister, brother, aunt, uncle, grandparents, cousin; if they are deceased, at what age and the cause of death

You will be asked to confirm that all the information the office or physician has for you is correct at every appointment. Always read through all the paperwork carefully each time, and promptly bring any incorrect information to the attention of the appropriate party.

Remember when going to an appointment to take your latest test results in whatever form they are: written, disks, films or slides. Keep the original versions, and give the copy to your doctor. Ask for your films and disks back at the end of the appointment. They are yours, and the cost of having multiple copies made for several doctors can add up.

Medical portals

Some larger facilities have patient medical portals that allow patients to manage some of their information electronically. A medical portal is a secure online website that allows patients access to their personal health information. They are set up and managed by hospitals and medical consortiums. The portal will allow a patient to communicate with their doctor, access test results, update information, request prescription refills, schedule an appointment and pay a bill.

A patient signs up for an account by providing the hospital or doctor's office with an email address and authorizes the facility to communicate with them electronically. A new patient may be initially required to provide all their information manually or on an electronic device at the doctor's office at their first appointment. For follow-up appointments, they will be able to manage the information online.

Myth
Regular mammograms
prevent cancer.

Truth
Mammograms do not prevent
breast cancer, but they can
save lives by finding it early.

—BREASTCANCER.ORG

When signing up for an account, choose the email you provide carefully. It is not recommended you use an account that others have access to such as the one you use at work. Anyone who can open your email will be able to see the information the hospital sends you. It will not include diagnostic information about your health—that will be available only once you log into the medical portal—but everyone will know the hospital is contacting you.

The hospital or doctor's office will usually send you an email with a link to its medical portal a week in advance of your appointment to remind you of the date and time and ask you to review your information. Always read all the details provided, confirm what is accurate and update anything that is wrong. Do not take for granted that the information will be correct in the system. I had to correct our insurance information with the hospital my surgeon worked at before every appointment even though our policy remained the same and I had been seeing her there for more than ten years.

Each institution has its own medical portal, but the data it requires is basically the same. Here is the information it will ask you to verify:

- Insurance information
- Allergies to medication
- Medications and over-the-counter supplements
- Health issues and medical history
- Pharmacy phone number and address

In addition, you will be able to do the following:

- Get test results
- Send and receive messages from your doctor
- Make a co-payment
- Check your account balance for any outstanding payments

Always call your doctor's office directly if you have an emergency. Do not communicate through the medical portal. It can take a doctor or her office up to forty-eight hours to respond to a question sent to her electronically.

Whom to bring

It is comforting to have a familiar and friendly face sitting next to you when the doctor uses terminology or asks questions you were not expecting. It is easy to get frightened by a word or phrase and miss the rest of what is being said. Having someone with you at appointments to take notes also allows you to stay focused on what you are hearing without being distracted by writing. Prior to asking someone to accompany you, check with your doctor or the hospital regarding Covid protocols.

Your companion may hear what the doctor says more clearly or objectively, which may help you better understand the information. Many times, I thought I understood everything in the appointment only to have no idea what was said as soon as I left. Or I thought I heard one thing when I was told another. Having Michael or a friend accompany me to the appointment helped me keep straight what I heard versus what was said.

When possible, bring someone who fills the following criteria:

- Someone who is willing to be a member of your team
- Someone who takes good notes
- Someone who will remain calm

I spoke to a woman who told me about taking her daughter with her to an appointment for support. Her daughter became so upset that she got up and ran from the room crying. The woman was too distracted to listen to her doctor, and she ended up having to leave and reschedule her appointment.

Cancer can be frightful and hard for a loved one to hear about. Make sure the person who goes with

Tip

Having someone with you at appointments to take notes allows you to stay focused on what you are hearing without being distracted by writing.

you is prepared. Let them know what the appointment is for: discuss treatment options, test results, next steps, etc. Tell them what you know about your diagnosis and prognosis. Also, let them know what you do not understand about your disease or the protocol to treat it. They do not have to know every detail, but your companion will be in a better position to listen, take notes and ask questions if they have an understanding of your diagnosis and concerns before the appointment.

If the person you want with you at an appointment is out of town or otherwise engaged, you have other options. Tell your doctor your companion is not available to come to the appointment, but you would like her to call and be put on speakerphone so she can still participate.

Recording your appointment is also a possibility. You can tape the conversation on your phone or other electronic device. It allows you to share what you have heard with others as well as pick up anything you may have missed later. Just be respectful and tell your doctor ahead of time you want to tape what she says.

What to wear

When dressing for appointments, tests or procedures, keep it comfortable and simple.

- Two-piece garments—top and bottom. Do not wear dresses, jumpsuits or one-piece outfits. You will feel more comfortable if you do not have to fully unclothe.
- Wear minimal jewelry.
- Wear shoes that are easy to slip on and off.
- Do not wear oils, lotions, powder or deodorant.
- Bring socks if you do not wear them with your shoes; you cannot walk around barefoot and they will be more comfortable than what the hospital provides.
- Bring a sweater or scarf to throw over your shoulders. Some imaging rooms are cold.
- If you wear hearing aids, put them in and bring extra batteries.

Tests and procedures

Some tests and procedures will require more than your just showing up. Ask the following questions when setting up an appointment:

- Will I need to abstain from food or drink before the appointment? If so, for how long?
- Will I need to take medication prior to the test?
- Will I need someone to pick me up?
- Can I have medication to help with anxiety for a test that may be stressful for me (for example, an MRI)?

A technician or nurse will ask you the following before performing the test:

- If you have any tattoos or piercings
- If you have any metal implants in your body
- If you have any allergies to medication and what your allergic reactions are: hives, rashes, throat tightening
- What medications you are on—the number of milligrams, the number of times per day and the reason for taking them
- The last time you had anything to eat or drink

Always follow up with your doctor for test results. Do not assume that because you have not heard from her that everything is okay. People get busy and things can slip through the cracks.

If tests are done at the hospital, the doctor will usually be able to look up your latest test results in the hospital computer system. If you choose to have your tests done at an outside facility, the results will be forwarded to the doctor who requested them, but the results may not be entered into the hospital system for other doctors to see.

Any doctors not associated with the hospital will have results only for the tests they ordered. If you have your tests done at an

> **Tip**
>
> *Always follow up with your doctor for test results. Do not assume that because you have not heard from her that everything is okay.*

outside lab or facility, ask for a release form at the time of your test so copies of the results can be mailed to your home to ensure you get a copy. If the tests were done at a hospital or doctor's office that has a patient portal, you can log into the portal and access or download your test results at any time.

Always indicate that you want your primary care physician to get a copy. She may not be involved with your health care right now, but at some point, you will switch back to her or she will become actively involved in your care. It will help this transition if she is up to date on test results and has been kept informed on your health from your initial diagnosis.

This task can easily be accomplished by requesting copies of all test results and doctors' notes taken while you are going through cancer treatment be sent to her office. The forms you fill out at the doctor's office and when getting tests will ask if you want other physicians to get a copy of the test results. Check in periodically to confirm she is receiving your test results. When you switch back, she will be fully informed and know how to proceed with your health care from there.

It is advantageous for your overall health to ensure that all your doctors have a copy of your current test results whether they requested them or not. It is best for you when everybody is working with the most up-to-date information.

There are additional reasons it is a good practice to have copies of your test results even if all your doctors are in the same hospital. You may decide to get another opinion, in which case the doctor will need to see a copy of everything to accurately assess your situation. If you are switching to a new doctor, you will need to have your latest test results. Having these records will give the new doctor current information and may enable you to avoid unnecessary and costly tests. If you move to another city or state, you will have all your medical records current and on hand, making the changeover to another physician easier.

Pre-op tests

Your doctor will require you to have pre-op (short for "preoperative") tests done to confirm you are healthy enough to undergo surgery. They are done no more than four weeks prior to your operation. They usually involve an electrocardiogram, lung X-ray and complete blood workup. Your surgeon may request additional tests such as a urine test or stress test to assess your health.

You can have pre-op tests done at the hospital, an independent facility or your primary doctor's office if it is set up to do them. Check with a lab about the costs for a procedure prior to making an appointment. Independent facilities can be less expensive than the hospital for these tests. Always confirm that an outside lab is in your network and takes your insurance and that the hospital recognizes the facility and will accept its test results.

Referrals

A medical referral is a form a primary care physician fills out when sending a patient to a specialist or when requesting tests. Most insurance companies require a doctor's referral before they pay for or reimburse you for fees and expenses. Your doctor will either send an electronic referral to the specialist or fax it to the specialist's office. A doctor's referral does not guarantee that insurance will cover whatever procedure or test is being requested. Before you make the appointment, check with your insurance company to confirm it will cover the tests. If it does not, discuss your options with your doctor.

A referral can be written for a single appointment or several if you will be having ongoing treatment or physical therapy. A referral is not open-ended and will need to be updated periodically, at which time you need to contact your primary care physician or another authorized doctor to write a new one. Not having a current referral in place can result in an appointment being canceled or postponed to a later date until you have obtained the necessary referral, or you might be billed for the full cost of the appointment. An expired referral can also cause a payment for a procedure to be denied or delay a reimbursement from your insurance company.

You will need to have a current referral in place for each doctor and for each test and procedure requested. Do not depend on the specialist's office to keep you informed when your referral will expire. Some may let you know when your referral is about to expire, but many do not. The easiest way to track each referral is to write down in your notebook the number of appointments it covers, which doctor referred it and the date it needs to be renewed. You can also set up a countdown calendar that indicates the number of visits remaining with each doctor before a new referral is required. Check with your doctor's office how much lead time is necessary to write one, and factor that in to your timeline. Some require seven to ten days' notice. Circle in red the date on your calendar when you need to request a new referral.

A referral will typically include the following information:
- Referring doctor's name, phone number, address
- The diagnosis
- The number of appointments you can have
- What is being requested—consultation, testing, follow-up, treatment
- Area of the body to be tested
- Type of test—X-ray, scan, image or others such as blood, urine

Review your referral with your doctor or her office before she sends it to anyone. Make sure you understand what you are having done and what she expects from the tests. Ask for a copy of the referral for your records, so you always have one on hand should you get to an appointment and there is not one on file. More than once I avoided grief because I was timely with a renewal or had a copy of the referral with me.

Pre-certification and pre-authorization

Pre-certification is a review process insurance companies use to determine the eligibility, level of benefits and medical necessity of a test, procedure or medication. Once an approval is obtained, a pre-certification number is provided and submitted with the claim. Pre-authorization is when a doctor must get permission from the insurance company to provide a service. This is to determine if the service she is prescribing is covered under your plan. It is also to ensure you have enough coverage for what she is recommending—for example, your plan may limit you to twelve physical therapy visits in a calendar year.

Your doctor's office will contact your insurance company directly with the request. Once it is approved, her office will contact the lab, pharmacy or hospital with the paperwork. Pre-authorization and pre-certification can take several days or as long as a month. Keep that in mind for anything that is time-sensitive such as medication.

Simply because your doctor wants a test, and the status of your health warrants it, the insurance company may not agree to pay for any or all of it. If your insurance company denies a procedure, it means it will not pay for it. It does not mean you cannot have it; you may need to find the means to cover the expense.

Do not panic if you are denied a procedure. You still have options.

- Discuss your situation with your doctor and see how she can help you.
- Ask if the hospital has a financial guidance counselor to assist you.
- Appeal the decision.
- Negotiate with the hospital to reduce the cost.
- Look for programs that provide a reduced fee or free services. (See Badass Cancer Resources, Financial Assistance, page 247.)
- Apply for financial assistance to help with the costs. (See Badass Cancer Resources, Financial Assistance, page 247.)
- Contact a patient advocate to assist and guide you with your options. (See Badass Cancer Resources, Patient Advocate, page 254.)

Being denied a procedure can be frightening, but do not let it stop you from getting the medical attention you need. Lean on others for help and guidance.

Care bag for appointments

You will spend a lot of time in waiting rooms of your doctors' offices and hospital. It can be boring, nerve-racking and difficult to pass the time. A care bag that you take to every appointment can help keep you comfortable and occupied. It should contain anything that makes you feel relaxed or happy. Mine included a bottle of my favorite iced tea, a snack, a magazine, headphones, music, tissues, a book, peppermint candy, knitting supplies, a sweater, socks and a small stone with the word "courage" cut into it that I held in my hand when I was anxious.

My care bag had everything I wanted or needed close at hand and brought me comfort and reduced my anxiety. When out running errands, I would look for items, like a new magazine, activity or snack to switch things up or add to my bag. That gave me something to look forward to the next time I sat in a waiting room. Pinterest, a free website where people share images and ideas around a theme, has several examples of care bags to help inspire you. In the search bar of a search engine—for example, Google or Yahoo!—type in Pinterest.com. In the search bar at the top of the Pinterest website, type in *cancer care bags*.

A care bag is a simple way to take care of your comfort and make a difference in your day as you wait for appointments, tests or procedures.

CHAPTER 6

Surgery

The days or weeks leading up to surgery can be fretful. It is hard to find things that lessen your fear, but there are ways to reduce your stress the day of the operation and promote your comfort and well-being after. Here are tips to help keep you busy and distracted yet prepared for the surgery.

Before surgery

A hospital can be an intimidating place, especially if you have not spent much time in one. One way to make it less scary is to go to the hospital before your operation and become familiar with your surroundings, Covid protocols permitting. You do not need a grand tour, just a bit of familiarity. Locate the registration desk, see the waiting room where your family will be and go to the floor where you will have surgery. If you are going to stay in the hospital, take a walk around a patient floor. Ask at the information desk any questions you may have about out-patient care or staying in the hospital.

There are also a few details you can take care of before surgery to avoid any confusion or complications later.

- When you get a surgical date, confirm with your surgeon's office that everyone involved in your surgery takes your insurance. The hospital and your surgeon may accept your plan, but

Tip

A hospital can be an intimidating place, especially if you have not spent much time in one. One way to make it less scary is to go to the hospital before your operation and become familiar with your surroundings.

the anesthesiologist may not. Most likely no one will tell you this critical information unless you ask. You will find out when you receive her bill. If the anesthesiologist is not on your plan, discuss with your surgeon if she can use one that is in your network.

- If the anesthesiologist is not in-network or does not take your plan, see if she is willing to negotiate her fee.
- Follow up with your doctor's billing department to confirm it has everything it needs from you and your insurance company. Even if you have already done this, it is best to do it again a week before your operation.
- Review all medications, supplements, herbs and over-the-counter medication you are taking with your doctor or surgical nurse. Discuss if there are ones you must stop prior to surgery and, if so, how many days ahead of time.

Planning for your comfort when you return home will allow you to come back to a relaxing environment and put your energy into recuperation. Below are some ideas you can do that will benefit you after surgery. Consider reaching out to an available member of your team to help you.

- Clean your house.
- Arrange your favorite things by your bed: books, lotion, lip balm, magazines, photos.
- Move snacks, food or other items on high shelves down to lower levels.
- Place necessities in easy-to-reach places.
- Prepare and freeze a couple of meals.
- Buy a sports bra or other supportive undergarments your surgeon recommends.
- Get an extra set of house keys made for your caregivers so they can let themselves in without disturbing you.
- Line up a couple of things to look forward to after your surgery: a book by a favorite author, relaxing activities such as puzzles, painting or coloring books.
- Get new loungewear or pajamas for yourself.

After you have gathered all the documents, signed any paperwork, had your pre-op tests, packed your bag and taken care of logistics, focus on creating peace around you. Take deep breaths often, calm your mind and visualize healing. There is no perfect state of mind for surgery, but the calmer you are before your operation, and the day of your surgery, the better it is for your overall well-being. It will benefit you mentally and spiritually if you find moments to take care of and pamper yourself prior to surgery.

- Get a manicure and pedicure with clear polish or no polish at all. Your doctor can monitor oxygen flow by observing the color of your fingernails. If you wear a dark polish, she cannot see if your nails are changing colors.
- Wash and blow-dry your hair the day before surgery; you will not be able to wash or style it for several days afterward.
- Get a massage or reflexology, or have a spa day.
- Get medication to help with anxiety if needed.
- Practice visualization, meditation or yoga.
- Find out if your hospital offers a preoperative program on therapeutic healing.
- Ask your surgeon if you can bring your iPod or MP3 player and headphones into surgery; if yes, you can download uplifting or healing music.
- Jot down words you want your surgical team to say as you are being sedated.

At Michael's urging, I booked a massage late Sunday afternoon the day before my surgery early Monday morning. Normally, I love them, but this day I sat in the waiting room of the spa fidgety over the thought of lying quietly for an hour. I was anxious about my operation, and

Tip

There is no perfect state of mind for surgery, but the calmer you are before your operation, the better it is for your overall well-being.

I did not think I could relax enough to enjoy a massage. I was about to cancel the appointment and leave when the therapist called my name.

When we got to the massage room she handed me a robe, instructed me to undress and to lie facedown on the table. As she turned to leave, she stopped and asked if I was okay. I quickly responded, "Yes." Then said, "No. I lied. I'm not fine. I'm having surgery for breast cancer tomorrow morning, and I'm terrified. I don't know if I can relax enough to get a massage."

She walked over to me, put her arms around me and in a calm and direct voice said, "Yes, you can. Give your worries to me for the next hour. I will hold on to them for you." She put out her hands as if she was accepting a package from me. She directed me to take a deep breath, exhale and transfer my anxiety into her hands. I did as she said and visualized my troubled thoughts leaving my body and moving to her. I took several deep breaths, and each time I exhaled, I unloaded a little more into her hands. I was surprised that it worked. I relaxed and felt calmer and was able to enjoy the massage.

When it was over and I was dressed, she held out her hands as if to give me a package. I looked at her confused, and she said, "Your worries." I smiled and thanked her for holding them but declined to take them back. I told her, "I will figure out which ones I want on my walk home." I was still scared about my surgery in the morning, but I was not as tense.

Paperwork and essentials to take to the hospital

There are several items you will need to take with you the day of your surgery. Gathering them ahead of time will make certain you are prepared.

Health-care proxy

A health-care proxy allows you to appoint someone to become your health-care agent. This person is responsible for making all your health-care decisions should you lose the ability to do so for yourself. You will need to have one on file with the hospital prior to surgery. The hospital can provide you with the forms, or you can get them online. (See Badass Cancer Resources, Legal Information and Documents, page 251.)

You should appoint someone you trust, such as a family member or close friend, as the agent for your health-care proxy. This individual will make sure the health-care providers follow your wishes as it relates to the care and well-being of your health. You may allow the agent to make all the health-care decisions for you or just some of them. You can also write into the health-care proxy instructions for this person to follow.

Have the following ready to take with you:

- Identification card—driver's license, passport, state/government ID
- Insurance card
- Name, phone number and relation of the contact person the doctor can speak with after your surgery
- Name, phone number and the relation of the person who will be taking you home if it is not the same as your contact person
- Cases or containers for eyeglasses, dentures, hearing aid(s), contacts, wig, and prosthetics. You will need to remove all these items before going into the operating room.
- Breathing machine for apnea, if you use one

Keep paper in a secure folder or large resealable bag, such as a plastic freezer bag, so nothing gets separated or lost. Take a small bag for the other items. It is not advisable to wear or take anything valuable such as jewelry with you to the hospital. You will not be able to wear it during surgery.

Overnight bag

Below are helpful items to include in your overnight bag if you are going to stay in the hospital:

- Your notebook
- Contact list
- Medications. You can take your own medication to the hospital. Inform your doctor if you will be doing so.
- Socks, slippers or flip-flops
- Comfy pajamas and robe
- Eye mask for sleeping

- Ear plugs for sleeping, if you are a light sleeper
- Underwear
- Toiletries. The hospital will provide toiletries, but you might prefer your own.
- Book
- Phone and charger
- Cases for eyeglasses, hearing aid(s), dentures, contacts, wig, prosthetics, and jewelry
- iPod, tablet, MP3 player (Check the hospital policy on electronics.)
- Headphones and charger for electronics

Surgery day

Get rest the night before, and follow your doctor's instructions for fasting before surgery. Remember the following:

- Wear your glasses instead of contacts.
- Remove all body piercings before going to the hospital.
- Wear loose clothing: button-down shirt; bottoms and shoes that are easy to slip into.
- Bring a sports bra to wear after surgery.
- Do not wear deodorant, lotions, creams, oils, powders, makeup or perfume.
- Do not bring a lot of cash or credit cards.

Intake

When you arrive at the hospital, you first go through intake. An administrator will give you consent forms to fill out and sign, take your insurance card, confirm your personal data and ask for your health-care proxy and information about the person picking you up. If you have not been given a Patient's Bill of Rights, you will be given one at this time. This document is a list of guarantees the patient can expect when receiving medical care such as information, fair treatment, autonomy over medical decisions and confidentiality.

Myth
Surgery causes cancer to spread.

Truth
Surgery cannot cause cancer to spread. Surgically removing cancer is often the first and most important treatment.

—MAYOCLINIC.ORG

Once you are through intake, a nurse will take your vital signs and ask if you followed the fasting schedule. She will ask you to verify your surgeon's name and the procedure you are having done. She will review prescribed and over-the-counter medication and supplements you take and ask you about any allergies you have and the reaction they cause. Make sure she is aware of any implants and tattoos as well as previous illnesses, aliments, surgeries or hospitalizations you have had. Let her know the outcome of any prior operations and if you incurred any complications.

The surgeon, anesthesiologist and surgical nurse will speak to you individually and ask you many of the same questions as the nurse did. This procedure is not redundant; you want everyone to hear your answers from you and not from a second or third party or by reading them off your chart.

Each individual will explain her role in your procedure. She may initial your breast in magic marker, confirming she has met with you and understands which breast will undergo surgery. All of this helps avoids any miscommunication or misunderstandings.

As you meet with each doctor and nurse, you need to let them know the following:

- Any allergies to latex or anesthesia and the type of reaction they cause
- If you have sleep apnea
- Any prior procedures and if you experienced any complications

Be honest with everyone about your alcohol, tobacco and recreational drug use. No one is there to judge you; the goal is to get you safely through the surgery. Holding back or not telling them everything could put you at risk of complications.

It is calming to have support throughout the day. It is not necessary to have someone take you to the hospital, the way you must have someone pick you up, but it is reassuring to have someone by your side. Ask a member of your team to be with you that day. She does not have to do anything except be a friend and provide company.

My surgery was scheduled for Monday morning at 8 o'clock. I had to be at the hospital at 6 o'clock to go through intake, change clothes and have a wire location procedure done. The hospital was quiet when we arrived, but as the morning went on it got busy. Michael sat next to me as I filled out paperwork and went into the dressing room with me while I changed. We made small talk and joked about the hospital décor, the gown and socks I had to wear and the morning entertainment on TV. I complained I could not have coffee before the operation and that the lights were too bright in the waiting room. He promised to write a letter to the president of the hospital about my grievances while I was in surgery. Chatting and joking with him kept my mind off my impending surgery.

My appointment for the wire localization placement was at 7 o'clock in radiology. For this procedure, wires are placed in your breast to mark the area of abnormal tissue, so it can be removed in surgery. I did not know what the procedure involved but soon found out it was very similar to the core biopsy: I was facedown on a table with my breast through a hole and in a mammogram machine. Images were taken to locate the suspicious spots, then two wires were inserted, and their exposed ends were taped to my chest. The experience triggered the feeling of powerlessness and panic I felt two weeks prior in that room. I left the procedure room shaking. When I saw Michael in the waiting room, I started crying. I was very grateful to have him with me as company and comfort.

Recovery

After surgery, you will be in the recovery area while you come out of anesthesia. Usually this is when your doctor will speak with you to see how you are and let you know how the surgery went.

If you are going home the same day as your surgery, you will be in recovery for a few hours until your vital signs are normal. If you are staying in the hospital, you will be transported to your room from the recovery area after a few hours of observation.

Visitors can come to the recovery room to see you after you wake up. It can take as long as ninety minutes after your surgery before you are well enough to greet anyone. To promote quiet and healing—even prior to the Covid pandemic—most hospitals limit the number of guests a patient can receive.

Going home

When someone picks you up after surgery, it is more than a drive-by to get you home. You will not be discharged until the medical personnel have shown you—and the person taking you home—how to manage your aftercare, such as how to empty your surgical drain, if you have one, and care for your incision.

You want someone who will pay attention to your discharge and medication instructions and next steps. Have the person picking you up write down what you are told or record what is being said on your, or their, phone or other device. It is important that you have correct information when you get home. Ask for a copy of the discharge summary and the results of tests and labs that were done while in the hospital. Get your chaperone to fill any prescriptions you are given at the hospital pharmacy. The person who picks you up should also be able to help you get dressed, carry anything you brought with you and get you settled when you return home.

Post-op appointment

Your surgeon's office will set up a post-op appointment for you for several days after your surgery. Your surgeon will go over any reports that are back, examine your incision and take out the drain. Make sure to ask for copies of these pathology reports for your records.

Following are post-op questions to discuss with your doctor:

- What size was the tumor?
- Were the margins clear, positive or close? What does that mean for me?

- Has the stage of my cancer changed since the original diagnosis?
- What grade is my cancer? The grade is how the cancer cells look under a microscope.
- How many lymph nodes were removed?
- Has the cancer spread to any of the lymph nodes? If so, how many? What does that mean for the rest of my body?
- Will I need more surgery?
- What is my prognosis?
- What are my next steps?

Your health prior to surgery will affect how much recovery time you need afterward. The best way to recuperate is to take the time you need to rest and relax. Your body will heal at its own pace; you cannot rush it. I did not heed that advice and paid for it in the long run.

The day after my surgery, I felt good, much more so than I anticipated. I had the drain under my left arm, my chest and left side were sore and bandaged, and I felt a little tired, but I was up and around. If it were not for fear that I would damage the drain or hurt myself, I would have been out running errands.

Three days after my surgery, I had the drain taken out in the afternoon and that evening went to a drawing class I had been attending. I felt fine, so I thought, *Why not?* It took about a week of my running on my old schedule before I crashed hard. I became exhausted, and my recovery took longer than if I had simply rested after my surgery. I complained to my surgeon about how tired I felt. She explained to me that even though the surgery was only on my left breast, my entire body and system experienced a very traumatic event.

If there is ever a time in your life to relax and focus on taking care of yourself, this is it. But not

Tip

It is not selfish to take your time to get back into your life; it is self-preservation. The more you rush to return to your pre-surgery schedule, the longer it will take for you to get there.

everyone can take all the time they want or need to convalesce. If your recovery time is limited, then pace yourself and put limits on what you are willing to do. Prioritize your list of tasks, and ask family and friends for their help and support while you go back to your responsibilities. It is not selfish to take your time to get back into your life; it is self-preservation. The more you rush to return to your pre-surgery schedule, the longer it will take for you to get there.

Chapter 7

Treatment

Just as many women want to know what to expect with surgery, even more want to know what will happen to them in treatment. Many have heard stories of what other people have gone through with chemotherapy, radiation and medications and can only imagine what is in front of them. How someone will react to these forms of treatment cannot be predicted. Everyone's cancer and bodies are different.

When I asked one oncologist about side effects, she told me she does not discuss them with patients. Instead she prefers to review how they are feeling at each appointment. She said that some women have certain side effects because they know about them. I do not know whether that is true or not, but I understood her point: Do not expect or dwell on them; it is better to address the side effects if you have them.

What to ask about treatment

The options and choices of cancer treatment are based on several factors. The type, stage and grade of the cancer as well as the health of the patient are taken into consideration when determining the form, type and length of treatment.

Before you determine how to proceed, review the following questions with your oncologist and radiologist. When discussing your options and next steps, ask your doctor how much time you have to make a decision.

Questions for your oncologist
- What are my treatment options?
- How many treatments will I need to have?

- What are the side effects of the different treatments? Short term? Long term?
- How will I know if the treatments are working?
- Will I need any scans prior to treatment?
- How is my health monitored during treatment?
- What symptoms or signs should I look out for?
- Is there medication to help me with side effects? Do they have side effects as well? If so, what are they?
- Should I consider genetic testing?

Questions for your radiologist

- How many treatments will I need to have?
- Will radiation cause my skin to burn? Is there medication to help with that?
- If the cancer recurs, can I have radiation treatment a second time?
- If I want to have reconstruction, how would that affect my treatment?

Additional questions to ask both your oncologist and radiologist

- What is expected from treatment? Will it eliminate my cancer, manage it or keep me comfortable?
- Who from her team will be involved in my treatment?
- Who will be coordinating my overall care?
- When will I be able to resume my daily activities?
- Will any of my supplements or medications interfere with my cancer medication?
- Are there lifestyle changes I should make while undergoing treatment?
- Can the treatment be delayed for a personal reason? If you have a special event such as a wedding or a long-planned-for vacation coming up soon, ask if you can wait and start treatment after.

If you are young and planned on having or growing your family, consult with a fertility specialist about your options before you start treatment. Discuss any recommendations from the fertility specialist with your oncologist. (See Badass Cancer Resources, Fertility, page 247.)

Help your doctor help you

Side effects of cancer treatment can be difficult for some women to manage. Your oncologist and radiologist can help you with this if you maintain consistent communication and are honest with them.

Keep a diary of how you are feeling physically, emotionally and mentally, and go over it with her at each appointment. Be clear and specific about any symptoms you are experiencing and when and how often they happen. Let her know if you have lost your appetite, feel pain or cannot sleep. Tell her if something changes, tingles, aches or is numb. Tell your doctors everything you are feeling whether you think it has anything to do with your cancer or not. You do not know what information can be very useful for them to help you. The more details you share, the easier it will be for them to make a connection between what is happening and how they can help you.

I worried about the radiation treatments burning my skin. I have a fair complexion and as a child would burn and blister easily when I went in the sun. I told my radiologist about my concern and history. He told me he would keep an eye on it and schedule a day off for me on a Friday or Monday as way to give my skin a three-day rest if needed.

By week three of treatment my left breast felt very heavy, as if a bowling ball were attached to my chest. I told him I had stopped wearing a bra because the fabric chafed my sensitive skin and started wearing soft camisoles. He suggested I get a soft supportive bra without underwire to lift my breast. It helped reduce the sensation some. I told him I was a swimmer, and he advised me to put

> *Tip*
>
> *Tell your doctors everything you are feeling whether you think it has anything to do with your cancer or not. You do not know what information can be very useful for them to help you.*

petroleum jelly on my breast before I got in the pool to help protect it from the chlorine. He also recommended that I keep my skin moisturized to prevent itching and cracking. I let him know about a couple of suggestions I had been given by people to help with the burning sensation after radiation, and he agreed they might help. One was a tea soak: Steep three bags of a black tea in a cup of hot water for about thirty minutes, add ice to cool it down, then soak a cloth in the tea for a few minutes. Loosely ring out the cloth so the tea does not drip down your body, and lay it over your breast for fifteen minutes. The tannin in tea is said to reduce the burning sensation and inflammation. Caution: Tea stains fabric. Use an old cloth you do not mind permanently discoloring. Additional suggestions: Refrigerate aloe vera gel and apply as a cool balm after treatment; use calendula cream or marigold cream to help heal the skin.

Before I left for treatment every morning, I put three tea bags in hot water. When I got home, I soaked a washcloth in the tea and lay it over my breast. I followed it with the cool aloe vera gel. The soak and aloe gel reduced the sting of the burn. I also slathered different nonfragrant creams and gels I found at the pharmacy on my breast throughout the day. My radiology doctor checked my breasts once a week during treatment to see how I was doing. My skin did burn but not enough to take a break from treatment. I was grateful I spoke up about my concerns.

I spoke with a woman who had a recurrence and was on her second course of chemo treatment. "I've never had a problem with chemotherapy. I tolerate it well," she said. "I get really sick some days, but I think that's the antidepressants I'm on."

"Did this happen the last time you had treatment?" I asked.

"I did get sick sometimes," she answered, "but it didn't happen on the days I had chemo. It was always later."

We discussed the idea of her keeping a diary to determine if there was a pattern of illness. After several weeks, she realized she was always very sick for twenty-four hours three days after her chemotherapy treatment. She was surprised because she thought she would be sick on the day of her treatment, not days later. At her next oncology appointment, she went through her notes with her doctor, who was able to see that the woman's bouts of illness were directly related to her chemotherapy treatment and prescribed medications to help her.

Another woman I spoke with who got very sick from chemo was given medication to ease her discomfort. She refused to take it, which made the treatment that much more difficult and put more stress and strain on her body. She viewed taking additional medication as a sign of weakness. She became depressed because she was so uncomfortable all the time. This made her time in treatment more difficult than it needed to be.

If you are having trouble managing the side effects of your treatment tell your doctor. This is not a time to hold back or show how tough you are. Taking medication to help with side effects is not a reflection of who you are or what you can withstand; it is how you help yourself get better.

Make a note of how you are feeling every day. Be specific about anything new that arises. If you are unsure about something, let your doctor know right away. Do not wait for your next appointment. Your doctor is depending on you to keep her up-to-date and communicate with her how you are doing.

Do not worry about telling your doctor too much. She will discard anything she thinks is irrelevant. Always be completely truthful, and let her know if something hurts and where. She needs to know if you are not taking your medications as prescribed. Let her know if you are taking herbal supplements, using alternative therapies, drinking or indulging in recreational drugs. She cannot help you if she does not know everything you are doing or experiencing.

When doctors have conflicting opinions

Some treatment options are clear and straightforward, and others less so, making decisions more difficult. After seeing three highly regarded oncologists, I had three different opinions on what to do about treatment.

My surgical pathology consultation report stated the following: *Final Diagnosis: Multifocal infiltrating, poorly differentiated duct cell carcinoma, of high nuclear grade. Level 1 Sentinel Node: lymph node free of metastases. Left Axillary Contents: four lymph nodes free of metastases.*

The only thing the oncologists agreed on was that my cancer was caught early. They differed on what treatment I should undergo to address it. The first one prescribed a very aggressive treatment of chemo, radiation and tamoxifen. The second one thought a more conservative plan of only radiation and tamoxifen was better.

The last one said, "I don't know if chemotherapy is necessary or not, or if it would benefit or harm you, so I leave it to you to decide what to do." When I pressed him, he finally said, "I would probably do it, but I don't know. Get back to me about what you want to do."

I was angry and frustrated by his lack of helpful information and guidance on such a monumental decision.

Several times I asked Michael, "What should I do?"

"I won't tell you what to do, but I will support your decision," he always replied.

One day I persisted, "Ugh! *Please* just tell me, what would *you* do?"

"I honestly don't know what I would do," he said. "But to ask me to make a decision about what *you* should do about something that will affect the rest of your life puts me in a precarious position. It is your body, and you will have to live with the outcome of this decision. I won't make that decision for you for both our sake."

I understood his position and did not blame him. It was not fair to put him in the position to make such a life-altering decision on my behalf. But I was distraught at having to make such a big decision on my own. I knew it was too great a responsibility to give to someone else, and it was something I needed to own, but I hated having to do it.

For the next two weeks, I agonized over what to do. The thought of being wrong on this, either way, paralyzed me. While doing research, I went to a breast cancer conference and heard a doctor discuss medical studies and the likelihood of getting a disease based on behaviors. She said there is a difference between absolute and relative risks. The percentages

Myth
Everyone with the same
kind of cancer gets the same kind
of treatment.

Truth
Your doctor tailors your
treatment to you. What
treatment you receive depends
on where your cancer is, whether
or how much it has spread, and
how it is affecting your body
functions and general health.

—MAYOCLINIC.ORG

were established using your current chances of being diagnosed with something. She explained that if your chances of getting pancreatic cancer, for example, were 2 percent, then an increased risk of 50 percent would raise it to a 3 percent. You would not have a 50 percent chance of being diagnosed with pancreatic cancer.

That information helped me come up with a way to decide what to do. I took the emotional aspect out of the decision and just focused on the facts. I used my business skills and created a spreadsheet that compared the pros, cons, possible short and long-term side effects of chemotherapy and the probabilities of each, from high to low against the likely chances of my having a recurrence based on my early-stage diagnosis and family history.

I found my chances of long-term negative side effects from the chemotherapy were much higher than my chances of a recurrence if I went with only radiation and tamoxifen. I had seven weeks of radiation and five years of tamoxifen. Even with the amount of information I found to support my decision, my choice to not have chemotherapy was one of the most difficult ones I have ever had to make.

Make a list of pros and cons for each treatment option. Discuss the list only with a small group of people whose opinions you value and trust. Bringing too many people and opinions into the conversation will complicate matters, not make them easier. But it helps to discuss the pros and cons with others to give you a different perspective.

Take your time, do research, gather the information and think through what is best for you. Give yourself all the tools you need to make an informed choice. Use charts, graphs, drawings and pictures. Meditate, visualize, light candles, pray, call a helpline and ask all the questions you have before you decide. Nothing should be off-limits or considered too crazy if it helps you come to a decision you are satisfied with.

Once you have made a decision, own it and move on. For several years after I chose not to have chemotherapy, I tortured myself every time I went for a mammogram. I worried that if they found something suspicious, it would be because I decided not to have chemotherapy. You cannot decide a year or two after the fact to have treatment because you do not know if you made the right decision. To second-guess yourself—or look back and wonder, *What if?*—is painful and unproductive. Trust the decisions you have made and move on.

Clinical trials

Clinical trials are research studies that involve volunteers to test new drugs, procedures and devices. These research studies help doctors detect new ways to treat, prevent, diagnose and screen for cancer as well as improve quality of life for the patient. A drug, procedure or device must go through years of rigorous studies and testing before it is given to patients. The trials take place in hospitals, doctors' offices, cancer centers, clinics and medical centers across the country.

Many think clinical trials are for those who have advanced cancer that is not responding to treatment. Others think patients are guinea pigs for doctors or laboratories. The truth is that trials are available for different types and stages of cancer, and only treatments that show promise are used in clinical trials.

Before someone can be considered for a trial, they have to meet certain requirements called eligibility criteria. They vary depending on the study but can include age, gender, medical history and status of the patient's health.

Tip

To second-guess yourself— or look back and wonder, What if?*—is painful and unproductive. Trust the decisions you have made and move on.*

The conditions for treatment studies often require that the volunteer have a specific type or stage of cancer. Volunteers are informed of benefits and risks before entering a trial and can choose to leave a study at any point for any reason.

Clinical trials are usually associated with cancer, but all drugs and procedures for any disease must go through years of research study before they are approved for the public. The trials are typically federally funded or paid for by private institutions, so there is usually little or no cost for the trial to the patient. Health plans are not required to pay for the research costs of a clinical trial. Often, the trial sponsor will cover the expenses, such as extra blood tests or scans that are done solely for research purposes.

If being a part of a clinical trial is of interest to you, discuss your options with your doctor, and see if she feels you would be a good candidate. There are websites and online directories that provide information, education, videos and databases of clinical trials taking place across the country and around the world. (See Badass Cancer Resources, Clinical Trials, page 245.)

CHAPTER 8

Rights, Responsibilities and Privacy

As much as we would like to be bystanders in this situation, as a patient you just cannot. You have a responsibility to yourself and your medical team to know what is expected of you and what you can ask of them.

You are entitled to information, fair treatment and the freedom to make your own medical decisions. You have rights and responsibilities, and it is in the best interest of your health and well-being to know them.

Patient's Bill of Rights

A Patient's Bill of Rights lists what you have the right to expect with your medical care and outlines the rules of conduct between the patient and medical personnel, caregivers, hospitals and institutions. The language may vary slightly, but the basic rights remain the same. Copies of a Patient's Bill of Rights should be given to you at your doctor's office or during registration at the hospital.

You have the right to expect the following:

- To be treated with respect and confidentiality
- To receive treatment without discrimination as to race, color, religion, sex, national origin, disability, sexual orientation or source of payment
- The freedom to consult with the physician of your choice
- Clear and accurate information concerning your diagnosis, treatment and prognosis
- Information on specific procedures and treatments and any pros, cons, risks, options and alternatives

- To understand the immediate and long-term financial costs of treatment choices
- To know the identity of everyone involved in your care
- To make decisions about your care without retribution
- To refuse to take part in research
- To refuse medical treatment even if your doctors recommend it
- To use your own money to seek the care of your choice
- To refuse third-party interference in your medical care
- To have access to your medical records and images
- Full disclosure and clear explanation of the insurance policy
- An itemized bill with an explanation of all charges

Patient's responsibilities

Just as the health-care workers and hospital have responsibilities to you, you must engage and participate with them. Doctors and hospitals have the right to expect the following from you:

- Accurate and complete information about your present condition, past illnesses and hospitalizations, medications and other matters relating to your health
- Confirmation that you understand your diagnosis, the intended course of action and what is expected of you
- Your intention to follow the agreed-upon treatment plan that your doctors, nurses and other health-care professionals provide
- That if you choose not to go with the recommended treatment, you take responsibility for the results of your actions
- That you are considerate of the rights of other patients and hospital personnel
- That you update all appropriate parties if there are changes in your insurance plan or another source of payment
- That you settle bills in a timely manner, and communicate any concerns regarding payments

If for any reason you do not understand your rights or responsibilities, it is up to you to get clarification. If you need an interpreter to further explain them, the hospital is obligated to provide you with one. It is your responsibility to speak up about your medical care, or everyone will assume you understand and are in agreement.

If you have questions, contact the social worker or patient navigator at the hospital to assist you. You can also reach out to a patient advocate organization for additional information and assistance. (See Badass Cancer Resources, Patient Advocates, page 254.)

Patient's right to confidentiality

Health Insurance Portability and Accountability Act, or HIPPA, is a law that was put in place in 1996 to protect patients' medical records and how their personal health information is handled as it relates to medical care, health-care providers, health plans, billing services, repricing companies and other health-care clearing houses.

HIPPA ensures you have access to copies of all your health-care information. It gives you the right to know how it is used, an accounting of who, when, why and how it was disclosed, and the right to decline permission for it to be used for marketing purposes. A copy of HIPPA guidelines should be given to you at your doctor's office or during registration at the hospital.

Given everything else you have to do, adding on knowing rights, responsibilities and privacy protections might not feel necessary or significant right now. But it is a good idea to understand them, so you can manage your expectations.

CHAPTER 9

Dealing With the Bureaucracy of Cancer

There are several issues you should know *before* you get sick, but who really plans ahead for getting a deadly disease? You do not think about the fine print of your insurance plan or the details for extended sick pay because you do not think you will ever need them.

Organizing paperwork, understanding your insurance and learning how to take useful notes are probably the last thing you want to do right now. I get it, but you will thank yourself that you did prepare, stayed organized and kept on top of paperwork if you are ever denied a claim, overcharged, double-billed or told your referral has expired. These are only some of the annoying incidents that can easily happen multiple times when dealing with the administrative part of the disease.

Until I was diagnosed with cancer, I had never paid much attention to the details of our insurance policy. I knew basic points: our co-pay and out-of-pocket deductibles and that my doctor accepted it. I did not know what to do if I changed to COBRA or how to use it for anything out of the ordinary.

Not long after my diagnosis, we started receiving bills for tests and procedures, and I could not figure out why. We were always prompt with our monthly premium, our reduced bank account was evidence we had met the deductibles and I knew my surgeon and hospital were in network. The insurance company did not have an explanation for the bills but said it would get back to me.

After about three months of almost daily phone calls, speaking to a different representative each time and being told, "I will get back to you,"

I finally got the same representative for the third time. I burst into tears and became hysterical when she said, "I will call you back."

"No, you won't," I choked out. "Let's just be honest here. Not one person in all the months I have been calling has called me back. Not *one* person. I am so done with all this! It would be easier for me to just die from the cancer than to deal with this insurance shit anymore!"

Two hours later, she did call me back. The problem was with me. When I left my last employer and transitioned my health coverage to COBRA insurance, I proceeded to use it as if nothing had changed. The insurance card, the benefits and the address to send claims to remained the same, but the department they went to changed. It was in the fine print, but I had not read the policy or called and asked the insurance company if there were any changes to the way I needed to file a claim since I went on COBRA. Consequently, I did not update this information at the doctor's office or hospital.

This inaction on my part started the chain of events that led to the insurance company having two separate files on me in two departments that never overlapped or communicated with each other about anything. Our bank account showed we had met the in-network deductible, but the company's accounting department did not. The invoices that somehow got to the COBRA department, about 15 percent, were put toward that deductible and paid. Those that went to the other department were not.

There was more confusion. I did not understand the referrals and pre-certifications protocol well either. Some of my referrals should have been written by my primary care doctor, who did not even know I had cancer, not my gynecologist, who wrote them for me. Therefore, many of the claims were denied because the wrong physician had written them. I had to backtrack every appointment when I had used an incorrect referral and get a predated corrected one and hope it would be accepted.

It took me almost a year to straighten out this mess. Meanwhile, we received persistent letters from collection agencies threatening to take

Myth
Drug companies, the government and the medical establishment are hiding a cure for cancer.

Truth
No one is withholding miracle treatment. The truth is, there will not be a single cure for cancer. Hundreds of types of cancer exist, and they respond differently to various types of treatment.

—CANCER.NET

us to court. The financial outlay and anxiety this caused kept me up at night and, at times, literally made me sick. That is not what you need or want when you are dealing with cancer.

In the end, we were reimbursed for some expenses but still lost thousands of dollars. All this angst and financial drain could easily have been avoided if I had slowed down in the beginning and paid attention to the fine points. I assumed if there were problems, someone would tell me. That is *not* how things work. It was up to me to be familiar with all the requirements of our insurance plan. I am the one who needed to be proactive, follow up, manage and communicate so everyone had what they needed. It makes sense, but it was hell to realize that after the fact.

It does feel like insult added to injury that you have to deal with insurance paperwork and money at all as you cope with your cancer. It can be hard to stay on top of all the paperwork, but the more you know, the quicker you will be able to spot errors and fix them. Read the fine print and understand your policy before you get started. Confirm that the doctor, hospital, test facility and pharmacy all take your insurance and have the most current policy details. If you change carriers or plans, update your records immediately. Ask someone on your team to assist you if you need help with any of this.

It is so much harder to go back and straighten things out, and you rarely come out even. This insurance debacle was a painful and expensive lesson for me. However, I learned to read the fine print on everything— medical and nonmedical—and it has saved me grief more than once.

Getting organized

The easiest and best way to stay on top of paperwork, bills and information is to be organized. Not everyone is orderly, knows how to become methodical or cares to be so. But when dealing with a major illness, being organized will save you time and money and free you to focus on your cancer and health.

Do not let the idea of getting organized intimidate you. You do not need an elaborate plan. It can be as simple as having a few boxes or folders with a sign or Post-it note on each one to identify the contents. It can also be something as detailed as color-coded folders, kept in chronological order by doctor, hospital, test and procedure. If you do not have a system or method of organization, then set up something that is comfortable and makes sense to you. Now is not the time to break in a new system or method. You just need to be able to easily access information at any given time.

If you are hopeless with organization, ask a friend who has offered support to help you. It is best if you ask someone who is organized or knows how to do it. Just make sure the person sets up a system that is easy for you. Someone else's way may look neat and precise, but if you cannot put a finger on what you need easily and quickly, then the system is pointless. It is also as important to stay organized—something you are more likely to do if you understand the system.

Begin by setting up a place for all things cancer such as a drawer, box, shelf, cabinet, etc. Communication and information will come in both paper form and electronically. Establish the same system of organization for both.

Everyone has a way that works for them. For me to get—and stay—on top of the insurance mess I created, I became very detail-driven and organized. I kept a copy

> **Tip**
>
> *Communication and information will come in both paper form and electronically. Establish the same system of organization for both.*

of current referrals, pre-authorizations, pre-certifications and test results in my notebook that I took with me to appointments, and I also stashed a copy of them in my files.

Below is how I systematized all my information.

- Referrals, pre-certifications and test results:
  - Set up in color-coded folders by:
    - Doctor
    - Treatment
    - Tests and procedures
  - In each folder and in chronological order:
    - Copies of referrals or pre-certification for each appointment:
      - On each form was written the date they expired and when I needed to request a new one. I also wrote this date on my calendar.
    - Stapled or paper-clipped to the referral or pre-certification the following:
      - Copies of the test results, written reports, DVDs and slides or film for which a request was written
- Bills and invoices:
  - Set up by doctor, hospital and labs in colored folders as follows:
    - Paid bills
    - Copy of the invoice:
      - Date paid written on the retained portion of the bill
      - Explanation of benefits outlining patient responsibility attached to the bill
    - If paid by check:
      - Check number written on the retained portion of the bill
      - To whom I wrote the check
    - If paid by credit card:
      - Copy of credit card statement attached to the bill
      - Payment highlighted in yellow
      - Date credit card was paid written on the bill

- Unpaid bills:
  - Note on the bill why it was not paid:
    - Double- or triple-billed
    - Needed a correct referral
    - Waiting on insurance payments
    - Not our responsibility
- Note on the bill any correspondence about why it was unpaid:
  - Verbal communication:
    - Note the date, time, name, and ID or badge number of the person with whom I spoke and a few words to recap the conversation
  - Written communication:
    - Kept a copy of the letter and noted the date it was mailed and to whom it was mailed
    - Included a copy of the explanation of benefits and highlighted in yellow what was and was not our responsibility to pay

Create a filing schedule. All this paper and electronic correspondence can quickly accumulate and become overwhelming. Once you have a system in place to handle it, staying on top of it is easier.

When you speak to someone over the phone about anything, always write down the following on the bill, on the explanation of benefits or in your notebook.

- Name of the person
- The person's badge number
- Date of phone call
- Time of phone call
- Your questions and the answers
- A case or reference number if you are given one

The more detail you have from the call, the better chance you have of getting a positive response on your follow-up. You are more likely to get action if you say, "I spoke to Ms. Danielle Smith, badge number 14356, on August 15th at 9:43 a.m., and she said…" than if you say, "I spoke to someone a couple of weeks ago, and they said…."

Understand your health insurance policy

It is helpful to know the following about your insurance policy:

- The correct address and department for all claims
- Your co-pay
- If you need referrals
- The doctor who should write a referral
- The exact costs that are covered: blood tests, exams, scans, surgery, treatment, chemotherapy, transportation, psychotherapy, physical therapy, home health care
- The prescription drug coverage
- The coverage for inpatient and outpatient hospital care
- If out-of-network providers are covered
- Your calendar year deductible for in-network and out-of-network providers
- The expenses that do not count toward deductibles
- If a pre-certification is needed for tests or medication

You may have additional questions. Do not hesitate to call your insurance company and ask them. It is its obligation to explain to you in detail what you want to know.

Consolidated Omnibus Budget Reconciliation Act, or COBRA

COBRA is a supplemental insurance policy that is offered to workers who become unemployed. It temporarily extends the most recent employer's coverage, but the worker pays the cost. It is not offered to every employee or their family. To find out whether someone is eligible, you need to check with the human resources department at the most recent employer.

Even though COBRA is an extension of previous coverage, the benefits do not always remain the same. If you have COBRA insurance, find out the policy differences and details by reviewing the plan you had prior to switching over and what you have now. If you need help understanding the changes, call the insurance company and ask a representative to go over the plan with you. (See Badass Cancer Resources, Legal Information and Documents, U.S. Department of Labor, page 251.)

Explanation of Benefits (EOB)

An explanation of benefits is not a bill. It is a statement sent by your insurance company explaining what medical treatments and/or services were paid on your behalf. Both you and the service provider will get a copy explaining the payment.

EOBs vary between insurance companies, but most will include the following information:

- Claim number
- Service date(s)
- Service provider
- Billed charges
- Discount amount
- Other adjustments
- Other plan payments (if you have more than one insurance plan)
- Patient's responsibility:
  - Co-pay—the amount paid for each appointment
  - Co-insurance—the amount a patient is responsible for until she meets the deductible
  - Deductible
  - Amount ineligible for payment
- Plan benefit—the dollar amount insurance paid
- Percentage of balance due paid
- Reason code—a code that references why a claim was denied or how payment was determined
- A section that explains each code

Review each EOB when you receive it. Note that multiple service dates can be on one EOB. If you are being reimbursed for a service, a check will accompany the explanation. Make sure you understand what the payment covers. If you make this an ongoing practice, you will stay ahead of your financial obligations and be ready to address any issues early.

If your expense for a test or procedure was denied, do not panic. Look at the codes on the explanation of benefits you received for clarification. There are many reasons a claim can be sent back to you as denied: The doctor billed the wrong insurance company, she has not updated her notes with them, your birthdate is incorrect on the form, the doctor entered the wrong diagnosis code or the specialist is out of network. If it is still not clear, contact the insurance company and request an explanation for the denial.

Health-care providers negotiate with insurance companies an amount they will accept as payment for the services they provide. As long as your doctor and hospital are in network, and you have paid your co-pay, met your deductible and insurance has paid the agreed-upon amount, the health-care provider cannot come back to you for the difference between what the insurance reimbursed them and what they choose to charge. If your doctor or hospital is out of network or you have a procedure that your insurance plan does not cover, you will be responsible for the bill.

There is a statute of limitations defined by local law on how long after a service the provider can sue you to collect on a bill. Check the laws in your state. The provider may continue to send you a bill after that time has expired. Always keep good notes, and do not throw away anything. (See Badass Cancer Resources, Legal Information and Documents, page 251.)

Understanding how you can negotiate your way through insurance and bills can be daunting. Consult with a patient advocate or patient navigator at the hospital to help you understand and resolve outstanding medical bills. You can also seek guidance from a national patient advocate foundation or contact a patient navigator at different organizations to help you. (See Badass Cancer Resources, Patient Advocates, page 254; Patient Navigators, page 254.)

The one smart thing I did with insurance and medical bills was to put it all in a box and put it in the back of our closet after my last treatment, instead of shredding the information. I kept copies of everything for at least a year after my last correspondence on it, which meant I held on to the records for about five years.

For three years after I finished treatment, we still received bills for appointments and tests I'd had. Some bills had already been paid, and some had balances not covered by insurance and not our responsibility because of the hospital and insurance company's negotiated rate. We continued to get threatening letters from collection agencies informing us we were being sued for the balances. Fortunately, I had records to back us up and continually sent proof until eventually everything stopped.

Unexpected medical bills

If you receive a medical bill for a procedure or medication you thought your insurance covered, your first course of action is to ask your doctor's accounting department for a detailed or itemized bill, so you can see what the charges relate to. The initial bill is usually a summary and will not have a breakdown of services.

- Compare your medical record to what you are being charged. Look for discrepancies such as a service or medication you did not receive.
- Review your EOB to see if it was something your insurance company turned down because of a coding error.
- If it is a code error, ask you doctor's office to resubmit a bill with the correct ones.
- Call your insurance company and review the services provided versus what the EOB says.

How to make an appeal

You can appeal to your health insurance company to review or reverse a decision if it denies, reduces or suspends a health insurance benefit or if it makes a decision to terminate or cancel your health insurance coverage.

There are two types of appeals: internal and external. An internal appeal is a review the insurance company does. An external appeal is one done by an independent organization that is not associated with the insurance company.

An external appeal is filed when a member has exhausted the internal appeal process but still disagrees with the insurance company's decision. It is typically only available for services or treatments that are medically necessary. Some insurance companies require you go through two internal reviews before you can file an external appeal. The decision from an external appeal is final.

Before you file an appeal, review your EOB and understand why your claim was denied. Review the itemized bill and look for errors first. If you need clarification, call your insurance company for an explanation.

Easy fixes:

- If it is an insurance company error, call the insurer and ask that it correct it.
- If it is an error on the part of the medical provider, contact the provider and request the claim be resubmitted.

If it is not a simple error, you will need to provide the insurance company with evidence that shows the services you want are medically necessary. This would include referrals and prescriptions from your doctor and notes with any relevant medical history.

Whenever you speak with the insurance company about the appeal process, note the date and time of your phone call and the person with whom you spoke. Often the insurer will generate a reference number when you call about an error. Make sure to ask for it. If you call to find out the appeals process, clarify with the representative that the phone call is to gather information and not a call to submit an appeal. The clock starts ticking on the timeline for an appeal as soon as you start

Tip

You can appeal to your health insurance company to review or reverse a decision if it denies, reduces or suspends a health insurance benefit or if it makes a decision to terminate or cancel your health insurance coverage.

communicating about it. It is critical that you take accurate notes on all correspondence.

Ask your insurance company the following:

- What is the time line for appeals? When does that start?
- What is the process?
- Does the insurer have a standard appeal form to send me?
- Does the insurer require more than the appeals form?
- Does the insurer require one or two internal appeals before I can go to an external appeal?
- Whom do I contact about an external appeal? Most insurance companies are required to offer this information.

If you need to write a letter or email, make sure to include the following information:

- Patient's name
- Type of coverage: individual, group
- Group number/policy number
- Name and ID number of contact person at the insurance company
- Date and reference numbers from any phone calls
- The name of the specific procedure denied
- Claim number
- Date of the denial
- The specific reason for the denial stated in the denial letter
- Your physician's name requesting the procedure and why
- The name of the specialist and treatment facility your doctor is recommending
- Any medical history that can support the need for the procedure

Ask your physician to write an appeal letter for you as well; it will help support your case. The Patient Advocate Foundation (https://www.patientadvocate.org/) provides examples of appeal letters you can follow.

Appeals must be made within certain time periods and the insurer must also respond within specified time periods. Always make sure to note *your* exact time frame and stay on top of it. Note when you send something out and how long you are told it will take to get an answer, then follow up accordingly. If you are told it will take a week, make sure to follow up at the end of the week.

If the situation is urgent, and your health condition cannot wait for the appeals process to run its course, you can file an expedited appeal. Most health insurers are required to offer an expedited appeals procedure if the standard appeal process time puts your life in jeopardy or would seriously hinder your ability to function again. If this is the case, you can file both an internal and external appeal at the same time. Your doctor may need to authorize your request for an urgent, expedited appeal.

In the end, if your appeal is rejected and you still have a bill, negotiate with your doctor's office or hospital to reduce it. Find out if the doctor or institution has a payment plan or will give you a discount if you pay it quickly or all at once. Look for an organization that can help you with financial aid. (See Badass Cancer Resources, Financial Assistance, page 247.)

Consider reaching out to a patient advocate to help you find financial aid or guide you through an appeal. If you want the assistance of a patient advocate for an appeal, to ensure you handle it correctly, contact her before you start the process. Backtracking because of incorrect paperwork or missed due dates can jeopardize your case. (See Badass Cancer Resources, Patient Advocates, page 254.)

You do not have insurance, or it is not enough

Not having health insurance or being on a plan that does not cover all your needs does not mean you cannot receive care. A number of places can provide help:

- Patient advocates: Several organizations offer patient assistance programs for the underinsured and uninsured. (See Badass Cancer Resources, Patient Advocates, page 254.)
- Health Resources and Services Administration—Hill-Burton Program: provides a list of free and reduced-cost health-care

facilities. (See Badass Cancer Resources, Financial Assistance: Underinsured or Uninsured, page 247.)

- Cancer and health organizations: Many have a database of places offering free or low-cost care. (See Badass Cancer Resources, Financial Assistance: Underinsured or Uninsured, page 247; Mammograms and Health Screenings—Low-Cost or Free, page 252.)

- Low-cost and free health clinics in your area: In the search bar of a search engine—for example, Google or Yahoo!—type in your city and *low-cost health services* or *low-cost mammograms* for information on locations in your area. Some examples: Chicago low-cost health care, New Orleans low-cost mammograms, Nashville free health clinics.

- State government health agencies: For information on hospitals with free or low-cost services. On the home page of your state's website—for example, www.ny.gov.com, www.idaho.gov, www.az.gov—type *low-cost health services* or *low-cost mammograms* in the search bar for a list of services and facilities in your area.

- Local government health agencies: For information on hospitals with free or low-cost services. On the home page of your city's website—for example, www.phoenix.gov, www.seattle.gov, www.houstontx.gov—type *low-cost health services* or *low-cost mammograms* in the search bar for a list of services and facilities in your area.

- Pharmaceutical companies: Some have patient assistance programs to help with the cost of medications. (See Badass Cancer Resources, Financial Assistance: Costs and Co-pays, page 247; Prescription Assistance Programs, page 247.)

- Medicaid: A state and federal program that provides health coverage if your income is very low. (See Badass Cancer Resources, Financial Assistance: Underinsured or Uninsured, page 247.)

- Social Security Disability Insurance: A federal insurance program that provides benefits to retired people and those who are unemployed or disabled. (See Badass Cancer Resources, Financial Assistance: Underinsured or Uninsured, page 247.)

• Social workers and patient navigators at your hospital

It is unfortunate that insurance, paperwork and bills need to be dealt with while you are going through cancer and not at a later date. Money mixed with cancer can be an emotional hurricane. Whether you are financially comfortable or not, when coupled with a life-threatening disease, money can take on a life of its own. It causes people to make decisions based on finances rather than necessity.

As tough as it may be, you must speak up. Be frank and upfront with hospitals and treatment centers if you have financial difficulties. They know all too well how expensive cancer treatment is. Most have financial counselors who can help you with your insurance, guide you to financial help if needed and possibly work out a payment plan for you. Many have programs that can help pay for tests, procedures and treatments. In some cases, institutions may reduce or waive some of the costs.

The one thing you should not do is ignore this part of cancer and hope it takes care of itself. It will not disappear just because you do not deal with it. Reach out and ask for help, and lean on your team to start dealing with the financial obligations sooner rather than later.

CHAPTER 10

Family, Friends and Illness

There is no easy way to tell someone about your diagnosis. The words "I have cancer" are hard to say. Most people do not look or feel sick when they are diagnosed, which makes it that much more of a shock for loved ones. Letting people know you have cancer can be as difficult and as emotional as when you first heard it. Fear of how they will react and how you will handle it can add stress to the situation.

I dreaded telling my sister I had cancer. We lost both our parents and several members of our extended family and friends to the disease, and I knew my diagnosis was going to be very hard for her.

On a Friday evening, two days after I was diagnosed, I called her in Arizona where she lives.

"Hey, Bonnie," I said when she answered the phone.

"Hey, what's up?" she replied.

"Well, I'm just going to blurt it out. I had a mammogram last week and a biopsy on Monday, and results came back positive for breast cancer."

She was silent for a long moment before she said, "They're sure?"

"Yes."

"What did they tell you?" she asked.

I told her what the pathology report said and my doctor's thoughts and recommendation and that I was going for a second opinion. She asked about my prognosis and when and where I was getting the second opinion. She wanted to know how Michael took the news. I told her, "He is still too stunned to say much yet."

She was quiet, and I could feel her distress through the phone. I wanted to tell her everything would be okay, but I did not know if it would be. There

Myth
If you have a family history of cancer, you will get it too; there is nothing you can do about it.

Truth
Having a family history of cancer increases your risk of developing the disease. It is not a definite prediction of your future health.

—CANCER.NET

was nothing I could do to relieve her anguish or make her feel better.

After a few moments she said, "Okay. Can we talk later?"

"Yeah. Sure," I said, and we hung up. I learned over the years that my sister reacts to bad news in one of two ways: She tries to fix what is wrong, or she needs to be left alone with the information to work out how she feels by herself. I found out later she sat on her kitchen floor and sobbed.

Most will react to your news based on their experience with it. Michael's mother was diagnosed with breast cancer two years before I was. It was caught early, she went through treatment and a year later she was cancer-free. He was terrified by my diagnosis but optimistic about a good outcome. Bonnie, on the other hand, witnessed many people she loved suffer and die from the disease. It was harder for her to feel as hopeful about my future. Knowing her past with the disease helped me anticipate her reaction and understand she was not abruptly hanging up on me after I told her I had cancer. It was hard not to talk about it, but pushing her to have a conversation at that moment would have been more difficult.

Everyone listens and takes in information in their own way. When it comes to big news, some prefer to hear it one-on-one or over the phone, so they can have their reaction in private. Others want to be surrounded by family members and friends for support.

Because you are the patient, and having a hard enough time dealing with your own emotions, it can be difficult to be sensitive to others and consider how to communicate with them. Keep in mind this is not about them; this is about you. You have a better chance of getting the help you need if you communicate with family and friends in a way they can hear you.

It took me a while to accept that Michael and I hear and respond to information differently. He hears me best when he is driving, washing dishes or cleaning the cat litter box. The distraction of doing an activity helps him focus on what I am saying. If I wanted to recap a doctor's appointment, discuss test results or get his thoughts on next steps, I had his full attention when he was busy with one of his routine activities. After telling him, I had to give him time to absorb the information and mull it over before I could expect a response. It could take an hour or a day.

I am exactly the opposite of that. I take in information and decide quickly what my next steps will be. Pushing him to respond the way I do caused frustration and conflicts and did not give me the desired response. He either shut down or said the first thing that came to mind. Later, after he had time to consider the information, he would tell me his true thoughts. If they were different than his original response, I got upset. This accomplished nothing. Our communication became more productive when I allowed him to hear and respond to information *his* way. It required patience on my part, but it was how I gained the support I wanted and needed.

I also needed to be specific in my requests for help from Michael. Making him, or anyone, guess my needs was wasted time of trial and error and caused friction. His tendency is to fix whatever is wrong. Sometimes I just desired a good listener. I did not always need him, or anyone, to say anything, give me their thoughts, make calls, bring food, go with me to an appointment, or be my cheerleader. Every now and then all I wanted was to unload the million thoughts running through my head. I had to be specific that was all I wanted. When that was the case I said, "I need a good listener right now. I don't need advice, help or ideas. I just want to talk. I know you have heard some of it before, but I need to talk about it again."

Telling loved ones

You can relieve some of the pressure and anxiety you feel about telling people by thinking through in advance what you want to say, whom you want to tell, and how much you want people to know. It is helpful to write down what you want to say then read it out loud a couple of times. Hearing yourself say it can take the initial emotional charge out of the words and allow you to remain calm when talking about it.

There will be those you wish to inform right away and others whom you can tell later. The ones you are closest to you will want to share details, but with people you are not as close with, you might want to give less information. Before you start telling people, make sure you have the correct diagnosis. It will help minimize inaccurate details from being communicated among family and friends. You do not have to share everything, just the final diagnosis. You can find the information on your surgical pathology consultation report. This is the report given to your doctor after your surgery with the definitive diagnosis. Ask her for a copy if she did not already give it to you.

Once you know what you are going to tell loved ones, the next step is to begin prioritizing a list of people you want to tell. As you write down names, think about why you are letting this person know. Is it to just to inform the individual, or do you want help and support? A good understanding of your intentions will help you communicate more clearly and get the desired results.

Think about if you are the right person to share the news. You may be too emotional to tell certain family members or your children. If that is the case, consider carefully about who would be the best person to tell them. It should be someone they are comfortable with and trust, such as another family member or close family friend. Also, think about where to tell them and when the most appropriate time would be. Cancer is big news and not something to share nonchalantly as you are getting out of your car or saying goodbye to someone after lunch.

After the initial shock of your diagnosis sinks in, people who are closest to you are going to ask questions. They will want to know what kind of cancer it is and the stage you were diagnosed. They may ask if you have positive lymph nodes and are having chemotherapy, or what your prognosis is. Some may show concern about your diet and nutrition and want to know the steps you are taking to care for yourself. It will be easier on you if they believe you understand your situation and have a plan to address it. You do not need to have a detailed strategy, just an idea of how you are going to proceed. In the absence of any course of action, they might feel the need to step in and provide one, inviting people to get more involved than you want.

If you have more help or advice than you would like, a polite way to handle it is to say, "Thank you for your advice and support. I have all I need right now. Too much information or help can be overwhelming and tiring for me to sort out. I will let you know if, and when, I need more. I appreciate your understanding."

Or "I appreciate your advice, but what I really need right now is a friend who will just listen and be with me, not fix my situation. If I do need more, though, I will let you know. Thank you for understanding."

Always be prepared to end a conversation if it becomes too much. You can say, "Thank you for asking about my cancer, but I need to discuss something else. I'm usually fine talking about it, but I'm tired today. I'm sure you understand." That is a respectful way to shut down the conversation and move on.

Sometimes a well-intentioned family member or friend can usurp your role in communication. They want to be the first to tell people news. Keep in mind that your cancer is your story to tell. If you have a special relationship with someone and want that person to hear about your diagnosis from you, let it be known. Speak up and be clear about how you feel. Let people know it is important to you to be the one to tell this special someone about your diagnosis. No one has the right to take this from you no matter what relationship you or these people have with the person. It should be handled in the manner you wish.

After you share your news, you will find there will be loved ones who immediately step up and get involved and help you. They will volunteer to run errands, bring you food, go to the doctor with you or take your kids for the evening. There will also be those who check in but have little time to help or support you, and ones who will retreat into the background and you may not hear from them again.

It is hard to understand how or why someone would disappear in your time of need. For some, cancer is too frightening or uncomfortable to be around, so they withdraw. Others feel helpless and do not know what to say or do. In most cases, you will never know the reason, which only adds to the confusion and sadness.

I had relationships that I thought could withstand my diagnosis but found cancer was a taller order than some could handle. It was painful and upsetting when people I was certain were my friends no longer returned phone calls, were not available to meet for coffee or never inquired how I was doing. As hurtful and unfortunate as this kind of reaction is, there is nothing you can do about people who will not support or be there for you. Manipulating or otherwise trying to force the situation will not give you the results you want. Arguing will not do it, either. Do not take it personally. It is not your fault they disappeared; it is cancer's. As hard as it is to do, it is best to let go of your hurt, confusion and anger and move on. Focus on your strength and the gratitude you feel for the loved ones who are there for you.

A difficult step I had to take was to let go of toxic relationships. There were a couple of people in my life who were critical, jealous or self-centered and did not have my best interests at heart. These unpredictable friendships caused knots in my stomach whenever we were together. I walked on eggshells when I was with them because I never knew what to expect. I did not know how to keep these relationships from being destructive, so I focused on the good times and made excuses for the bad ones. After I received my diagnosis, I had less endurance for the negative behavior.

A voice message from someone I knew more than half my life pushed me to finally act. I returned the call and said, "I never know if you are going to love me or hate me when I see or hear from you. It is too exhausting and emotional for me to live with that right now. I need to take a break from us. I will call you in a few months."

"Fine," was the response.

I hung up the phone, amazed and frightened by my actions. What if we never spoke again? What would our friends say? What if we ran into each other? Each month that went by, I found I was calmer and more relaxed. I felt liberated. I had not realized the negative affect this relationship had on my life. I never picked up the phone and called. Nor did she.

I lost a few friends when I got my cancer diagnosis. Once I got through my initial disbelief of their behavior, I redirected my attention to the people who were supportive and showed up for me and away from the ones who did not. It helped me let go of the hurt. I also met new friends through the experience and gained a deeper connection with old ones. When I look at the kind of relationships I had before I got cancer and the ones I have now, I came out ahead.

Not telling loved ones

"Why are you sitting in New York when your mother is in the hospital having cancer surgery in Arizona?!" an aunt yelled at me as soon as I picked up the phone. I had no idea my mother had a recurrence and was having surgery. I was surprised, angry and concerned. I immediately hung up the phone and called my mom.

"I didn't want to worry you," she said when I asked why she, or my sister, had not called me. She felt she was doing me a favor by handling it on her own.

Her reasoning made me angry at the time, but when I first heard my diagnosis, my thoughts were not to share it with Bonnie. I would tell her I had cancer when I was done with treatment. With her in Arizona and me in New York, I could conceivably keep her from knowing about it as long as things turned out okay. Then I thought about our parents, who believed shielding us from my dad's diagnosis, when we were in our twenties, would keep us from worrying about him. I remembered how livid I was when a relative slipped and inadvertently revealed that my dad had terminal cancer less than two months before he died.

I spoke to a single mother who would not tell her teenage daughters about her diagnosis. She explained her oldest was in her last year of college, and her youngest was just starting.

"I don't want them to have any worries as they are starting something new," she said. "Someday I will tell them I had breast cancer, but they should enjoy their life as much as possible for as long as possible. All my friends think I am crazy and tell me it's the wrong way to handle it, but my girls have been through enough. I just want them to be happy."

I understand. Not telling someone you have cancer or deciding not to share bad news comes from a loving place. It crossed my mind many times not to let Michael know when a doctor requested additional tests or when results were not as we hoped. I wanted to take care of it and let him know when I learned more. I thought, *There is no point in both of us worrying.* But I have been on both the delivering and receiving end of cancer news and updates. It is more painful to be kept in the dark than to receive or relay upsetting news. It also invites questions if there are other things you have not shared.

Not telling loved ones about the status of your health can have unanticipated long-term consequences. I no longer trusted my parents after they kept my dad's lung cancer from my sister and me. I did not feel protected by their silence; I felt betrayed when I found out. After the phone call from my aunt about my mother, I felt hurt and angry that after so many years, my mom still did not want to include me in such a huge part of her life. I also worried she would die and no one would tell me she was sick until shortly before she was gone. Once my mother died, I realized how tense I had been for years over her health and the secrecy surrounding it. I did not feel kindly toward her for it, which was the opposite of her intention.

> **Tip**
>
> *I have been on both the delivering and receiving end of cancer news and updates. It is more painful to be kept in the dark than to receive or relay upsetting news.*

Loved ones are going to find out about your diagnosis. If they hear about it through rumors or gossip, are told years after you have recovered or first learn about it when you are dying, they will be angry and hurt. They will question and challenge your motives. Your intentions may be compassionate, but that is not necessarily how they will take it. It will be far better for your relationships if you inform family and friends of your diagnosis and let them support you through it. They will be in a better position to manage their fear and grief if they are a part of your experience. Let them in, share information, support them with resources that can help them cope and trust that they are going to be able to handle everything. (See Badass Cancer Resources, Cancer Information, page 244; Caregiver Support—Helplines, Peer-to-Peer, Live Chats, page 244.)

Sharing your diagnosis with someone can also deepen your relationship and bring an intimacy to it in a way little else can. People feel a bond with someone who entrusts them with personal and vulnerable news. Tell people you care about that you have cancer, and allow them to be a part of your life as you go through it.

Managing family, friends and commitments

Family and friends will appreciate when you communicate clearly how they can best support you and when to back off. They will be more comfortable around you if they know what you expect of them and how they can best be there for you. It also allows them to manage their time and know where to put their energy when giving you support.

Family and friends mean well, but they can be taxing in their concern without planning to be or realizing it. After my surgery, a well-intentioned friend offered to take me on a weekend spa getaway before I started treatment. She was very health-conscious and insisted I needed to clear the toxins from my body to heal properly. It sounded lovely, but I did not want to go. My diagnosis had rattled me, and the thought of being away in unfamiliar surroundings made me anxious. The only place I felt safe was at home with Michael and our cats. She called several times and tried to talk me into it. She could not accept that I just did not want to go. "Who does not want an all-expense paid spa weekend?" I could not find the right words to communicate the fear I felt about being away from home. I thought my reason seemed childish, and I was embarrassed to express it. I kept putting her off until I started treatment. I knew her persistence was out of love and worry for me, but it was an emotionally draining experience.

Unlike me in that instance, do not be afraid to say no and set clear boundaries for loved ones to follow. It is beneficial if you have a ready response for things you do not want to do. It would have been less stressful for me if I had said to my friend, "Thanks for your concern. In an ideal world I would love to take you up on that. Right now, I have a lot on my plate to sort through. I'm saving my energy to stay focused on what I need to do. I am sure you understand."

It is up to you to draw the line on what you are *willing* to do while you have cancer. When we cross the invisible line of being willing to do something, and our involvement becomes an obligation, our enthusiasm can diminish, and the activity becomes drudgery.

A month before I was diagnosed, I agreed to be a part of a tenant association in our apartment building to get the landlord to address complaints he ignored. I was one of several people nominated to take complaints, contact the landlord and follow up with tenants. The list of unanswered grievances about the building was long, and once I was diagnosed, it was a bigger job than I wanted to do. When I told the members of the association I had breast cancer, they offered their good wishes, but none asked if I wanted, or was able, to continue taking calls.

I wanted to back away from the commitment but felt guilty about doing so. It had taken six months to organize the tenants, and I discovered I was one of only three who answered their phone if someone called with a complaint. I rarely go back on my word, and I felt bad about letting people down. I wanted the group to take the commitment off my hands. I realized no one was going to do that if I kept doing the job. It was another month before I finally wrote a letter informing the tenant association I was stepping away for personal reasons. It was possible for me to continue to take calls and follow up for people, but I did not want to once I was diagnosed.

People will take from you as much as you allow. It is up to you to tell them what you are—and are not—willing to do. To preserve your strength, learn to be selfish with time and commitments. Do not push yourself to keep going or feel guilty if you are not able to do all your usual things. It is okay to back out of a commitment you made prior to your diagnosis, change your schedule, drop out of the car pool or cancel plans if you are not up for them. What is important is that you are not exhausted from managing family and friends. It is not self-indulgent or self-centered to be judicious with your time and energy when you are sick. That is the way you hold on to the health you have and improve from there.

Sharing information

The information you share about your diagnosis is up to you. It should be sufficient to inform but not overwhelm loved ones. You can let them know your diagnosis and what you are doing to treat it, but too many complicated details are as hard for them to take in as it was for you and invite more conversation, which can be tiring.

Below are three ways you can make sure people receive sufficient details on a consistent basis and support you without exhausting yourself in the process.

- Pick a point person for communication. Ask a friend or family member you trust, who is calm and a good communicator. This person will be responsible for updating everyone on your behalf. Let your family

Tip

It is not self-indulgent or self-centered to be judicious with your time and energy when you are sick. That is the way you hold on to the health you have and improve from there.

and friends know who will be supplying the updates and where to direct their questions.

- Use an online personal health journal or care calendar. Several websites have simple, secure, private personal calendars or allow you to build a free website where you can post your needs, such as a ride to the doctor, a meal drop-off, or a grocery or prescription delivery. Only family and friends with whom you share the password have access to your journal. (See Badass Cancer Resources, Care Calendars, page 244.)
- Set a schedule to communicate. Let everyone know you will send out information once a week via text, email or whatever method you choose. Tell them that if you get any big news, you will let them know at the time.

Understand and accept that whatever you do about communication, you are never going to satisfy everyone. Some loved ones will not be happy if they do not have direct access to you all the time; they will not want to go through a point person or check a website. There are those who will expect a reply to every email or tweet. It is up to you to decide how important your boundaries are and how flexible you are willing to be if people ask you to change them.

Stupid and insensitive things people say

Truly, it is hard to imagine how someone would think any of the insensitive comments people make to a cancer patient could be helpful or productive. Below are a few I and others have heard:

"Oh, my God! You're going to die!"

"My friend's mother had that. She's dead now."

"Oh, gosh, that's a painful death."

"How much time did they give you?"

People are not thinking of you and what you are going through when they blurt out these thoughts. Often what you hear is their fear and lack of knowledge about the disease. It is not their intention to hurt you. They are shocked and do not filter their first reaction. Sometimes their thoughts are of what your news means for them. They are not being selfish, but humans are survivalists in love and life.

One way to handle insensitive statements is to know which ones trigger a painful response in you and prepare a comeback that cuts off the conversation. "God doesn't give you more than you can handle" was the comment I heard most often from people who did not really know me. I know people think they are actually being sensitive when they say that, and I am not even weighing in on my feelings about God here, but I found it too trite and beside the point, and it made me angry. I either said nothing and stewed about it or was not kind in my response.

A better way to handle it would have been for me to have a prepared rejoinder that moved the conversation in another direction such as, "Speaking of things I could handle, I am going to get a cup of coffee," or "Thanks. I don't always know my own capabilities."

You do not have to stay silent if someone's words hurt or offend you. There is no need to protect other people's feelings at the expense of your own. You can tell them, "Thank you. I would appreciate only helpful or comforting comments," or, if you know they have a sense of humor, "Seriously? You thought that would make me feel better?"

The more you speak your mind, the easier it gets and the more emboldened you feel to protect yourself from hurtful comments.

Handling judgments

Family, friends and complete strangers are going to have an opinion about how you handle your diagnosis. They will judge everything including what you eat and drink, the lifestyle choices you make, which hospital you are going to and what protocol you are following. They are

Tip

You do not have to stay silent if someone's words hurt or offend you. There is no need to protect other people's feelings at the expense of your own.

judging your choices against their value system and standards and what they think they would do.

If they would not go to the hospital of your choice, they will question the quality of care you are receiving. If they would not add alternative medicine to a traditional protocol, they will criticize your doctor for allowing it. It is not right or wrong; it is just their thoughts, ideas and philosophies. That is all. But cancer is out of our realm of experience, so we question ourselves and take these judgments more seriously. It is hard to not justify our thinking or explain our actions, especially about something as big as cancer.

Their thoughts and how they would handle a diagnosis should have no bearing on you. It is not your responsibility to make others understand your choices. What matters is that *you* understand and are happy with your choices and approach. You are the one who will live with the outcome of each decision.

A helpful way to stay calm in the face of judgment is to educate yourself on the disease and be informed. It will increase your self-confidence and help you hold fast to your decisions when others challenge your choices. You have the responsibility—and power—to do what feels right for you. Make no apologies or excuses for it.

As difficult as handling the judgment of others can be, managing your own can be just as hard. People are complicated, and cancer can make them act in unfamiliar ways. It is inevitable that some friends and family will mess up along the way. They are concerned about you and want to help, but they will miss the mark, forget and not follow through or just be jerks about something. To say they are not doing their best is you measuring their behavior against your beliefs and standards. Sometimes they line up, and sometimes they do not. Expecting a certain behavior based on past experience with someone seems reasonable, but cancer changes things. Fear and uncertainty cause people to react in unpredictable ways. It goes with the territory.

Tip

A helpful way to stay calm in the face of judgment is to educate yourself on the disease and be informed.

If people do not support you how you want them to, do not judge. Accept their responses as something that works for you or does not and forgive their indiscretion. This does not mean you accept their behavior; forgiveness means letting go of the emotional charge attached to an act. You do not have to like or condone or tolerate someone's bad or hurtful conduct; but you can let go of the pain that comes with it. Holding on to the frustration and anger that someone's judgment causes does not help or change your situation. Instead, it puts limitations on you.

Managing your loved ones while coping with cancer can test or deepen the strongest of bonds. A diagnosis emphasizes the good, the bad and the ugly in any relationship. It does not create these behaviors; it just puts a spotlight on them. You cannot fix how someone else feels about or responds to your cancer. Nor is it your job to handle a person's emotions regarding the disease. Family and friends have to work out how they feel about your diagnosis for themselves.

Patience, understanding and love help smooth the rough spots you inevitably will encounter. People are figuring out life as they go, and they have their own road to travel. You can support them by being forthcoming with information and honest in what you tell them and by providing resources for information and caregiver support. Encourage them to take the help, and be accepting if they do not. This is the thought to keep in mind: The reason everyone has gathered around to support you is because they love you and are concerned for your welfare.

The best thing you can do for yourself, your family and friends is to have truly meaningful relationships. Life becomes easier if you accept what is in front of you and go from there. Appreciate people's behavior for what it is: an opportunity to get to know them better. The knowledge you have gained about loved ones can strengthen and deepen your relationships. Do not hold on to lapses in judgment. Let go of the trivial. Enjoy the good you have with family and friends. You will be rewarded more than you can imagine.

CHAPTER 11

Telling Children About Cancer

The worst way to find out someone you love has cancer is to overhear it. Children know when things are not right, no matter how normal you try to make everything seem. They can feel when you are anxious or hurt and know when you are hiding something. They know when you do not feel well. A modification in their routine without an explanation will concern them. Eventually they will notice a change in your appearance. They may think whatever is wrong is so bad you cannot talk about it. The American Cancer Society (https://www.cancer.org/) cautions that it is impossible to keep cancer a secret.

I knew something was very wrong with my mom when she was diagnosed with breast cancer. There was too much tension and anxiety and too many quiet conversations among the adults for everything to be fine. I found out she had cancer when I overheard my dad talking about it on the phone with someone. When I asked him what it was, he said, "It's nothing for you to worry about." With no one to turn to and nothing to go on, I was left with my imagination to figure out what it was. Everything I came up with always ended with my parents dying and Bonnie and I left homeless with no one to help us.

My parents did not tell us my mom was sick or talk about her illness in an effort to protect me and my sister, but their silence only made matters worse. It exacerbated my nightmares and heightened my fears. I no longer felt safe or secure anywhere, and I lost trust in the people around me. It was the beginning of my lifelong panic attacks.

For many diagnosed with cancer, telling their children, along with concerns about how the disease will affect them, is their number-one worry.

Parents naturally want to protect their kids from things that are scary or make them anxious. At some point, they will find out you have cancer. You do not want them to learn about it by overhearing a conversation or being told by a neighbor or friend. It will be more frightening for them that way. They will question why you did not tell them. They may lose confidence in your ability to be straightforward with them about information in the future.

Your children should hear about your diagnosis from you or, if you are not able, from someone they trust such as a grandparent, an aunt, or a close family friend. Try to have another adult with you when you tell them. If you are in a relationship, ask your partner to be with you. If you are single, have a relative or close family friend they trust join you. It will help you to have the support, and it will comfort them to know there is another adult they can turn to.

The National Cancer Institute (https://www.cancer.gov/) advises openness and honesty when speaking with children. If you are uncertain about what to say, speak with your doctor and ask her for advice about what and when to tell them. You can also ask her if she has other cancer patients who are parents who would be willing to share their experience. If you need someone to help guide you through such a conversation, a cancer helpline is a good resource. (See Badass Cancer Resources, Patient Support—Helplines, Peer-to-Peer, Live Chats, page 254.)

What to prepare in advance

Prepare before you talk to your children. Decide in advance how much you want them to know, and consider what you think they can handle. Some experts recommend waiting to tell children until you have a final diagnosis and treatment plan in place. It is easier for kids to understand a situation when you give them all the information at once, not in bits and pieces.

It is helpful in a situation such as this to write down what

> *Tip*
>
> *Your children should hear about your diagnosis from you or someone they trust.*

Myth
Cancer is always painful.

Truth
Some cancers never cause pain.

—MAYOCLINIC.ORG

you want to say and role-play with your partner or a friend. Walking through the conversation in advance can release some of the anxiety you attach to the words and help you stay calm when talking about your illness.

The American Society of Clinical Oncology and Cancer.Net (https://www.asco.org/, https://www.cancer.net) advise using the word "cancer" when speaking to children. They caution against using words such as "boo-boo" or "lump" to describe it. Euphemisms can be confusing or cause misunderstandings. They may think all boo-boos or lumps will become cancer.

A good place to start is to ask them what they know about cancer. This will help guide you on what to say and allow you to straighten out any misunderstandings quickly. Then explain what cancer is. Depending on their age, you can say, "Cancer is a disease in which unusual body cells begin to divide without stopping and crowd out normal cells. This makes it difficult for the body to function normally. Some cancers grow slowly, and others grow and spread quickly. The doctor told me the type of cancer I have…" Tell them about your cancer and where it is. Talk about treatment: what it does and what kind you will be having. Let them know the side effects you might experience, and prepare them for any physical changes such as hair loss. Keep it simple and straightforward so the information does not overwhelm them. There are several online booklets and websites to help guide you through the conversation and offer advice and age-appropriate language you can use when talking with children. (See Badass Cancer Resources, Telling Kids About Cancer, page 257.) Do not leave cancer to their imagination or assume they know what it is or how treatments for it work. An explanation about how you and your doctor are addressing it will help them manage their fears and feelings of helplessness.

Consider when and where you want to talk to them. Arrange to have time when you will not be interrupted and can focus. Mute cell phones, and turn off other distractions such as the TV or computer. Sometimes talking to them while doing a simple, routine activity such as going to the park, walking the dog or folding laundry can help them concentrate on the conversation and reduce everyone's anxiety. Address their concerns directly and with confidence. They will feel more safe and secure in the situation if you show strength and optimism when speaking with them. If they ask questions for which you do not have an answer you can say, "That is a very good question and one I would like to know the answer to as well. I will find out so we both know." Get back to them with the answer in a timely manner. It will help you gain their trust and confidence.

When speaking with them, make sure they understand the following:

- Cancer is not contagious.
- It is not something they did or caused.
- They can still touch, hug and cuddle with you.
- Not everyone dies from cancer.
- It is okay to be angry.
- They will always be taken care of.
- They can come to you with questions anytime.

Tips parents have found helpful:

- Tell them separately, especially if there is a big age difference or they have very different personalities.
- Let your older children know first, then the younger ones.
- Give each of them the time and attention they need to understand, ask questions and express their emotions.
- Depending on how old they are and the age difference, consider asking an older child to help you talk with a younger one.
- Do not overexplain; too much information can overwhelm them.
- Engage them in a distracting activity before you tell them. They will feel calmer if they can direct their energy into something that absorbs their attention.

- Ask them to come to you with questions and not do research on the internet about cancer. There is a lot of information online, and it can be confusing or even inaccurate.

Manage their expectations

Children do best with routine and when they know what is going to happen. Help them accept variations in their schedule by putting a plan in place before you tell them about these changes. For example, "I'm going to have an operation and have to rest afterward. I will not be able to drive for a while, so Kevin's mom will take you to school and bring you home until I feel better."

If you are not sure if you are going to make it to a basketball game or school play, tell them so. You can say, "I know you have a basketball game on Friday at 6 o'clock. I plan on being there, but I can't promise. If I'm not going to make it, I'll let you know in advance."

Tell them who else knows about your cancer and who you are still planning to tell. Ask if they have friends they wish to know and if they want to tell them or want you to. Let them know you are going to tell the principal of their school, their teacher and school counselor. Assure them they can talk to these adults as well if that would make them feel more comfortable. Sometimes it is easier for them to talk with someone whom they are not intimately connected. This is a good way to let them know there are additional adults they can turn to. It also informs school administrators about the circumstances going on at home. The professionals will be able to keep an eye out for any changes in behavior and alert you if problems start to arise. Also notify the school of any changes to your children's routine such as someone else dropping them off and picking them up from school.

You know your children and how much they can handle. If you see their attention start to wane, you can say, "Thank you for letting me talk to you about this. We will stop for now and pick up the conversation later. Know you can come to me anytime if you have any questions."

Have a way to end the conversation. You can say, "If you don't have any more questions, it looks as if we have covered everything for now. I'll keep you informed as I learn more. If you want to know anything, remember that you can come to me anytime." When you are done, do something easy to change the mood such as going out for a treat or to the park.

If you are going to be admitted to the hospital, consider taking them there before your operation to have a look around and get familiar with the surroundings. Show them the patient waiting room so they can see where loved ones will be while you are in surgery. Prepare them in advance about what to expect before they visit. Tell them there is medical equipment in the hallways and doctors and nurses in and out of patients' rooms. Let them know in advance if you are hooked up to a machine such as a heart monitor or an intravenous drip; explain what they do and how they are helping you. This way they will not be surprised when they see you.

If possible, before you start treatment, take them to the area or facility where you will be. It will help them visualize where you are and what you are doing when you are not home. They may see other patients who look very ill. Let them know that the treatment for cancer is different for everyone, and it does not mean you are going to be that sick or look like them.

Additional tips parents have found helpful:

- Maintain boundaries. It may be tempting to relax rules, but that adds more disruption to their routine.
- Do not lean on children too heavily for chores you are unable to do. Allow them to pick up tasks that make them feel useful and not overwhelmed.
- Stick to their routine and schedule as much as possible. If something is going to change, have an alternate plan before you tell them. For example, "I'm not going to be able to take you shopping for a prom dress, so Grandma will go with you."
- Encourage them to ask you questions. Do not assume that because they are not saying anything, they do not want to know something. They may think it will cause you stress if they bring it up.

- Help them through observation. You can say, "You look worried. Is that how you are feeling?" or "You seem angry. What's going on?"
- Post a weekly schedule of appointments and activities, so they always know what is happening.
- Keep an open line of communication through treatment and recovery.
- Express optimism. Make sure they know that not everyone dies from cancer. Unless your doctor told you your time is limited, remind them of the people you know who had cancer and are now fine. They can be family or friends or someone famous.
- Do not make promises you cannot keep. If your prognosis is not good, do not promise them you will not die. They might feel betrayed when you do.

Keep your kids active and engaged. Give them easy activities that make them feel useful and helpful. You can ask them to do something to cheer you up. Below are some suggestions:

- Draw pictures to decorate your room at home or in the hospital.
- Create a treatment countdown calendar and help you mark off each day. Help them with ideas. In the search bar of a search engine—for example, Google or Yahoo!—type in *cancer countdown calendar* for websites with images and directions.
- Make a scarf for you to wear if you lose your hair.
- Send you motivational quotes or funny pictures of animals.
- Read a book to you.
- Play cards or color with you.

Children do not always want to talk about what they are feeling. For some, it is easier to express their emotions through art. Below are activities to help them cope:

- Write a story. It can be about your cancer or something else.
- Draw their feelings to help express difficult emotions.
- Keep a journal to write down what they are experiencing.
- Create a collage using pictures that express how they feel.

Make sure your kids stay active with physical pursuits such as swimming, bike riding or playing ball. It will help release some of the excess energy they have and reduce their anxiety. If they are involved in after-school activities such as team sports, encourage them to continue, and make arrangements for other parents to pick them up and drop them off if you are unable.

Set aside time to do fun things with your children that do not involve cancer. Enjoy easy activities that allow you to laugh, joke and relax. Play games, go to the park or movies, or work on a puzzle. Simply taking a walk and spending time talking about subjects other than cancer can be uplifting for everyone.

If you see your children are not coping well, speak to your doctor about support groups for children with a parent or caregiver who has cancer. Find out if your hospital has programs to support the emotional needs of children such as The Children's Treehouse Foundation (https://childrenstreehousefdn.org/). Also, cancer helplines can guide you to additional resources. (See Badass Cancer Resources, Children, page 245; Patient Support—Helplines, Peer-to-Peer, Live Chats, page 254.)

Cancer is a family experience. It is important to make sure children are included because a diagnosis affects everyone. Kids are smart, understanding and accepting. They love you and want to be there when you need them. Include them in this part of your life. Support them with information, and allow them to express their emotions. The more communication they have, the better they will handle your cancer.

CHAPTER 12

Cancer and Work

Telling your employer you have cancer is a personal decision. Generally, you are not required to share information about your health at work. You may want people in the company to know, or you may choose to keep the information private.

Your work setting may dictate how much you share. If you are in a small office or department where everyone talks about her life, you may feel support and free to open up. Large corporations are less likely to have that kind of environment, so you may want to keep it private there. It also depends on your needs. If you request any accommodations, such as a reduced workload or time off, or need to take medical leave, you will have to let your employer know, but you may not need to be specific about your disease.

What to do before you tell your employer

Before you start telling co-workers about your cancer, first understand your diagnosis and treatment protocol. The place to start is with your doctor. Talk to her about your job. Tell her what it involves, what your schedule is and what your responsibilities are. Question her about what you can expect from surgery and how long it will take for you to recover and return to work. Talk to her about your treatments; ask if you can schedule them at the end of the day or week to give yourself time to recover. Discuss what you can expect from the medication and if the side effects will become easier or more intense over time or will begin to affect your ability to concentrate or do your job. Let her know if you travel and where you go. Ask her if you should be aware of any restrictions. Gather

Myth
Men do not get breast cancer; it affects only women.

Truth
Each year, it is estimated that approximately 2,190 men will be diagnosed with breast cancer and about 410 will die.

—NATIONAL BREAST CANCER FOUNDATION

as much information as possible. It will help you formulate a plan to manage your workload and allow you to control the dialogue about your disease at work.

Once you understand what to anticipate with surgery and treatment, review your workload and agenda and have a plan for your work assignments. Outline a strategy for who will handle the work in your absence, and plan how to communicate that strategy to your co-workers. Your boss will be less likely to panic over your absence if you present a plan to keep your workload moving.

Should you decide to tell people at work, your boss or supervisor should hear your diagnosis directly from you and not through the rumor mill. It is also not advisable to stop your boss in the hallway or mention it in passing while walking out of a meeting. The person might be confused about what happens next and might become angry with you. Make an appointment to see your manager or someone in the human resources department.

Decide which co-workers you will tell and how much you want them to know. Determine which questions you are willing to answer, and have a reply prepared for the ones you are not. For anything you do not want to talk about you can simply say, "Thank you for asking. I prefer not to talk about the details of my cancer at work. It is distracting to talk about it so much. I would rather focus on my job. I am sure you understand."

Think about how you will share your news and what you will do to handle different reactions. Some co-workers will be understanding and supportive, and others will not. You may find that everyone at work is a friend until you have cancer and they might have to pick up your work. Be prepared for the possibility that some will think you will not be up to the job while you are ill. Determine in advance how you want to deal with any negative reactions, and have a response ready. You can say, "I appreciate your concern. I know you heard I have breast cancer. It hasn't affected my ability to think or work. If it does, I have a plan in place to ensure I do not neglect my responsibilities and everything continues to run smoothly. But if you're bringing it up to offer your help in the future, thank you. I'll let you know if and when I need it."

Lean on your co-workers, and delegate when you can. Be specific about where you will need their help, and assist them with a plan to accomplish it. You will be more successful in keeping your job running smoothly if you are clear with your colleagues and give them all the information they will need in your absence.

There will be those who will be willing to pick up some of your workload and others who will not. Decide in advance how you want to deal with uncooperative co-workers, and consider other alternatives. The goal is to manage your stress. If you have a plan to ensure your work continues to move smoothly, you will feel less anxiety about being absent.

Learn about your workplace policies regarding sick leave and sick pay

Understanding your sick pay benefits, as well as short- and long-term disability policies, before you inform your employer of your illness puts you at an advantage when discussing the situation. It will also help you plan for your recovery.

Sick pay and sick leave are not mandatory, but many employers offer these benefits. A few states require employers to offer short-term disability policies. This pays you a portion of your income for a short period of time after you run out of sick leave. Some employers offer long-term disability, which will pay you a portion of your income for the duration of your illness or until you retire.

Asking for details about sick pay and disability plans out of the blue can be a red flag. If you do not know your employer's policy on sick leave or personal days, first, go through your benefits handbook or any employee guidelines to get the information. See if your company has an intranet where you can access material that covers employee benefits.

Knowing the following can help you plan accordingly:

- The total amount of sick days you get per year
- Whether sick days can get carried over to the next year
- If vacation days are deducted for time out before sick or personal days are used
- Whether you need a doctor's note to be out of work
- What information the note should contain
- How often the note needs to be updated

Disability questions (if necessary):

- What is the length of my short-term disability insurance?
- When does short-term disability insurance start?
- What medical documentation is required?
- When does long-term disability insurance start?
- What percentage of my salary is paid if I am out on long-term disability? What it is based on? Does it change over time?

Additional questions for your employer:

- Can I still take advantage of any services or benefits my company offers such as child care while I am out?
- Is there an employee assistance program to help with personal issues such as financial planning or crisis support?
- Is there an employee assistance hotline to help with medical emergencies?

Worrying about your job or the consequences of being out of work because of illness is not something anyone should have to worry about. Unfortunately, that is not always the case for everyone. It is wise to keep track of conversations you have with your boss or anyone in human resources. Make a copy of reviews, emails with correspondence about your performance or illness, and requests, if any, you have made for accommodations. Keep the copies at home. Make note of any changes you experience in the workplace such as meetings being moved to a time you are not available or a change in responsibility. Write down the date, time and with whom you speak on the phone about your illness and what you discussed. It will be helpful to have these notes and records to support you if you need to defend your rights in the workplace.

Questions about employment cause many who have cancer to become anxious and afraid to ask for information or help. The American With Disabilities Act, which Congress signed in 1990, was passed to protect workers from discrimination in employment, public services, public accommodations and telecommunication. It defends your right as a cancer patient to continue working during or after treatment, as long as you can still do the basics of your job.

There are several organizations that can answer legal questions on your rights and provide information on job and career-related issues such as insurance, legal and financial matters, self-employment with cancer, networking and getting back to work after cancer. (See Badass Cancer Resources, Employment and Careers, page 246; Patient Advocates, page 254.)

CHAPTER 13

Identity Crisis

Charting a path through unfamiliar territory with a new identity as a cancer patient can be hell on your self-confidence. The decisions you make on how to manage cancer are questioned by family and friends, long-held beliefs come into question and your confidence can get beaten up, by both yourself and others. People do not do it intentionally, but your cancer takes center stage, and *you* get pushed aside.

With this new identity comes a sharp awareness of what is truly important to you. You may think you know, but when your very existence is put into question, some matters rise to the top. You can be left feeling adrift, swirling with unfamiliar emotions, uncertain what to do or feel. You are not alone in this emotional turmoil; it happens to everyone.

Many scientific studies support the belief that your personality is shaped by the time you are as young as five or seven. The environment where you lived and how people treated you—what they said and thought about you— provides the "stuff" that creates who and what you are and how you think about yourself. You then spend the rest of your life confirming they were correct or working to prove they were wrong, whether consciously or unconsciously.

By the time you are diagnosed with cancer, you are committed to your self-image, good or bad. When that rug of certainty gets yanked out from underneath you, you can hit the ground hard. Hair loss, scars, skin problems, body changes, loss of sensation, early menopause, memory loss, diminished libido and fertility issues all test your confidence. Who you are at work, your ability to be a capable parent or a skilled lover, your position as the breadwinner, your hobbies or independence are also a part of your identity. When these things are threatened or stripped away, who are you?

Myth
Doctors can tell if a lump is cancerous just by feeling it.

Truth
Neither you nor your health-care provider—no matter how good he or she is—can tell whether a lump is cancer without diagnostic imaging.

—CLEVELAND CLINIC

How do you prove yourself? You, like everyone else, will have your moment of understanding when you realize that an intrinsic part of your identity has changed forever.

I spoke with a woman about her 84-year-old mother, who had a bilateral mastectomy about a year ago.

"My mother sank into a deep depression after her surgery and has lost her will to live," she said. "All she says is 'I am not a woman anymore.'"

The daughter had taken her mother to a psychiatrist, who prescribed medication, but nothing was helping. The woman explained that she and her mother's surgeon made the decision that her mother should have a bilateral mastectomy, but they did not discuss it with her. She could have had a lumpectomy, but her daughter and doctor both felt that the mastectomy would be simpler. Neither one of them thought about or understood the magnitude of that decision.

Losing her breasts broke her spirit, and she had no will to get it back. Distressed, the daughter said, "She's in her eighties. What does she need them for?" Her mother felt her breasts were what made her a woman, no matter her age. Without them she had lost her identity.

Another woman identified with her career. "I tried to work after chemo treatments, but my memory wasn't the same, and I couldn't focus or concentrate on the job anymore. After a year of struggling, I quit. Now I am lost. I thought I would have figured it out by now, but I still have no clue what to do with myself. I worked my whole life climbing up the ladder to corporate success. I miss the adrenaline rush of being a high-powered executive, but I don't have the desire and energy for it anymore. I keep describing to people what I used to do for a living and who I used to be, because I don't feel like I am anything now.

I am fifty-two and floating without an anchor or idea about what to do with the rest of my life."

My challenge was my hair. About three weeks after my surgery, a friend called to see how I was faring. He knew I was unsure about what to do about chemotherapy and said, "Don't worry, your hair will grow back." Several people had already said that, but this time it triggered something deep inside me. Out of my mouth came a torrent from someone I did not recognize. "But it may not come back red!" I cried. "Don't you *see*? It's not my hair—it's the *color*! It is who I *am*!!!" Then words just started tumbling out. "Cancer can't take my height, but it can take my red hair! The only compliments anyone ever pays me are "You are so tall and thin—how nice that must be" and "You have beautiful red hair." I started choking and crying harder. "My whole life, my red hair has been the only physical trait that made me different and the one fucking thing people thought was beautiful about me. If I lose that, then what?!"

Wow! Where did *that* come from? I sat on the bedroom floor and sobbed that gut-wrenching, heart-pounding, breathtaking cry I had been holding in since I was diagnosed.

Until that moment I did not fully understand or admit what the color of my hair meant to me. It is what made me *me*. Dying it would not be the same. My body image, my self-worth and how I value myself all rested on the natural color of my hair. It could grow back another color, change texture, come back straight or stay curly. My red wavy hair was my identity. Now that could all be taken away, and no one really understood what it symbolized to me. I felt my sense of self was slipping away, and no one cared. I felt like a nobody.

We all have features, traits, characteristics, jobs and hobbies that influence and contribute to who we are. To have them torn from you is painful. Physical changes are the obvious scars from the cancer experience, but what goes on inside your mind is where significant change and damage can happen and where negative thinking can begin.

Victim versus fighter

There is a difference between feeling bad *for* yourself and feeling bad *about* yourself. When you feel bad for yourself, your circumstances are generating your emotion. When you feel bad about yourself, that comes from thoughts of feeling unworthy, flawed and defective.

Feeling sorry for yourself because you got breast cancer is part of the emotional roller coaster of a diagnosis. It is normal to have moments of anger, exasperation and feeling unjustly put upon by the disease. Life is not fine. It is frantic and confusing. Expect meltdowns and outbursts—they are normal.

When you begin to believe you are worthless, less than, damaged or diminished after cancer surgery, though, you are harming your mental health and self-esteem. That has deeper and more far-reaching effects on your life. Self-esteem comes from confidence in your abilities and how you value and respect yourself. When you do not think you matter, you become more apathetic, depressed and less likely to make an effort. Those emotions are on display every day in the way you walk, talk, stand and engage with others.

This dark thinking influences your choices and the decisions you make for yourself, and it is detrimental to your overall well-being. It can lead you—or allow you—to identify as a victim. It is understandable that you could believe you are a casualty in this situation. Cancer happened to you; it was not your fault. But there is a difference between acceptance and resignation. If you recognize you are a victim of circumstances, you will look for a way to improve your situation.

When you resign yourself to something, you give up on what you thought was possible. A victim mentality is a habit and can be used as a fallback plan to address unpleasantness in life. Identifying yourself as a victim can bring you attention and validation and allow you to avoid risks and responsibility. Cancer does not cause this thinking. The way people act and behave indicates how they view the world. If you saw

> *Tip*
>
> *There is a difference between feeling bad* for *yourself and feeling bad* about *yourself.*

life as futile and dreary before you got sick, then a diagnosis fits right into your point of view.

It is not a conscious decision to become a victim but choosing to remain one is. The good news is you can change your approach to life. There is no question cancer is awful. It is wrong, and it is unfair, and you should acknowledge it as such. Then let it go and not let it influence your behavior. There are many people to support, help and guide you, but it is your disease and your responsibility to take care of yourself. Decide if you want to have the mindset of cancer victim and hold firm to negative thinking or see yourself as a victim of circumstances and live like a fighter. The former will keep you living in the past; the latter will have you living for the future.

You do not have control over your diagnosis, but you always have power over yourself. Below are ways to help you improve your outlook:

- Commit to being the person you want the world to know regardless of cancer.
- Take responsibility for your choices and actions.
- Become informed so you can make sound decisions.
- Be grateful for all the positive aspects of your life that are still possible: enjoying friends, listening to music, going to work or the gym, driving, reading.
- Write down what you are giving up on—a relationship, having a voice, your body—and decide if you really want to lose them
- Take the focus off yourself and help someone else: volunteer at a charity, give someone flowers, write uplifting notes to other cancer patients.
- Forgive and let go; do not hold on to feelings of being slighted.
- Stand straight and present yourself to the world as someone who is in charge of your life.

Be kind and understanding with yourself. It is okay to feel what

Tip

You do not have control over your diagnosis, but you always have power over yourself.

you feel. A victim mentality is a difficult and scary rut to get out of. It takes effort and patience to change your way of thinking. Slipping back into the habit will happen. The important part is to recognize it, accept it and pick up and move forward again. The more you practice getting out of that thinking the easier it becomes.

Regaining your identity

It is important to remember that you are *not* your cancer. Cancer is something that happened to you. You are still the person you were before you were diagnosed; you just need help getting back to that person or creating the one you want to be.

When everything you know is challenged or stripped away, it is hard to regain your sense of self. Here are some steps to help you recover your identity:

- Maintain as much of your routine as possible: Wake up and go to bed at your usual times, go to the gym, shop at the same places, take care of pets, clean your house.
- Give yourself time to remember all your talents; cancer has shifted your focus: Write them down and look at them often.
- Be around people who affirm who you are: If you are a painter, associate with artists; if you are an architect, socialize with builders and engineers; if you are a mom, stay involved with other guardians; if you have a good sense of humor, surround yourself with people who make you laugh; if you are a humanitarian, donate some time to a charity.
- Replace negative thoughts with positive affirmations: In the search bar type in *50 affirmations for breast cancer survivors.*
- Watch inspirational videos: INC. (https://www.inc. com/) has thirteen videos to

> **Tip**
>
> *It is important to remember that you are* not *your cancer. Cancer is something that happened to you.*

motivate and inspire you. In the search bar type in *these are the most inspirational videos ever made.*

- Focus on what grounds and balances you in your day-to-day life: family, friends, colleagues, pets, work or studies.
- Continue to socialize and engage with family and friends.

You will have a different take on life after getting cancer. Some thoughts such as *Life is short* are apparent right away. Others, such as who and how you want to be, come over time. I did not consciously reassess my goals and personal values after getting cancer, but I found, as time went on, that they had shifted. Prior to my diagnosis, all I knew was my job and how to work. After, I appreciated there was joy to be had in activities such as volunteering, dinner parties and swimming. Cancer gave me my voice, and I began to use it to empower others. I was sad at times and mourned the life I used to have but realized I could have another one that better fit the person I am now.

Caring for yourself

Making an effort in your appearance is a simple step that can make a big difference in how you feel about yourself. Looking good is essentially connected to feeling good; it is an important aspect of how we approach life. When you put on clothing you love and know you look good in, you feel more confident, beautiful and strong. You do not have to dress up or be formal; just be conscious of what you put on.

Feeling good about yourself also feeds your spirit, gives you energy and can bring you enormous benefits. You make healthier choices for yourself: You are more forgiving of yourself and others; you attract and can take advantage of opportunities; you laugh more. When you get rid of the darkness of negative thoughts, you start to light up from within. That is the most powerful place from which to rebuild.

Below are some steps you can take to help boost how you feel about yourself:

- Trust yourself to know what is best for you.
- Feel confident about your problem-solving abilities.

- Congratulate yourself for all you have accomplished in addressing your cancer.
- Be kind to yourself; do not say anything to yourself you would not say to someone else.

Additional ways to improve how you feel:

- Style your hair. Work with your hairdresser to fashion your hair or wig in a way that is flattering and easy for you to maintain.
- Put on makeup. It does not have to be much—something simple such as lipstick or blush can make you feel good and brighten your face.
- Pay attention to your wardrobe. Wear clothing that is clean and in good condition.
- Wear the special pieces in your closet. Do not wait for the right time to wear a particular dress, blouse or pair of shoes. Every day is the right time.
- Eat a nutritious diet, and focus following a healthy lifestyle.
- Do something special for yourself, such as a massage or a facial, or go to a concert, and indulge in a favorite activity.

When your confidence is strong and healthy, life is less threatening and you feel more satisfaction in what you do. Several companies and websites provide help for women working to regain their sense of self after getting breast cancer. They offer ideas and tips, sell practical and sexy clothing, provide free wigs and prostheses, and have suggestions for health and wellness specifically for breast cancer patients. Many were started by a woman diagnosed with breast cancer or those affected by the disease. (See Badass Cancer Resources, Clothing and Accessories, page 245; Nutrition and Lifestyle, page 253; Prosthesis, page 256; Self-care, page 256: Wigs, page 258.)

Our breasts, ourselves

Our breasts are connected to who we are as women. They feed our babies and fill out our clothing. They are sexy, sensitive, feminine and empowering. It does not matter if you are in a relationship, how old you are or what your sexual orientation is; losing one or both breasts can be

Myth
Using hair dye increases the risk of breast cancer.

Truth
There is no convincing scientific evidence that personal hair dye use increases the risk of cancer.

—NATIONAL CANCER INSTITUTE

traumatic and emotional. You do not owe anyone an explanation about why you mourn their loss. Only you know how you feel about them and what they mean to you mentally, physically and emotionally, and yours is the one voice that matters.

For several years after my initial diagnosis, I continued to have atypical cells appear in both breasts. Atypical cells are not necessarily cancerous, but they are abnormal and need to be checked out. Each time they appeared, I had to have a surgical biopsy. I was given the option to have a bilateral mastectomy to alleviate this emotional roller coaster. I was unwilling to have both breasts removed because I did not want to lose feeling in them, which would have happened if I had had them completely removed and reconstructed. Family, friends and people I barely knew felt no reservations about confronting me on my choice.

"They're just breasts. What's the big deal? I would just get rid of them if I were you."

"What do you need them for? You aren't going to be having kids now."

"You're playing with fire, keeping those breasts, you know."

"I don't understand why anyone who had cancer would keep having biopsies. Just cut them off already and be done with it."

Nine years after my initial diagnosis, I decided to have reconstructive surgery to fill in the areas I had lost each time they found atypical cells. By then I had had two lumpectomies and several surgical biopsies that left my breasts quite misshapen. The lower half of my left breast was missing, and my right breast was caved in around my nipple, among other scars. Prior to my diagnosis, I loved the way my breasts looked and felt and the pleasurable sensations they gave me. After so many procedures, they were no longer as beautiful, but I still had feeling in them, which was important to me.

I tried to make up for the missing areas with push-up pads under my breasts and on the sides of my bra, but I still had visible gaps. I bought expensive bras, ones with a smaller cup size, preshaped bras and padded bras, but nothing fit well. T-shirt bras were comfortable but did nothing for my shape. My clothing no longer fit the way it used to without my breasts to fill them out, so I started wearing loose blouses and sweaters. A few months after a surgical biopsy took more of my right breast, a woman at the gym said to me, "Wow, that breast looks very sad." I contacted my breast surgeon the next day. She recommended a plastic surgeon and called her for me. I saw her the following week and had breast reconstruction a month later.

I had fat grafting supported with silicone implants in both breasts. I did not have enough fat to completely fill the missing areas, so the implants were needed. The plastic surgeon used small silicone implants to fill in the biggest gaps and layered fat from my thighs over them. The silicone implants added stability and shape where I had none. She reconstructed my breasts back to the size I was prior to my diagnosis, 34B, and I maintained sensation in both. I was surprised by how much better I felt. Over the years, my self-esteem had been whittled away along with each procedure, but I did not realize how much until after my reconstruction.

Many women are choosing to "go flat" and not have reconstructive surgery after breast cancer. There are several possible reasons why they decide against it: They cannot imagine putting a foreign object in their body; they do not want to go through more surgery; they want to reduce their chances of recurrence; they just do not want breasts anymore. Some women have reconstruction at the time of their mastectomy, then years later change their mind and have the implants taken out. Do not feel pressured by your doctor, family, friends or social norms to have your breasts reconstructed or keep your

> **Tip**
>
> *It is not egotistical or vain to want your body back. You are not self-centered or shallow when you strive to look good and feel positive about yourself after cancer. You are human.*

implants. It is okay to not want breasts. Your breasts do not define who you are as a woman or a person. You do.

You do not have to live with the impaired self-esteem that comes with breast cancer. Talk to your doctor about seeing a therapist if you are struggling. Consider reconstruction if you had a lumpectomy or mastectomy that has left you feeling self-conscious. Most insurance plans will cover reconstruction for breast cancer patients. Also, consider working with a life coach to help guide you into your future if you feel lost. It is never too late to explore all your options. (See Badass Cancer Resources, Life Coaching, page 252.)

Having your breasts amputated was not a choice a long time ago. Now it is. It is not egotistical or vain to want your body back. You are not self-centered or shallow when you strive to look good and feel positive about yourself after cancer. You are human.

Whether you decide to have reconstruction or go flat, you do not owe anyone an explanation for your choices.

Many survivors share your experience and know all too well how damaging to one's self-confidence cancer can be. Call a helpline, connect with a peer, and reach out to online communities for ideas and tips others have used to cope with these issues. (See Badass Cancer Resources, Online Communities, page 253; Patient Support—Helplines, Peer-to-Peer, Live Chats, page 254.)

A challenge to your identity is only a crisis if you make it one. Your values and beliefs, cultural background and physical attributes are what give you your individuality. You have a choice in how you present yourself to the world and what you want everyone to know about you. A diagnosis will challenge you, but it cannot take from you who you are. On the contrary, it can actually strengthen your character and fortify your belief in yourself and what you stand for.

It is an opportunity to take the information you have acquired and build from there. You can let go of perceptions, judgments and ideas that no longer serve you and get comfortable in your own skin.

Chapter 14

Emotional Rescue

In the same way your identity defines who you are, your emotions influence your thoughts and behavior. They dictate how you behave through a good or bad situation. The emotional aspect of cancer can be a minefield of unexpected twists, turns and revelations that can pick you apart and leave you in pieces. Many patients experience post-traumatic stress disorder, a mental health condition that develops in response to a terrifying event. PTSD can cause severe anxiety and depression and last months or years. It can require the attention of medical professionals to address it. Doctors and other health-care providers are trained to focus on the area of their expertise—in this case, breast cancer—and you want that, but it is up to you to figure out how to put your emotional and mental health back together and feel whole again.

When you are diagnosed with cancer, you become so focused on fixing your body that you can forget or forfeit your emotional, spiritual and mental health needs. It is understandable why this happens, but those needs require as much attention and care as your body. Not addressing the emotional aspect of cancer leads to depression, anger, fear and pain.

Here are ways to help you deal with the nonphysical aspects of a cancer diagnosis.

Healing a weary spirit

Our spirit is the essence of who we are. It is what motivates us to get up every day and gives us the drive to take on life. Our mental muscle can push us forward, but it is our spirit that gives us energy. It gives us the strength to persevere and to get up and do it all again when we so badly want to stay under the covers until it is all over. When our spirit is broken, we feel emotionally defeated. The fight goes out of us, and we are just tired and depressed and apathetic.

It is easy to get so focused on mentally and physically dealing with your diagnosis that you do not realize your spirit is being worn down. Then one day you hit the wall and are done with all of it. The confusion and urgency you felt when first diagnosed has become routine, and you are just over this new version of your life.

Every cancer patient I have spoken with has felt her spirits sag at one point or another. What is important is to recognize that it has happened. Do not judge or dwell on it; accept that you feel broken and create a space to mend. It is possible to be exhausted from cancer but keep your spirit intact.

A way to begin healing a weary soul is by taking moments to just be *you*. Not a wife, mother, grandmother, sister, father or brother, just you. Be who you are without all the influences, trappings or boundaries in your life. Let all that go, and start to indulge the whims and desires of *that* person or the person you want to be. Do not overthink it; simply let yourself enjoy.

- Do what you love to do every chance you get: Go out with friends, go to the movies, read books by favorite authors, play with your pets, enjoy your family.
- Be around people who make you laugh.
- Carry something such as a stone, coin or prayer beads in your bag or pocket that you can touch for courage or solace.
- Allow yourself to relax and trust again and follow your intuition.
- Surround yourself with positive, supportive people.

Make a point of doing something every day to boost your spirit. It keeps your mind actively engaged in the process. The more attention you give to positive behavior, the less time you have for thoughts that wear you down.

Sometimes what is best for your spirit is not what the doctor ordered but is exactly what you need. Four weeks into my radiation treatment, I woke up on a Sunday morning and felt done with illness hell. I was angry, tired and over everything cancer. I did not want to do anything about anything ever again.

I lay in bed and stared at the ceiling. I did not have a lot of energy, so doing something ambitious was out of the question. Instead, I chose to stay in bed all day and be self-indulgent. I ate junk food, drank coffee, smoked marijuana, read magazines and watched reruns of old sitcoms on TV. It was not the healthiest day for me physically, but mentally it was just the break I needed. It was not a pity party. I did not feel sorry for myself. It was a guilt-free effort to get out of cancer world for one day. The next day I stepped back into it with a renewed energy and drive.

I took another mental pause toward the end of my treatment. I began the morning as usual at the hospital for my daily radiation therapy, followed by some routine blood tests. I left feeling tired and over all of it. Instead of going back to my office, I went shopping for sexy underwear, then went to a coffee shop and ate cupcakes and read trashy magazines. It was only a couple of hours that afternoon, but for that short time, I felt in charge of my life again.

Those little breaks reminded me I was not cancer. I still had a say in my life. Take moments for yourself and do something that brings you joy and pleasure. Reward yourself with the time you need to mend your broken or worn-out spirit, even if it is only for an hour or two. It can give you the extra push you need to get through one more day or week. These diversions will also remind you of all the positive aspects of your life that have nothing to do with the disease.

Bolstering your mental reserves

Your mental strength is what marshals your physical self into action. It is also what gives you the resolve to make difficult decisions. The constant mental hoops you

Tip

Make a point of doing something every day to boost your spirit. It keeps your mind actively engaged in the process. The more attention you give to positive behavior, the less time you have for thoughts that wear you down.

jump through once diagnosed with cancer, however, decrease your ability to perform at your maximum. Your brain is overtaxed and tired, just when your life depends on you staying clear and sharp to handle the unknown.

Like your spirit, your brain needs to take a step back from everything cancer all the time. This is not a selfish or extravagant thing to do—it is a necessity. It is another way of taking care of your whole being. If you do not do something to help yourself mentally, you risk getting into a rut of negative thinking.

Consider doing some of these activities to bolster your mental reserves:

- Let go of low-priority tasks. (See MoSCow Method, page 424.)
- Make a decision, then let it go; second-guessing yourself is exhausting.
- Set short-term goals: Hop in the shower in the next thirty minutes; call your doctor to get or renew a referral by the end of the day; look into a cancer retreat by the end of the week.
- Take up a relaxing hobby that requires concentration and focus: knitting, embroidery, painting, coloring, drawing, gardening, puzzles, crafting.
- Journal everything you are feeling: what makes you sad and angry, what has surprised you, how cancer makes you feel, your biggest fear. When you get these thoughts on paper, it can ease your anxiety around them.
- Maintain a schedule: Eat, wake up and go to bed at your usual time.
- Delegate tasks to friends and family: paying bills, making phone calls, organizing support.
- Exercise: Take a yoga or tai chi class, swim, walk.
- Join an online community, and ask others for tips and ideas on how they cope with the mental exhaustion of cancer. (See Badass Cancer Resources, Online Communities, page 253.)
- Join a support group, or call a support helpline. (See Badass Cancer Resources, Patient Support—Helplines, Peer-to-Peer, Live Chats, page 254.)

When going through a crisis, it is valuable to have ideas to help you relax, get you through a rough moment or distract you. Below are techniques, tips and activities to support your mental health and help you deal effectively with a stressful situation.

Mantras

A mantra is a word, words or a sound you repeat, silently or aloud, to aid in meditation. Mantras originated in India more than 3,000 years ago and are a simple yet powerful way to soothe and silence your mind. Repeating a mantra silently or chanting it out loud can take your focus off your surroundings, center your thoughts and calm you down. Doctors encourage patients to find a saying or mantra to help them cope with the stressful situation of cancer.

My mantra was simply "I'll be okay." When I was in a doctor's office and felt panic coming on, I asked for a moment to gather myself. I closed my eyes, took deep breaths and repeated my mantra silently in my head while I rubbed a stone with the word *courage* cut into it. If I was in a waiting room and felt anxious, I went into the ladies' room and sat in a stall and said my mantra. It was usually quieter and less chaotic in there than the waiting room. When I was at home, I would sit on a pillow on the floor in our bedroom, hold my stone and repeat my chant out loud. Those three simple words calmed me down and saved me from a panic attack more than once.

Positive triggers

A positive trigger is something that elicits a response when emotional input becomes high. It is the one thing that makes you want to live no matter what. It is someone or something you hold dear and will do anything to always be there for. Triggers are very helpful in a fight; they are one of the ways a Navy SEAL prepares for battle.

A trigger can be a child, spouse, parent, pet or something else. When life looks grim and you are in an awful place, visualize that trigger for support. You can also carry a photo of your trigger to help you in tough times. It is an effective way to give yourself that extra push you need when feeling down and out.

The word *trigger* is also associated with the setting off of a trauma, but the definition of the word is *an action that brings on an immediate result.* The strength of your love for the person or creature you cherish will carry you through those hard moments.

Positive self-talk

Another way a Navy SEAL gets himself through a tough time is with positive self-talk. SEALs are taught to "self-hypnotize" themselves with positive words to keep their spirits up. They are trained to constantly remind themselves that no matter how difficult something is, it will be over.

Use positive self-talk to help get through moments that are trying and painful. Some examples: anticipating the beginning of a procedure; walking into a hospital for treatment; preparing for medical tests. Tell yourself, "I can do this," or "I might not like it, but I can get through this" or "I have done this before, I can do it again."

This technique will help you focus on your strengths and distract you from the psychological pain of what you are doing.

Minute-long meditation

Letting your mind completely escape, even for only a minute or two, can be restorative.

An easy practice you can do anywhere is to focus on a sound in your environment. It can be a bird chirping, the clicking of a radiator, the hum of an air-conditioner or cars driving by. Close your eyes and zero in on that sound until it is all you are aware of. Empty your brain of thoughts, and just listen.

Relax your shoulders, take slow deep breaths and concentrate on that one simple sound for as long as you can. This meditative technique will occupy your mind with something simple, instead of chaotic thoughts, and allow you to calm down and regroup.

Myth
Having an abortion raises your
risk of getting breast cancer.

Truth
Several studies have provided
very strong data that
neither induced abortions
nor spontaneous abortions
(miscarriages) have an overall
effect on the risk of breast cancer.

—AMERICAN CANCER
SOCIETY

Slow a mind spin

A mind spin is when your thoughts start to race, and fear and anxiety begin to take over rational thinking. To slow it down, you need to switch your attention from what is causing these thoughts to something less threatening.

A simple way to do that is to find something specific in your environment to focus on, then count how many there are. For example, think of the color red. Put all your attention on counting how many items in your environment are red. Concentrate on finding objects with even hints of red. If you run out of colors to tally, look for shapes and patterns: circular, triangular, stripes, dots.

Take deep breaths and keep counting colors or objects until you feel calm again. This action will disrupt the energy fueling the negative or scary thoughts leading to an anxiety attack and give your brain a moment to regroup.

Breathing exercises

Breathing exercises can aid in reducing your stress. They allow your muscles to relax, drop your blood pressure and increase the supply of oxygen to your body.

I used an easy exercise I called four in, five out. You begin by counting to four as you breathe in and five as you breathe out, then increase the count with the next breath: five as you breathe in, six as you breathe out. Breathe the air in through your nose and out through your mouth. Increase the numbers until you cannot take in any more air, then start over again: four in, five out. Relax your shoulders and listen to the sound of air entering and leaving your body. Continue this breathing exercise until you calm down or feel relaxed.

Vision board or dream board

A vision board serves as an image of the future you want to have. You design the life you aspire to on a poster board or an electronic device. They are easy to put together with images and mementos that inspire, uplift and encourage you.

There are two types of vision boards: digital and traditional. Digital vision boards are created on your computer or electronic device, with images and photos you have saved in files or downloaded from the internet. The benefit of a digital vision board is that it takes less time to create than a traditional board and you can have it wherever you go.

Traditional vision boards are constructed on foam board or cardboard. You tape, glue or tack your favorite pictures, magazine cutouts, mementos and keepsakes that embody the future you want to the board. The benefit of a traditional board is that you can make it more personal with tokens and remembrances. It also requires you to be more active as you collect images and supplies.

People create vision boards to focus on a specific goal or help clarify what they want in life. They are an ongoing project that you can continually build on and update as your desires for the future develop or change. Creating one is an activity you can do alone or with a gathering of friends.

Creating a vision board can be very therapeutic, relaxing and pleasurable. You can make your digital vision board a screen saver to inspire you and remind you of your goals. Hang a traditional board where you can see it in the morning when you get up and in the evening before you go to bed to encourage you as you start and end your day. Several apps and online tutorials are available to guide you step by step on how to create either type of board. (See Badass Cancer Resources, Vision Boards, page 258.)

Whether you choose to do any of the ideas above or already have a method to relax, it is important you do something regularly to quiet your mind. The constant barrage of information, changing priorities, uncertain next steps and emotional upheaval is exhausting to your mental well-being. You need your full brainpower as you make decisions and forge ahead. (See Badass Cancer Resources, Self-care, page 256.)

Recognizing depression

Not everyone is familiar with the feeling of depression and therefore cannot identify it when suffering from it.

Many women thought of it as just a mood swing, or the "blue devils" they got around their period. They were surprised when they found out it was the cause of their apathy, loss of energy, restlessness and agitation. They did not know depression could cause physical pain, impair their functioning or make them give up on their treatment plan.

According to the National Alliance on Mental Health (https://www.nami.org), there are two kinds of depression you can suffer from: situational depression and clinical. Situational depression is a short-term form of depression that a crisis or painful event such as a cancer diagnosis can cause. Some symptoms: feeling listless, trouble sleeping, bouts of crying, unfocused anxiety and the inability to concentrate. Because situational depression is usually short-term, once you are able to deal with the situation or it improves, it is possible to get through your depressed mood.

Clinical depression involves chemical imbalances in the brain and is classified as a mood disorder. It can have genetic origins or be activated by the enormity of a traumatic event such as a life-threatening illness like cancer. Medication, exhaustion and pain can also cause it. Indicators include loss of appetite, extreme fatigue, sleeping too much or too little and the reduced ability to function normally.

Additional signs of depression to look out for:

- Feeling worthless
- Major weight loss or weight gain
- An immense sense of futility
- Inability or lack of desire to socialize
- Difficulty getting out of bed
- Unable to concentrate or feeling confused
- Loss of interest in regular activities
- Thoughts of death or suicide

If any of these symptoms occur daily, or every other day, and go on for two weeks or more, speak with your doctor or someone on her team. Do not accept that these feelings are "just a side effect of having cancer." They may be, but they are unhealthy. Depression is harmful to your mental and spiritual stability. It threatens your quality of life and is detrimental to your overall well-being. It can also be one of the hardest challenges you will experience.

Your doctor and her team know very well how common depression is in cancer patients. Let your doctor know when you started feeling down and listless, how often you feel that way, if you suffered from depression prior to being diagnosed and how, or if, you addressed it. She may prescribe medication or recommend you seek professional help from a therapist. You do not have to take antidepressant medication for the rest of your life. Some women decide to take it temporarily to help them through a rough time, and others prefer to stay on medication longer. You and your doctor, together, will determine what is right for you.

It is easy to slip into isolation when you are suffering. Patients who have social support and interactions with others do better with depression and have a higher quality of life. It is important to have physical contact with people outside the hospital and cancer arena. Look for human contact, not only connections through the internet. Even going to a coffee shop and being with strangers is helpful. If you live in a remote area or do not live near other people, speak to someone at a cancer helpline or share your story with others through online communities. Video call a willing cancer survivor for support. (See Badass Cancer Resources, Online Communities, page 253; Patient Support—Helplines, Peer-to-Peer, Live Chats, page 254.)

Additional ways to deal with depression:

- Set up a routine, and add structure to your life; without them, you can lose track of time or days.
- Exercise. It does not have to be a rigorous workout routine: Take a walk; go for a swim; spend time outdoors.

- Set short-term goals: Make yourself a meal in the next hour; by the end of the day, make an appointment to get your hair cut by the end of the week; by the end of tomorrow, make a date to have lunch or dinner with a friend over the weekend.
- Try something new: Take a pottery class; volunteer to teach kids to read; join a book club.
- Invite family and friends over for a game night: bingo, charades, Pictionary, Uno.
- Keep a "grateful" journal: Every morning or evening write down three things you are grateful for in your life.

Consider going to a camp or retreat specifically for people diagnosed with cancer. Several are free or have minimal fees, and you can spend a few days or a week relaxing and connecting with other people who are living with cancer. These retreats are sponsored by different nonprofit organizations and are located across the United States. (See Badass Cancer Resources, Camps and Retreats, page 243.)

It is difficult to adequately describe how you feel when suffering from depression. It distorts your reality, and you can convince yourself of just about anything. There is help for it, but it takes effort. Reach out to someone on your support team to help motivate you or get you to your doctor if you cannot do it on your own. Medication and therapy are successful in treating it and have helped cancer patients feel like themselves again. Do not keep your suffering private or try to handle it by yourself.

Managing pain

It is very common after surgery or during treatment to feel pain. Doctors do not always ask about it or bring up the subject, so you *must*.

When you hurt, your whole body is stressed. Pain can cause your blood pressure to go up, diminish

Tip

It is important to have physical contact with people outside the hospital and cancer arena. Look for human contact, not only connections through the internet.

your appetite and take away your ability to rest or get quality sleep. It is also very distracting and can leave you feeling impatient, angry, frustrated and depressed. Pain does not have to go hand and hand with cancer. Your doctor knows her patients experience it, and she can help you.

Be as descriptive as possible when discussing where you hurt. Tell her if the pain is sharp or dull or if you have a burning sensation. Let her know where you feel it in your body and whether it travels to another area. Tell her if it comes and goes or is constant, when it started and if something makes it better or worse. Let her know if it is causing you to lose sleep or not eat. Use a scale of zero to ten when describing the level of distress you are feeling. Zero represents no pain, and ten is extreme pain. Everyone in the medical world understands this scale, so it quickly and clearly illustrates what you are experiencing. If you have debilitating pain it does not help your doctor to say, "On a scale of one to ten, my pain is a fifteen." She will understand you are in severe pain if you stay within the boundaries of one to ten.

Write in your notebook how you feel every day. If you were given medication to reduce pain, make note of the intensity before and after you take it. Communicate with your doctor if there was any change and to what degree. If the medication she prescribed is not working, be honest. There are different medications you can try. Even reducing the pain by 25 percent is that much less discomfort you are in and can help you get a good night's rest or eat a full meal.

Pain is scary when you have cancer. It can add to the fear and anxiety of a diagnosis. But it is your body crying out for help. You do not know what is causing it. It may be the cancer, in which case your doctor needs to know so she can determine the next steps. Or it may not be, and she can relieve your discomfort. Discussing it will not change your prognosis one way or another, but it can get you some relief.

"Have you told your doctor about your pain?" I asked one woman.

"No, I can't do that," she said.

"Why not?"

"If I tell him about my pain, he will tell me my cancer is getting worse, and I just can't hear him say that to me," she said.

Let your doctor and cancer team determine what is causing the pain. If you do not get satisfaction from your surgeon or oncologist, ask for a referral for a pain management doctor. Her primary concern is your ability to function. Her goal is to reduce your pain and make you comfortable.

On a first visit, a pain management doctor will ask you about your medical history and review the reports on your diagnosis and treatment plan. She will do a physical exam and ask you questions about when the pain started, where it is on your body and its intensity. She will then determine if she has enough information or if additional tests such as an X-ray or MRI are needed to establish a course of action.

She may prescribe medication or suggest interventional techniques such as nerve blockers, injections of medication into a specific area to relieve the pain. She may also recommend physical therapy to reduce your discomfort.

Below are some additional ways to alleviate pain and other symptoms:

- Acupuncture: a technique of complementary and alternative medicine that involves pricking the skin or tissues with needles
- Acupressure: a technique of complementary and alternative medicine that uses the fingers or thumbs on the same pressure points as acupuncture; also known as shiatsu
- Massage therapy: the manual manipulation of soft body tissue; also relieves tension and enhances health and well-being
- Physical therapy: treatment for a disease or injury with massage, exercises, heat and other means; also increases mobility
- Reflexology: application of pressure to the feet and hands with specific thumb, finger and hand techniques
- Stay hydrated, and get restorative sleep.

Pain caused by cancer has an emotional component other pain does not. It is helpful to talk with others who have experienced pain because of their cancer. It can reduce your cancer-related stress. Contact a helpline or connect with an online community and ask what others have found helpful when dealing with pain. Do not suffer with it in silence.

If you are given recommendations for alternative therapies, herbs or over-the-counter supplements, remember to always let your doctor know what you are considering before you take anything. Some integrative medicine can interfere with traditional protocols. (See Badass Cancer Resources, Online Communities, page 253; Patient Support—Helplines, Peer-to-Peer, Live Chats, page 254.)

Dealing with anger

You have every right to be angry about being diagnosed with cancer. It upended your whole life in a matter of seconds in a terrifying and dramatic way. It is understandable to be furious and try to figure out why it happened.

When a crisis hits, we want to put the blame somewhere. It feels better when we can focus our confusion and anger at a specific reason or hold someone accountable for our hell. We get a false sense of control that we can influence an outcome if we know why our predicament happened.

Cancer has no rhyme or reason. There is no logic to why someone gets cancer. I knew a woman who was very knowledgeable and diligent about living a healthy life. She was the first person I met who read food labels, juiced vegetables and exercised regularly. She was diagnosed with advanced breast cancer when she was in her early forties. Another woman I knew ate red meat every day, drank three fingers of scotch a night and from the time she was thirteen smoked two packs of Camel nonfilter cigarettes a day. She lived into her eighties and never had a cancer diagnosis. There is no way to make sense of who is diagnosed with cancer and who is left untouched.

Tip

Although you might find out the cause of your diagnosis, such as a mutated gene, there will never be a true reason you got cancer. It is not bad karma. God does not hate you. It is not anyone's fate or lot in life. It is just what happened.

Although you might find out the *cause* of your diagnosis, such as a mutated gene, there will never be a true *reason* you got cancer. It is not bad karma. God does not hate you. It is not anyone's fate or lot in life. It is just what happened.

This void of a reason can be hard to accept and can add more feelings of helplessness and fury to the diagnosis. To guess or speculate why you got cancer is a distraction that can add to your feeling of powerlessness over the situation. I have spoken with women who became so focused on where to put the blame for their cancer that they lost sight of the big picture: regaining their health.

"Do you know how much time and money I put into working out the anger I feel toward that man?" a woman fumed. "I guess not enough, because I have cancer. He wins again!" She believed holding on to anger caused cancer and blamed the volatile relationship with her father as the reason for her diagnosis.

"I just feel if I had stayed at the church this would not have happened," said a tearful woman who felt cancer was her punishment for leaving.

"My grandmother had breast cancer. We did not get along. She is dead now, but I know she gave me this cancer. It is her way of getting back at me for all the things I've said about her since she died," said another woman very matter-of-factly.

People can come up with all kinds of reasons for having cancer, but it is all irrelevant. Spending time trying to figure it out will not change where you are; it will only compound your feelings about it. There is no reason *why* anyone gets cancer.

Fury over a diagnosis, however, is real and can consume you. Holding on to it can become addictive and lead to depression. Anger is a controlling emotion that will negatively shape your narrative and how you approach life every day; it can give you permission to feel like a victim. To stay in this emotionally dark place is to give your power to cancer.

Do not bury or ignore anger or allow it to get out of control or turn into violence. None of these responses will help your situation.

Acknowledge how furious you are about it. Give it its due. Scream, cry and punch pillows to release some of your rage. Give yourself the time to feel your fury and fully express it. Discuss it with your doctor. Let her help you learn how to reduce your anger. Seek help from a therapist. Talk about it. Do not bottle it up or hold on to it.

Anger is powerful energy. Cancer can instigate this emotion, but you can redirect it to your benefit. Look for avenues to dispel or channel it in ways that support your overall health and well-being.

Doing physical activity helps make the energy more manageable and allows you to focus the energy. Below are ideas to put that power into something physical to reduce your ire.

- Start an exercise routine: running, walking, swimming.
- Take an exercise class: aerobics, Zumba, Spinning, boot camp.
- Start a project: Clean out the closets; wash the windows; organize your drawers; build a doghouse.
- Tackle your home: Rearrange furniture; hang pictures; alphabetize books; paint the kitchen or bathroom.
- Start a new hobby: drawing, painting, gardening, baking, scrapbooking, photography.

Additional ideas that are helpful:

- Write about anger in your journal: how it makes you feel— helpless, vulnerable, frustrated. Think about the cause of your anger. Is cancer motivating it, or are other factors—pain, loneliness, family or friends? Put it all down on paper. No one will read it but you.
- Draw an image of your cancer, then slowly tear it up or burn it. Visualize that it is your disease you are destroying.
- Blow up balloons and write thoughts about your cancer on each one. Pop them, and visualize the remnants as your disease destroyed.
- Listen to calming music or recordings of the ocean or rain. On a search engine—for example, Google or Yahoo!—type in *calming*

Myth
Antiperspirants cause
breast cancer.

Truth
There is no scientific evidence
to support the claim that
antiperspirants cause
breast cancer.

—SUSAN G. KOMEN

music or *music for medication* or *sounds of nature* for a selection of relaxing music.

- Take a warm bath with soothing bath salts to relax. Repeat a happy mantra while soaking.
- Carry a stress ball, and squeeze it when you feel moments of anger.
- Join a support group or call a helpline and connect with others who understand cancer anger. (See Badass Cancer Resources, Patient Support—Helplines, Peer-to-Peer, Live Chats, page 254.)

A productive approach to anger is to switch your thinking of it as a negative emotion to one that is positive. View it as a motivator for change. Use anger as a tool to energize you to achieve your goals. Make it an incentive to use your voice. Most important, do not let it take over your good judgment and limit your possibilities.

Addressing fear

Fear is a painful emotion that can be mild or paralyzing. It is driven by the unknown. Cancer creates the perfect scenario to push every fear button you have. It is easy to imagine all the awful, horrible things that can happen to you after a diagnosis. It does not matter if some—or all—of these ideas are not possible or applicable to you. They feel real, and the more fear you feel, the scarier things will be.

My usual first reaction to anything unfamiliar was to shut down in fear. I imagined everything that could go wrong in a situation, threw all those fears into one big pile and then jumped to conclusions for answers. The unknown was too uncomfortable for me. My actions helped me always have an explanation for everything. This behavior combined with my confusion and imagination took me to some very dark places.

A different fear over my cancer would arise every day, but three scenarios in particular haunted me and kept me up at night: We would go broke and become homeless because of my diagnosis; we would not be able to afford my treatment; a cure for cancer would be announced the day after I died. I was not fast enough or smart enough or I did not do enough in time to keep it from killing me.

Like anger, fear is a powerful emotion. A fear of failure, missing out on an opportunity or abandonment are situations that can either motivate you into action or shut you down. It is helpful to know what exactly is causing your panic. This will give you a starting place to find a way to reduce it. An understanding of each worry individually and a plan to address it will give you a sense of control over the painful emotion.

Here are some ways to help you handle your fears:

- In detail, write down every fear you have. Next to each one, describe what is real and what you have magnified. Do not judge your thoughts; just put them down on paper. Be honest—no one else will read them.

- Make a plan to address each one. Doing this will help you regain some of your power over them. You do not have to put each plan into action. You will be less vulnerable simply by having a plan.

- Write down your cancer experience, from how you heard about your diagnosis to the present. This will help you see the facts and dispel any unrelated fears you have added to the situation.

- Identify triggers that cause panic attacks or intensify your fears. Being aware of what sets off your fear can help you avoid the trigger or talk yourself through the fear. An example: "Getting a mammogram triggers my fear of finding a recurrence of breast cancer. I can't avoid this trigger, but I have support and am capable of dealing with the results."

- Do not ignore your fears; accept them. The more you push them away, the stronger they will feel.
- For every fear you feel, think of a positive thought. It does not have to offset the fear; it is a reminder that you have more in your life than what is causing the fear.
- Talk about your fears: Call a helpline; write a live chat; go to a support group; join an online community (See Badass Cancer Resources, Patient Support—Helplines, Peer-to-Peer, Live Chats, page 254.)
- Discuss your fears with your doctor. Let her know what is keeping you up at night. She can help you with some strategies and guide you to additional support if needed.

Additional steps to take:

- Acupuncture is a technique of complementary and alternative medicine that involves pricking the skin or tissues with needles to alleviate fear and anxiety.
- Acupressure is a technique of complementary and alternative medicine that uses the fingers or thumbs on the same pressure points as acupuncture to alleviate fear and anxiety. It is also known as shiatsu.
- Practice breathing exercises daily.
- Meditate regularly.

Nothing is more uncomfortable than fear, and there is no way to get rid of it completely. But you can learn to manage fear so it does not manage you. It is important not to judge your anxieties or yourself for being fearful. You may think some are rational and legitimate; others are not. It does not matter what they are. It is how you feel, and it is valid.

Do not let anyone diminish, negate, ridicule, judge or in any way

Tip

You can learn to manage fear so it does not manage you. It is important not to judge your anxieties or yourself for being fearful.

make you feel guilty, insignificant, weak or less than for how you experience cancer. You do not owe anyone an explanation for your thinking. There is no way to predict how something will make you feel, what will trigger an emotion or how you will react to information.

The real drain of cancer happens over time. When I first heard my diagnosis, I hit the ground running and did not think about how I was feeling. In the beginning I ran on adrenalin, but as the weeks and months wore on, exhaustion set in and everything became harder. I did not know how to take care of my emotional health without feeling as if I was selfish or slacking off on taking care of my cancer. Plus I had so many emotions going through me, I did not know what I was feeling. It was easier to keep moving than to figure it out. I paid for that thinking with bottled up emotions that convoluted my good judgment, caused me to lash out and melt down over trivial grievances. And it just wore me out.

It is possible to do both: take care of your cancer while seeing to your emotional needs. You must first concede there was a breakdown. If you do not acknowledge that your spirit is broken, or that you are bubbling with anger, or that you have shut down in fear or that you are depressed more days than not, then you cannot do something about them.

There is no dishonor in hitting the wall and having meltdowns or wanting to crawl into a corner and be left alone. It is when you do not recognize there is a problem or believe your emotional condition does not deserve as much attention as your physical well-being that your experience with cancer becomes that much more difficult. Give yourself a break from the physical aspect of cancer, and check in on your emotional, spiritual and mental state. They need to be healthy to put you in the best position to deal with your cancer.

CHAPTER 15

Cancer and Sex

Women know they may lose their breasts when diagnosed with breast cancer. What they do not know is that their sex life may be affected. How to begin engaging in intimacy again is one of those topics that leaves women bewildered or at a loss.

It is impossible to know how cancer will change your sex life. Some women do not feel any difference. Some feel an increased desire to engage in sexual relations. Others find that a diminished libido or physical changes have reduced their pleasure or deteriorated their self-esteem, making intimacy difficult and not enjoyable.

This subject comes up frequently on the helpline and in support groups. It is not typically the opening topic, but as soon as someone brings it up, it becomes apparent how many women experience a diminished sex life. Not everyone is comfortable talking about it, but many are interested and take notes on what to do.

It is a difficult topic for many to speak about openly. They feel self-conscious, awkward or guilty when talking about desire or the physical aspects of having sex. One woman I spoke with told me how her friends were astonished that she was pursuing a solution for her physical limitations and lack of desire.

"You have cancer and you are worried about sex?!" they said.

It is perfectly normal to want to feel desire and intimacy after a breast cancer diagnosis. You are still a woman. There is no shame in wanting a satisfying sex life. Physical relations with others is human nature and an important part of our quality of life. It is distressing when something has a negative impact on it.

Several factors can cause women to have trouble in the bedroom. Chemotherapy and other medications can induce menopausal symptoms, causing hot flashes, night sweats, vaginal dryness, lack of sexual desire and painful intercourse. Temporary numbness in their skin—or permanent if they had a mastectomy—can hamper their enthusiasm for sex. Fatigue, pain, depression, anxiety and loss of self-confidence can make getting in the mood feel like too much work.

Uncertainty about how to broach the topic, embarrassment over the subject or not knowing what questions to ask can keep patients from getting help. Typically, many sexual issues that cancer brings on will not go away on their own. But do not despair; there is help for it. Women and men can and do enjoy a satisfying sex life and reach a deep level of intimacy in a relationship after cancer. You can get your sex life back on track with help from a doctor: She can prescribe medications or recommend over-the-counter remedies. The most important factor is your willingness to do what it takes to reincorporate sex in your life.

It is possible to desire sex again

When I was first diagnosed, I did not even think about sex. I was too busy figuring out what to do about cancer. Once the newness and shock of my diagnosis wore off, I put effort into getting my life back to normal. I had always taken great pleasure in desire and the intimacy and physicality of sex and was ready to feel the comfort and closeness of Michael again.

In the beginning, I was surprised to find I had little desire for it. I reasoned that it must be exhaustion from coping with cancer and that I needed to give myself time. The situation was depressing, but I expected it to be temporary. A few weeks after I was done with radiation, I started tamoxifen. My libido further reduced, and the times I was aroused, intercourse was painful. Again, I thought it was temporary and did not address it. Instead of getting better, it got worse.

Several more months went by before I finally brought it up to my oncologist. She confirmed that many women suffer a diminished sex life and painful intercourse, but she had no recommendations or solutions. I asked if it would always be like this. She did not have a concrete answer. She said, "You'll know when you know." Her response was surprising, and I was angry she was so nonchalant about it. I brought it up to my radiologist and a hematologist, who both concurred with my oncologist on the issue. I could not believe this was a common occurrence for women and no one had a solution for it. It seemed no one thought a lost libido or painful sex was as grave a condition as I did. I also thought, *My concern is about sensual pleasure. What did couples planning a family do?*

No one told me problems in the bedroom were a possibility. When prescribed tamoxifen, I had been advised it could bring on menopausal symptoms, but the discussion was about hot flashes and weight gain. Nothing was ever said about libido or vaginal dryness. Michael and I had been married for only three years. We were still in our honeymoon phase, and my body's response was devastating to me. He was patient and understanding, but I knew how much he missed our pre-cancer sex life too. I did not know what to do.

I spent time online, went to the library and looked for magazines with articles, but the little information I found was not very helpful. I talked to my girlfriends about it, but they could not relate. Finally, I called a cancer helpline. I was relieved when the woman who answered the phone said she had a similar experience with medication.

Comfortable, I told her how prior to surgery, Michael and I had enjoyed an active sex life and my breasts were a big part of it. I explained that my right breast was still intact and sensitive. But on my left breast, I could feel only the pressure of touch; I could not feel the sensation of it. My skin was numb. It was a creepy feeling to me. My whole body felt queasy when Michael touched my left breast. I also told her how painful intercourse had become after tamoxifen and that it diminished my desire to have sex at all.

She told me my experience was common for women on medication for cancer. She counseled me not to despair; there were actions I could take to make it comfortable again. My first step was to get used to being touched. She told me that even if I felt desire, it was highly unlikely I was going to enjoy sex if physical contact was uncomfortable. She gave me tips: Caress the skin on my right breast; feel the pleasure it still could give me; recognize that I could still get aroused with only one breast. Move to my left one: Feel for areas where I still had some sensitivity; note the different sensations around my scar; stroke my breast and look for areas that retained some feeling. She instructed me to touch myself with the intent to find and feel pleasure, not to focus where I had numbness or pain.

She also recommended that I see my gynecologist for medication that would help with vaginal dryness. Surprisingly, my cancer doctors had not recommended this. After sharing some home remedies such as organic coconut oil as a lubricant, she told me to relax and not be discouraged or give up. If I kept at it, I would be able to have fun in the bedroom again.

I made an appointment with my gynecologist, who prescribed Estriol, a vaginal estrogen cream, three or four times a week, and told me to lubricate liberally. Within a few weeks, I felt relief, which increased over time. After addressing the physical hurdles to having sex again, I was still experiencing low libido. I ate foods that were touted as aphrodisiacs, and drank teas and herbs that were supposed to boost your libido. I took natural supplements and tinctures I found at a homeopathic store. Nothing helped me very much. I kept my oncologist informed about all the remedies I was trying to make sure nothing conflicted with my medication. After eight months of searching for a solution, help for my desire came in a surprising and unexpected way.

My favorite genres of books are biographies, autobiographies, and detective and murder mysteries. I regularly ordered books from the library's lending catalog to be delivered to our local branch. About a year after treatment, I was in a rush to order a book, and I saw one that looked interesting by an author who was unfamiliar. It had the words *murder* and *mystery* in the title, so I ordered it.

Tip

Many sexual problems can be solved or improved with communication, medication and determination.

There was a murder—two, in fact—and some mystery, but primarily it was an historical romance novel. I was annoyed because neither historical nor romance books appealed to me. I was going to return it but instead figured I might as well finish it while I waited for another book to come in. That book changed everything for me. Reading about romance and passion ignited my desire again.

The more romance novels I read, the more sex I desired. Reading about desire and being wanted was a turn-on. I became a regular reader of romance and erotica. The books also opened my eyes to other possibilities of gaining sexual satisfaction and made me rethink all the times I judged the women who read books with Fabio, the king of romance, on the cover.

Putting all the pieces together to regain our sex life took more than a year. That was because I did not address it as soon as I began to experience problems. The issues did not go away on their own as I had hoped they would. I had to talk about it, ask questions and actively look for ways to remedy the situation, then follow through on implementation. It took about two years for my left breast to regain some feeling. It is not as sensitive as it was prior to surgery, but I can feel touch now.

I never expected to have my sex life challenged. I was distressed when I lost my desire, but working to get it back brought me and Michael closer together and deepened our connection with each other.

If sex is important to you and it has been negatively affected by your diagnosis, know that there is help for it. Many sexual problems can be solved or improved with communication, medication and determination.

Spouses, lovers and significant others

Losing a body part does not diminish love, but spouses and significant others can feel an emotional and physical loss and difficulty with intimacy when a partner goes through cancer surgery and treatment. One man I spoke with was having a hard time with the idea of his wife having a bilateral mastectomy.

"I'm 38, and my wife is 33. We've been married five years," he said. "She's having a bilateral mastectomy. I'm calling because I'm having a hard time with that."

"Okay. In what way?" I asked.

"We have a very active, intimate life, and I'm struggling with the idea that she's losing her breasts."

"That's understandable," I said.

"I feel so damned guilty about how hard I'm taking this. I feel like such a shit about it."

"Is she having reconstruction?" I asked.

"Yes," he replied, "But they won't be hers. That's where my problem is. I love her breasts. When she has reconstruction, they won't be *hers* anymore. They won't be the real thing."

"Does she know how you feel?"

"No," he replied. "She doesn't know I'm calling you. I don't know how to talk to her about it, and she hasn't said anything. God, I feel awful."

"It's more than how they look or feel, though," he continued. "They are a part of her. They *connect* us."

Sex is more than a physical act in a loving relationship; it is knowing someone completely. Sex is something you do with someone. Sexuality is your connection with body image, eroticism, intimacy, love and affection. Intimacy is a shared connection of familiarity, comfort and trust. You can have sex without intimacy, and intimacy without sex, but when you experience sex and intimacy together, it is a deep emotional connection. When one partner loses an erogenous zone, sexual pleasure can be diminished for both. The anger and sadness he felt about possibly losing that union and not being able to give his wife pleasure in the same way he could before were deep and painful for him.

I shared with him what another man in his position told me he found helpful. Prior to speaking to his spouse, he went online and looked up before and after pictures of bilateral mastectomies. He viewed many images and became familiar with what women look like with no breasts and

Myth
If you have an adult relationship, you do not need masturbation.

Truth
Masturbation teaches you about your body. It is the fastest way to orgasm.

—WEBMD

reconstructed ones. He joined his wife at her appointment with her plastic surgeon and asked questions. Doing these things helped him manage his expectations. He also looked for new erogenous zones on his wife's body after her reconstruction. When a woman has a breast or both breasts amputated and reconstructed, they are numb, and her nipples lose their ability to be involved in sexual arousal.

Communication is key to getting through this traumatic event. I have spoken to women who were devastated by their surgery but did not know how their spouse felt about it and were hesitant to ask. Have a frank and open conversation with your significant other about what you both want to do about your situation. Let each other experience any uncomfortable moments in the exchange. Do not let cancer rob you of the closeness you feel with your partner. Let it bring you to new levels of intimacy through honest conversation.

If you are having problems being intimate again, or your partner is, consider speaking with a sex therapist. This person is a psychologist, therapist or psychiatrist who has additional training and expertise in sexual issues. The American Association of Sexuality Educators, Counselors and Therapists (https://www.aasect.org/) provides an online directory to help you locate a sex therapist in your area.

Talk to your doctor

Most cancer doctors do not talk about a reduced sex life brought on by surgery or treatment if a patient does not bring it up, and patients will not talk about it if the doctor does not.

Some women find it awkward to talk about what goes on in their bedroom with a doctor. Talking to your girlfriends about it is different from speaking with your physician. I found the best approach is to look at it as a fact-finding mission. Keep your attention on gathering information, and let go of any stigma you have about the subject.

Before you see your doctor, write down all your questions, so you feel less flustered. When you are at your appointment, pull out your notes and start going down your list. Take comfort in the knowledge that many women have been where you are and anything you bring up she will have heard before.

Tell your doctor about any physical concerns that are new and different for you. Let her know if your libido has diminished or intercourse has become painful. Talk to her about areas that have lost sensation or ones that are unusually sensitive. Tell her when they started and the severity. You can discuss these concerns with your gynecologist if you are more comfortable speaking with her about sexual matters or if your oncologist is not very helpful.

Additional points to discuss with your doctor:

- Any changes in your body: sensitivity to light; dry, itchy skin; loss of sensation in your breasts
- Changes in your sex life: lack of desire, trouble achieving orgasm
- Changes in your relationship: emotional distance, increased irritability, less communication
- Feelings of depression or sadness
- Stress or anxiety you feel about intimacy
- Any body image issues you are experiencing
- Birth control you are taking or are considering

Discuss the medications you are taking or any she may recommend. If you have been prescribed anti-anxiety or antidepressant medications, check to make sure they do not interfere with sexual desire.

Even if you are emotionally willing and ready to engage in intimacy again, it may be too uncomfortable physically. Medication can dry out your whole body, leaving you with problems such as vaginal dryness. Ask your gynecologist about prescription creams and discuss over-the-counter lubricants and moisturizers to reduce the discomfort.

Below will help you understand how they can help:

- Lubricants and moisturizers are sold directly to the consumer without a prescription and usually come in liquid form or a gel that you apply to the vagina or vulva. They are nonhormonal, and skin does not absorb them. They work by reducing the friction on thin, dry genital tissue.
  - Lubricants are fast-acting and offer temporary relief when engaging in sex. You apply them right before intercourse.
  - Moisturizers are designed to keep the vaginal lining moist. You apply them regularly during the week, not right before sex. Their effects can last three to four days.
- Estrogen creams restore vaginal health and require a prescription from your doctor because they contain hormones. Breast cancer patients can use them in small amounts. Vaginal tissues absorb these creams, reversing the thinning and dryness. These creams are prescribed in the lowest possible dose to be effective and to limit side effects elsewhere in your body. The long-term side effects are unknown, but your quality of life might outweigh them. Creams offer greater long-term relief than lubricants and moisturizers. They are available in the following forms:
  - Vaginal rings: You insert a plastic ring that contains estrogen inside the vagina for three weeks. You take it out for one week then insert a new one.
  - Vaginal tablets or suppositories: You insert a tablet or suppository into your vagina twice a week using an applicator or a finger.

Additional options to discuss with your doctor or gynecologist:

- Vaginal dilator therapy: Vaginal dilators are smooth cylinder-shaped devices to stretch the vagina. Chemotherapy and other medications reduce estrogen circulating through urinary and vaginal receptors; this can cause thinning and shrinking of vaginal tissues. A dilator helps women expand the vagina in width and depth and restore elasticity to have pain-free intercourse or pelvic exams. Dilators are made of plastic, rubber or glass and come in graduated sizes. Consult with your doctor about their use; she will modify the therapy to your personal situation. Vaginal dilators may be obtained by prescription or purchased over-the-counter. Your doctor's office may sell them, or she can recommend a place where you can purchase one. The difference between a vaginal dilator and a sex toy: A dilator is a therapeutic device that can be used without the need for sexual stimulation; a sex toy is designed to provide sexual stimulation. Many retailers that sell sex toys also offer vaginal dilators. (See Badass Cancer Resources, Sex, page 256.)

- Pelvic floor therapy: This therapy is provided by pelvic physical therapists who specialize in musculoskeletal areas associated with the pelvis, vulva and vagina. They perform internal evaluations and prescribe exercises to help strengthen and increase flexibility of pelvic floor muscles. Pelvic physical therapists require a referral from a doctor.
- Vibrators: These devices can increase blood flow to the genitals and help women with arousal or orgasm problems. Many gynecologists have vibrators for sale to patients at their office. If yours does not, ask if she can recommend where you can purchase one. You can locate a retailer near you by searching online. In the search bar of a search engine—for example, Google or Yahoo!—type in *sex toys* and your city. Some examples: Billings MT sex toys, sex toys Milwaukee, adult toys Portland Maine. In addition, the websites that provide information on sexual health have lists of places where

Tip

Fellow cancer patients and survivors can be very helpful by sharing creative and unique ways to enjoy sex again.

you can purchase vibrators, vaginal dilators and sex toys. (See Badass Cancer Resources, Sex, page 256.)

Ask your oncologist or her team if the hospital has any programs for sexual health. Fellow cancer patients and survivors can be very helpful by sharing creative and unique ways to enjoy sex again. If you are uncomfortable speaking in a support group about it, call a cancer helpline. The volunteer will not know who you are, and you can speak freely and confidentially. Join a cancer chat room and ask for ideas. (See Badass Cancer Resources, LGBT, page 251; Sex, page 256; Patient Support—Helplines, Peer-to-Peer, Live Chats, page 254; Online Communities, page 253.)

Working your way back to sex

The one thing to keep in mind as you rebuild your sexual life: The rest of the world is not having rocking, hot sex all the time the way it is portrayed on TV and in movies. It just is *not* happening that way. Take that pressure off yourself.

Relax and explore sex and intimacy at your own pace. It is not a good idea to discover what you can do, how you feel about your body or whether you like being touched by having sex. It is better to become familiar with the changes and comfortable with the notion of being intimate again first. Jumping in too quickly when you are not ready can make the moment uncomfortable for both you and your partner and could make getting in the mood again at a later time more difficult.

Begin getting close to your partner again with simple gestures such as kissing, holding hands, walking with your arms around each other and snuggling in bed or while watching TV. Become physically intimate by touching purely for pleasure. Slowly build desire and anticipation.

The buildup:

- Change your environment. Rent a house for the weekend; take a two-day cruise; camp out, even if it is in your own backyard.
- Plan outings for just the two of you: a hot-air balloon ride, an evening at a pool hall, miniature golf.
- Find a new activity to share. When you do new things together, you produce more feel-good brain chemicals. In the search bar of a search engine—for example, Google or Yahoo!—type in your city and *things to do*. Some examples: things to do Boise ID, indoor activities Springfield MO, outdoor activities Baltimore MD, hobbies and events Benson NC.
- Take a class or workshop together. In the search bar of a search engine—for example, Google or Yahoo!—type in *classes or workshops near me* or workshops Tucson, Chicago classes and workshops, workshops Cheyenne WY, classes for adults St. Paul MN.

Additional ideas:

- Have romantic dinners, picnics, nature walks.
- Send or email each other greeting cards.
- Text each other love notes during the day. For ideas to get you started, in the search bar of a search engine—for example, Google or Yahoo!—type in *love note ideas*. You will find hundreds of examples.
- Leave each other love notes in drawers, on the bathroom mirror, in a purse or briefcase.

Getting in the mood:

- Write down a sexy fantasy, and send it to your partner. For help with ideas on sexy fantasies, in the search bar of a search engine—for example, Google or Yahoo!—type in *sexual fantasies*. Also, YourTango.com (https://www.yourtango.com/2014206789/sex-valentines-day-30-sexual-fantasies-youll-both-love) offers thirty sexual fantasies for ideas to explore.
- Buy sexy lingerie as a teaser. Look for things that not only look good but also make you feel good. Examples: A silky slip can

make you feel silky; thigh-high stockings can make you feel sexy and desirable.

- Pleasure yourself to start feeling desire again. Use a sex toy to enhance your experience or if you are having trouble achieving an orgasm.
- Read romance novels and books on erotica. If you do not know where to begin or what might turn you on, *The Sexy Librarian's Big Book of Erotica* by Rose Caraway offers twenty-two short stories, including dirty fairy tales and a sexy dominatrix.
- Pick up magazines for ideas and tips. It does not matter what age you are; you can always try new things.

Engaging in sex again:

- Have your partner first touch you someplace other than your breasts.
- Explore new erogenous zones and areas on each other's body that have a heightened sensitivity.
- Add sex toys to enhance your pleasure; shop for them together.
- Have your partner buy something for you that is a turn-on: a sexy negligee, a corset, a garter belt and stockings
- Make sure you are physically comfortable. A mood killer for women is cold feet, literally. Get sexy thigh-high socks, and have your partner put them on you.
- Wear a camisole or lingerie if you are uncomfortable with the way your breasts look. Or find a new position for sex that does not have them front and center such as doggy-style.
- Sex first, then dinner. Eating a meal can make you sleepy or feel bloated, or can give you heartburn and make you less likely to be in the mood.
- Lubricate liberally.
- Make sure you are aroused before you engage in vaginal sex.

When you are ready to have sex again, just do it. Do not keep putting it off until you are in the mood. Desire and passion will come and build over time. Do not compare your sex life now with the one you had before cancer. Your experience with intimacy may feel different from the past.

Keep your focus on your pleasure, your partner and how to achieve satisfaction now. Start with the will, and a way will present itself.

The dating game

Dating can be a minefield of hits and misses that you maneuver with courage and tenacity. Finding that perfect mate can be hard enough without breast cancer. Once you add a diagnosis to the conversation, some relationships fall apart or never go anywhere. Wondering if a potential partner will appreciate your new body or accept your diagnosis can make dating feel particularly daunting. When to talk about your diagnosis, how to bring it up and what to say about it can make you question if dating is worth the bother.

Do not let these things stand in the way of socializing. It is important to regain as much of your life as possible after a cancer diagnosis. Flirting, dating and engaging with others are healthy and part of the human connection everyone needs. Let it be known when you are ready to date again. Tell your family and friends. Tell them your wish list of the type of person who interests you. Do not hesitate or be shy about it if you are genuinely interested in meeting someone. Take heart: There are quality people ready to meet the right person. It improves your chances to be ready, available and open to meeting them.

Below are tips for before your first date:

- Accept that cancer is something that happened to you; it is not who you are.
- Practice what you will say in the mirror or with a friend.
- Start socializing so you are comfortable being around people again.
- Do not automatically assume that a date will reject you upon learning that you have cancer.
- Understand that some will get past your diagnosis and others will not; do not take it personally or be discouraged.

Tip

It is important to regain as much of your life as possible after a cancer diagnosis.

- Do not compromise yourself or put up with someone who does not accept your diagnosis just to have a date.

How to talk about it:

- Wait to share your cancer news until you feel a level of trust and mutual attraction.
- Share minimal details of surgery and treatment; you want your date to see you as a woman, not a cancer patient.
- Be honest about your diagnosis and status. Most people know something about the disease, so it will not be an unfamiliar topic.

Covid has changed how we come together, but it has not stopped people from meeting and socializing. The most important point when meeting someone is to feel safe and comfortable. Below are some places to meet a potential date:

- Join a gym; meet people who are health-conscious.
- Take a class: wine tasting, dance lessons, drawing class, woodworking, magic, beer brewing.
- Spend time in a bookstore. Many having seating areas, and some have coffee bars.
- Read in a coffee shop. Make a point to frequent the location at the same time so someone knows how to find you.
- Volunteer for a cause. In the search bar of your search engine—for example, Google or Yahoo!—type in your city and *volunteer opportunities.* Some examples: Philadelphia volunteer opportunities, volunteer opportunities in Nashville, volunteer Chicago animals, volunteer Albuquerque homeless.
- Advocate for something you feel passionate about. In the search bar of your search engine—for example, Google or Yahoo!—type in your city and *advocate volunteer opportunities.* Some examples: volunteer advocate for child foster care Salt Lake City, breast cancer advocate volunteer events Atlanta, Alabama human rights advocate volunteer.
- Get involved in community events. In the search bar of your search engine—for example, Google or Yahoo!—type in

your city and *community events*. Some examples: Columbus community events, community events Wilmington NC, Las Vegas community events.

There is no one size fits all when it comes to sex. Everyone is different. Some people care very much about sex and intimacy, others have retired that part of their life and some never did have much desire for it. Only you know where you stand on this subject. If it is something that matters to you, take comfort in knowing that women—and men—have come back from a cancer diagnosis to enjoy a satisfying sex life and deep intimate relationships.

Nothing will change your cancer diagnosis. How you accept and deal with it will set the tone for how you interact with others and how they behave around you. Your experience with cancer has made you incredibly strong, capable and resilient. It has given you an exceptional insight into life, love and relationships and made you more aware of who you are and what you want. Remember those triumphs and how much you have to offer as you start dating again. Always remember, the sexiest thing a woman can wear is confidence.

Tip

Always remember, the sexiest thing a woman can wear is confidence.

CHAPTER 16

Getting Support

I was not aware that there was support for someone with a diagnosis of breast cancer. My breast surgeon handed me brochures for SHARE Cancer Support and the American Cancer Society after she gave me my diagnosis and told me to call them. She knew what I did not: Information and support are critical when going through the crisis of cancer. It was the most thoughtful and compassionate act a doctor had ever done for me.

I do not know that I would have researched support groups or called a helpline if she had not directed me to. I did not think I needed support but called the numbers the next morning anyway because I did not know where else to begin.

As soon as someone answered the phone, I blurted, "My name is Theresa. I have cancer."

"Hello, Theresa. My name is Caroline," she said. "When were you diagnosed?"

"Yesterday," I said.

"Which breast is it?" she asked.

"My left."

"How did you find it? Did you have a lump?"

"No. I had a mammogram that showed suspicious spots," I said. "Then I had an ultrasound and an MRI. Then I had a biopsy, which confirmed I had cancer."

"What did they tell you, or what do you know about your diagnosis?"

"Well, that I have it, and I have to have surgery," I said. "My doctor also told me I should get a second opinion. I'm working on that."

"Yes, that's a very smart thing to do," she said. "Anything else?"

"It was calcifications? Can that be right? My doctor referred to my cancer as lesions, but I think of lesions as cuts. I don't understand how you can have cuts inside your body," I said. "I always thought cancer was a lump."

She explained lesions—a term physicians use to explain an area of abnormal tissue, benign or malignant—and calcifications. We discussed what I knew about my diagnosis and cancer in general, which was not much but more than I realized. She explained the role of each of the doctors who would be a part of my care and walked me through step-by-step what to expect with a lumpectomy. She also gave me tips to take care of myself afterward: Use an electric razor instead of a straight-edge one when shaving under my arms to minimize nicks and cuts; take warm showers, not hot, which can be uncomfortable on your sensitive skin; wash with fragrance-free soap.

When we were done with the medical topics, she asked how I was handling my diagnosis emotionally. I said, "I'm good."

"Would you like information on support groups?" she asked.

"No, thanks. I'm good," I responded.

"Okay," she said. "If you change your mind, you can call this number again or go to our website for a schedule of meetings."

I thanked her and hung up. I was not ready to accept that I was now a cancer patient and could participate in a breast cancer support group. I thought, *Those meetings are for sick people. I am not sick.* And, *I'm fine. I can do this.*

Over the next couple of weeks, I called the helpline periodically but only when I had medical questions. I had paranoid, crazy cancer ideas that kept me up at night, but I did not think a helpline could do anything to help me with them. Plus, I was too embarrassed to share them. I would lie in bed at night and imagine every ache and pain was cancer. A headache meant the cancer had already shot to my brain. A cough meant it had filled my lungs. Common sense told me my foot going numb was because I was sitting on it, but a part of me was sure it was cancer and I would have to amputate my poor appendage. I was certain no one else felt the same way.

Myth
If a woman is pregnant, she
cannot get breast cancer.

Truth
Breast cancer is the most
common cancer in pregnant and
postpartum women.

—SUSAN G. KOMEN

I did not anticipate the irrational and isolating thoughts that come with cancer, nor did I think it would feel so lonely. I did not foresee just how deep and far-reaching an emotional impact the disease would have on me. I had no words to describe how I felt. Terrified, overwhelmed, running on adrenaline, yes, but it was so much more than that. I did not know what to say or how to talk about these feelings, so I did not.

The time span from diagnosis to surgery was eleven days, so there was not much time for me to reflect on the enormity of my situation or anticipate the emotional upheaval that would soon take a big toll on me. The week after my surgery, I met my first oncologist and radiologist and started discussing treatment options, medications, side effects, timelines and prognosis. That is when the magnitude of cancer hit me. It was more than a momentary crisis. Cancer treatment comes with a myriad of lifelong consequences such as chemo brain, congestive heart failure, lymphedema, cognitive issues and dental problems. Comprehending that I could have all these additional medical problems terrified me.

During my third week of daily radiation treatments, I was sitting on a table in the center of a treatment room. Three technicians were watching me through a thick, narrow window as another technician prepared me for treatment. He told me to pull my gown down around my waist and lie on my back. He put my left arm above my head in a cast formed to hold it and placed my right arm at my side. He positioned the pointed tips of the machines at the six marks tattooed on my chest. They were inked between my breasts and under my left one four weeks earlier as the precise locations to aim the radiation beams. When he was done, he left and pulled the thick metal door closed behind him. It made a deep booming sound followed by a quiet so still you could hear a feather float. As I waited for the whirring sound of the machines that told me the radiation beams were burning through me, tears rolled down the sides of my face. *How was this my life?* That afternoon, I signed up for a breast cancer support group and went to my first meeting a few days later.

I had never been to a support meeting of any kind and had no idea what to expect. There were about ten women in attendance, some newly diagnosed, others out of treatment. The facilitator, a breast cancer survivor, opened the meeting with a topic the women had said they wanted to discuss that evening. Then she turned the meeting over to the group to ask questions and share information. The women spoke openly and freely about milestones with their treatment, challenges with their medication and issues they faced with family, work, sex and appearance.

Everyone spoke the same language: breast cancer patient. It was more comforting than I could have imagined. It was the first time I could feel myself relax since I received my diagnosis. I did not participate much at first—I mainly listened—but as time went on, I began to contribute. Hearing other cancer patients talk about the very things that kept me up at night greatly improved my mental, emotional and spiritual health. I was not alone in my thinking. Everyone in the room had crazy cancer thoughts, dreams and ideas that kept them awake at night too.

It is more productive to speak with someone who is currently coping with cancer, or did in the past, than talking with friends, family or even physicians, nurses and patient advocates. It was a relief to be around people going through the same thing I was. Many cancer survivors volunteer to offer support, both emotional and informational, to those diagnosed. They do so for various and personal reasons, but they all share one objective: to help others get through a crisis they know too well. A fellow cancer patient does not need an explanation, she just *knows*.

Tip

It is more productive to speak with someone who is currently coping with cancer, or did in the past, than talking with friends, family or even physicians, nurses and patient advocates.

Helplines, peer referrals and support groups

There are several ways for you to get support: helplines, peer referrals and support groups. The first step is deciding how you would best receive it. Some people want one-on-one over the phone, whereas others like a group environment. Whatever approach you prefer or think will benefit you the most is the way you should go.

Here are some definitions to help you understand your options:

Cancer helplines

A cancer helpline is a service that has a staff of volunteer survivors. They listen and provide emotional and educational support to people diagnosed with the disease and to those who support them. The people who answer the phones have lived through the confusion, fear and frustration you are feeling and are experienced and trained to speak to you about your diagnosis. They can answer your questions, talk with you about treatments and help you sort through your options and make informed decisions. Or they can simply lend a compassionate ear.

Most helplines operate during regular business hours, Monday through Friday. Some have evening hours and volunteers who return messages at night and on weekends. Many helplines are very accommodating and try to make themselves available when you are. You can request to speak to someone during nonbusiness hours.

Helpline volunteers are not psychiatrists or therapists, so they cannot recommend doctors, hospitals or medication. A helpline is not a substitute for therapy and is not considered medical treatment. (See Badass Cancer Resources, Patient Support—Helplines, Peer-to-Peer, Live Chats, page 254.)

Peer referrals

Many cancer helplines have peers for cancer patients to speak with. Peers are volunteers whose disease or situation most closely aligns with yours. They will typically have had the same type or stage of cancer as you or have had the same type of surgery. They took the same medications or had a similar home life, such as young kids, single mom, etc. They can relate more personally with what you are going through.

A volunteer on a helpline may suggest you speak to a peer if the volunteer's experience does not support yours. Once you tell the person on the helpline what you want, the volunteer takes your number and will contact an appropriate peer, who will give you a call.

Helpline and peer volunteers know to be discreet. If you tell the person on the helpline that you need confidentiality, the peer will be mindful not to announce herself as being from a cancer organization or leave a message with such information.

Volunteers are advised not to give out their phone number and usually have blocked their home or mobile number if they are calling you from either. Do not take this personally. They need to be able to control calls. Many peers or facilitators have ignored this advice and receive calls in the middle of the night from women who have their number. This situation can become difficult for the helpline peer because it can create an unhealthy dependency on the part of the patient. If you really like a specific volunteer and want to speak with her again, ask for her name, and when you call the helpline, ask the helpline if she can she call you back.

When you contact a helpline, the conversations are confidential and anonymous. To get support, no one has to know who you are, where you live or what you do for yourself. When you call a helpline or speak to a peer, it is your conversation. The volunteer will know only what you choose to tell her. She may ask for your information to follow up with you, but you can decline to give it.

If you call a helpline more than once, you might not speak with the same volunteer. To make follow-up conversations easier on the caller, some cancer helplines will log the conversation between a volunteer and caller into a secure internal database for future reference. If that person calls back, a volunteer can quickly review previous conversations and find out the woman's diagnosis and status without making her repeat her story.

The organization will not share your information with anyone, and no one in your family or circle of friends will know you called a cancer helpline unless you tell them.

In addition, you can join online forums, ask questions and contribute anonymously. You can participate in webinars without revealing who you are by blocking your photo. Do not let the fear that someone may find out who you are keep you from getting support. You are in control of how you get help and what information is shared.

Support groups

A support group is a gathering of patients who are either dealing with cancer or have completed their treatment but still want support. The groups are formed, managed and run by facilitators who were also patients at one time. Support groups are different from group therapy in that medical professionals such as therapists and social workers run the latter.

Support groups are an open place to discuss your disease, ask questions or express your feelings without any influences from family, friends or doctors. Because of this, cancer support groups are usually limited to patients and survivors. There are groups in which both the patient and her family and friends can attend, but the groups will always make it clear if they welcome other people.

Support groups are available face-to-face, over the phone with group calling or online. (See Badass Cancer Resources, Online Communities, page 253; Patient Support—Helplines, Peer-to-Peer, Live Chats, page 254.)

How to find support that fits you

Before going to a support group, there are questions you can ask to determine if it is the right one for you. What kind of support group is it, emotional or informational? You will get information in an emotional support group, but you may not get emotional support if you are a part of a group that focuses on education and information.

Below are additional questions to ask when evaluating a group:

- Is it only for breast cancer patients, or can people with any cancer attend?
- Are men with breast cancer allowed, or is it specifically for women?
- Is it only for patients, or can survivors attend as well?
- What kind of group is it? Young women? Newly diagnosed? Metastatic cancer?
- Does this group run for a limited number of weeks, or is it ongoing?
- Is the facilitator of this group a former patient?
- Does a psychiatrist or social worker run this group? Did this person have cancer? (If that matters to you.)

The organization sponsoring the support group will typically provide the facilitator's name and contact information next to the time and date of the meeting. Many groups request that you register for a meeting rather than just showing up. Always check before you go to see if you need to sign up and to confirm the time and location.

Like any group environment, the dynamic works for some and not for others. Do not be frustrated or give up if the first meeting you attend does not meet your needs. Determine what you did not like about it: Was it the way the facilitator ran the meeting? How the participants interacted? The focus of the meeting? Understanding why you did not like the meeting will help you formulate questions to ask if you decide to look for another one.

Where to find support

Like any group environment, the dynamic works for some and not for others. Do not be frustrated or give up if the first meeting you attend does not meet your needs. Determine what you did not like about it: Was it the way the facilitator ran the meeting? How the participants interacted? The focus of the meeting? Understanding why you did not like the meeting will help you formulate questions to ask if you decide to look for another one.

Where to find support

The first place to start looking for a group is at the hospital or clinic with which your doctor is affiliated. Ask her or her office for information, or look on the hospital website for support groups.

Information on locations of support groups is also available from other sources:

- Hospital social workers
- Patient representatives, coordinators or navigators
- Physician's assistants
- Cancer organizations: The websites will inform you how they offer support, whether it is in the form of helplines, support groups or peer referrals. Some also offer live chats, teleconferences, online forums and webinars. Many also have resource guides and can let you know what is available in your area. (See Badass Cancer Resources, Patient Support—Helplines, Peer-to-Peer, Live Chats, page 254.)
- Other patients: Ask your doctor if she has other patients who would be willing to speak with you.
- State-, city- and community-sponsored support groups. In the search bar of your search engine—for example, Google or Yahoo!—type in your city and *breast cancer support groups* or *moms with breast cancer* or *breast cancer survivor support groups* for meetings in your area. Some examples: Denver breast cancer support groups, moms with breast cancer Atlanta, breast cancer survivor groups Phoenix.

Many women call the helpline or attend a support group long after they finish treatment. Someone they know had a recurrence and it produced old memories; a new study has them anxious; long-term side effects of treatment still affect their quality of life; they are struggling with PTSD (post-traumatic stress syndrome) from their diagnosis. Some women are living with cancer and want the continuous support. The fear and anxiety of a diagnosis can linger for years. Know that you will always have support and be welcomed no matter when you were diagnosed.

Accepting support

Asking for help can be very difficult for many people. For some, they have always been the caregiver or breadwinner, or they like their position as boss. For others, fear of losing their cherished independence will keep them from reaching out for assistance.

I did not accept help and support very well. It made me feel too vulnerable. My role with loved ones was bossy caregiver. I am the one everyone turned to in a time of need. I felt good about that position. My ego disintegrated at the thought of asking for help and showing any weakness to my family and friends—the very people I should have trusted enough to still love me no matter what I was going through.

It is hard on your family and friends if you try to go it alone. Your diagnosis has affected them as well, and they will cope with it better if they feel they are doing something to help you. When you have cancer, loved ones do not see your need for support as a flaw or negative reflection of who you are. They see someone they care about who needs a helping hand while facing a life-threatening disease. Family and friends want to be there for you and be a part of your team. They feel useful and can better cope with your diagnosis. This involvement brings them comfort.

Why you need support

Cancer is out of your area of expertise.

Your diagnosis thrusts you into a situation in which you have little or no experience. It upends your home and work life, forces you to make life-altering decisions, pushes your body to its limits and challenges you to confront your mortality. These are monumental undertakings. It makes sense that you would need help to get through it.

Do not despair if family members or friends are not willing or able to always step up. There are people ready and prepared to help you if you reach out. You may meet them in a support group, a hospital patient program, a community center, your church or through a friend of a friend. It does not matter if you hardly know someone or do not know someone at all. Incredible friendships have formed between strangers in a crisis. What is important is that you get the support you need. Let people help you or point you in a direction to get whatever assistance you require.

It is not a sign of failing to need support with your diagnosis. In fact, winging it through cancer on your own is not smart and can be detrimental to your well-being. Accepting support does not diminish who you are. It strengthens you. It allows you to focus your energy on what you can easily do and not spend time on tasks that are draining. The strongest and smartest people in the world know when they are out of their depth and need help. They reach out to others for their knowledge and guidance. It is how they become successful.

CHAPTER 17

Caregivers and Supporters

It makes all the difference in the world when someone is there for you in your time of need, even if it is just to hold your hand. Caregivers and supporters can make the road less difficult to manage at a time when you feel most vulnerable. They provide comfort and familiarity when everything is strange, new and scary. They are invaluable to a cancer patient.

It is not always easy, though, for family and friends to know what to say or do for you. Cancer is not a person's disease; it is a family's disease. Everyone is affected when you are diagnosed with an all-consuming illness. As quickly as you are thrown into the chaos of a diagnosis, your family is propelled into duty, with little knowledge and no experience.

Spouses and significant others can become overwhelmed by the responsibilities that are quickly thrust upon them. They are at a loss over how to manage children and family, run a household and handle financial obligations while continuing at their job and coping with fear for their loved one. This onslaught of additional duties can cause anger, depression, anxiety, loneliness and isolation on the part of the caregiver.

I have spoken with many spouses and significant others who felt their emotions did not matter because they were not the one with cancer. They thought they did not have a right to their feelings because they were not the one suffering. They may not have cancer, but they are hurting nonetheless. The anger and frustration they experience is not over you, their loved one, but what has happened to you. There is no fault in that. It *is* an awful situation.

Caregiving is one of the most stressful roles a person can ever take on. Caregivers are on an emotional roller coaster as well, and sometimes they need someone to hold their hand too. Your team will need direction on how to best aid you. The following will help you guide the people taking care of you to also take care of themselves.

Supporting caregivers and supporters

People perform one of two roles when caring for a patient: caregiver and supporter.

A caregiver is more involved with the day-to-day care of a patient, such as administering drugs and managing side effects. They help determine if something is working or not, and they communicate with doctors.

Supporters are family and friends who give support such as visiting, running errands or doing chores for both the patient and the caregiver.

Many people who suddenly find themselves in the position of caregiver will hit the ground running and start taking care of things as soon as they hear the news. They will maintain that pace despite what they are feeling or what their body is telling them.

When they overlook their own needs, both they and the patient suffer. If they are exhausted or hungry, they may be less willing to be helpful, and that can cause hurt feelings and resentment or poor care. It is not selfish to take care of oneself before taking care of someone else. The best thing caregivers and supporters can do for a cancer patient is to take care of themselves. It is how they will have the energy and strength to give you the support you need. When caregivers tend to their needs first, then they can give someone undivided time and attention and the best care.

Suggest that they let go of the thoughts that no one will be able to take care of you or handle your responsibilities as well as they can. Others might not be as capable, but that is all the more reason for them to delegate and take care of themselves, so they do not get burned out and become unable to take good care of you at all.

Here is a list to give your caregivers to help them take good care of themselves and you:

- Maintain as much of your own schedule and routine as possible: Eat well; get enough sleep; go to the gym, church or work.
- Do not isolate yourself with me. Engage with people outside a cancer center environment, and take time for yourself: Go to a coffee shop and read; join a cycling class or do some other form of exercise; take a writing class; set aside quiet time for yourself to do a whole lot of nothing.
- Get together with friends, and talk about subjects other than cancer. When cancer becomes the only topic of conversation, depression can creep in.
- Do not pretend you always know what to do; ask me what I need or how I would like something done.
- Talk about it: Join a support group; call a helpline; or join a chat room for caregivers and supporters. (See Badass Cancer Resources, Caregiver Support—Helpline, Peer-to-Peer, Live Chats, page 244.)
- Journal thoughts on being a caregiver: Write down fears about the situation and what you would change if you could.
- Set up a caregiver calendar, and post my needs. (See Badass Cancer Resources, Care Calendars, page 244.)

Build a team to support yourself. Delegate responsibilities such as these: picking up the kids from school, cleaning the house, grocery shopping, preparing meals.

If friends or family members want to pitch in, let them know not to wait to be asked; they can just do it. Some examples: When at the grocery store, they can call and ask what you need; they can surprise you with a meal for your family; they can give you some time off and take your kids to the movies, dinner or a ball game. Or they can simply show up at your home for a visit and unload your dishwasher. Every little bit helps.

Below are some additional ideas for your support team to help you:

- Go to an appointment with you: Take notes; arrange for transportation; provide companionship.
- Organize paperwork: medical bills, household bills, mail.
- Run errands: Pick up a prescription; mail a package; drop off dry-cleaning.
- Be the point person for communication: Take charge of health updates with friends and family.
- Assist you in gathering and preparing things for your stay in the hospital: paperwork, toiletries, entertainment.

Below are more ideas to support a patient:

- Be company for you: Take a walk; go for a cup of coffee; go to the movies.
- Household chores: Water the plants; do a load of laundry; sweep the kitchen; vacuum the living room.
- Help with meals: Cook a breakfast, lunch or dinner; prepare and freeze snacks; organize weekly meal deliveries among friends.
- Pet care: Pick up food; take my pet to the groomer; walk my dog.

End-of-life support:

- Help you with end-of-life paperwork. (See Badass Cancer Resources, End-of-Life Planning, page 246; Legal Information and Documents, page 251.)
- Help you understand the options for end-of-life support. (See Badass Cancer Resources, Hospice and Palliative Care, page 248.)

A thoughtful way to be considerate of your caregivers and supporters is to set aside a kitty of cash in small bills so family and friends can reimburse themselves for expenses. This gives you both the freedom to request and fulfill a favor anytime.

Support from afar

Family and friends who do not live near you can still help and support you. Below are some ideas to give them:

- Be a good listener; do not try to fix things or be a cheerleader.
- Provide emotional support: Call; send notes, uplifting cards, inspirational texts.
- Do research and report back to you: clinical trials, support groups near you, financial relief.
- Send meals: Arrange to have your favorite lunch or dinner sent to you through a meal service. (See Badass Cancer Resources, Nutrition and Lifestyle, page 253.)
- Send you goodies every other week or once a month. Give them a list of things you can use: socks, scarves, books, coloring books, teas.
- Support the caregivers helping you: Have them send a card or a gift certificate for coffee to friends who are helping you.

It is difficult for family and friends who live far away to help when a loved one is in crisis. They will be grateful, and feel less helpless, if you let them be there for you in a manner that works for them.

If you do not have a caregiver

For several reasons, some people do not want to be or are unable to be the caregiver. Some examples: They are not well themselves; they cannot commit the time; they barely know the person—they are a distant relative or are not related. These situations are less than ideal for all involved.

Below are additional places to look for support:

- Consult with your physician for services the hospital may provide.
- Reach out to your community for services. The American Cancer Society (https://www.cancer.org/) provides a state-by-state directory of the services and programs it offers.

- Speak with a social worker, patient representative or patient navigator at the hospital.
- Reach out to a patient advocate organization for information on free and fee-based services. (See Badass Cancer Resources, Patient Advocate, page 254.)
- Talk to a clergyperson. Many churches have parishioners who volunteer to help and support those in need.
- Reach out to the cancer community for a list of organizations that offer support. (See Badass Cancer Resources, Caregiver Support—Helplines, Peer-to-Peer, Live Chats, page 244; Hospice and Palliative Care, page 248.)

Illness can put a strain on both patient and caregiver, and they can take their anger and frustration out on unintended targets. It is not deliberate, but fear, frustration and pain can push people to the edge of their good judgment, testing their kindness and compassion. Understanding is necessary, but tolerating abuse, verbal or otherwise, is not. If things are going in that direction, take action. You can say, "I'm scared too. Directing our anger at each other is getting us nowhere. More will get accomplished if we work together as a team. Everyone needs patience and understanding."

Communication between family and friends is key. Accept that there will be moments when you, family and friends reach a breaking point with one another. When that happens, talk about it. Take time out to calm down. Give one another space, and do not judge. Remember: No one is a bad person in this situation for how she feels.

CHAPTER 18

Remission, Recurrence, Survivor

The one word everyone wants to hear regarding her cancer is "cured." That term means the cancer is gone and there is no chance it will return. The longer someone goes without a recurrence, the higher the chance it will not return, but doctors are hard-pressed to tell a patient their cancer is cured. You are more likely to hear, "Go enjoy your life. I'll see you on your next follow-up visit."

The week after I finished my radiation treatment, I had an appointment with my oncologist. She was the doctor who prescribed the tamoxifen and the one who would monitor my health for the next five years while I was on the drug. At the end of the appointment, she stood up, reached out and shook my hand and said, "Okay, everything looks good. I'll see you for a follow-up in three months."

"Am I in remission?" I asked as I shook her hand.

"You could say that," she replied.

"Well, either I am or I'm not," I said.

"There is no sign of cancer, is what I tell patients," she said.

"So that means the cancer is gone," I said.

"It means there is no sign of it at this time," she replied.

"But it could still be there or come back."

"Your test results show no evidence of cancer in your body. It can always come back," she said. "Your prognosis is good. Your cancer was caught early. Don't obsess over it. Enjoy the results."

I stood on the sidewalk in front of the hospital and thought, *So, is no sign of cancer better or worse than being in remission? Or is it the same thing?* I knew the term "survivor" did not describe my health; that word defines someone who endured a difficult experience. I did not know what explained the status of my cancer.

There are several terms that describe cancer and a patient's health after her diagnosis. Below are different classifications of the disease.

Remission

There are two types of cancer remission: complete remission and partial remission (or partial response). Complete remission means all tests and screenings such as blood tumor markers, CT, MRI, bone or PET scans show there is no cancer present. Another term used to describe complete remission: no evidence of disease (NED). It does not mean the cancer is cured or will not return, but there is no indication the patient has any cancer in her body at that time. A patient in complete remission still needs to stay on top of her health and get regular checkups and screenings.

Partial remission means the cancer partially responded to treatment but not completely. It is still present, but the tumor is smaller. The tumor will need to be observed and monitored on a regular basis to confirm it does not spread or get bigger. As long as the tumor does not grow, the patient may be able to take a break from treatment. If it starts to spread or grow, it is called "cancer progression" or a "recurrence," at which point the patient may need to undergo treatment again to get the cancer back into remission.

A patient who has cancer in partial remission must stay on top of her health, see her doctor regularly and undergo routine tests and physical exams. When cancer is in partial remission, it is also called "chronic"—a condition that persists or recurs and needs to be monitored—or "stable"— the tumor has stayed the same and not grown bigger. Some liken this condition to a patient who has heart disease: an ongoing situation that needs to be monitored regularly but it is not progressing at this time.

The treatment options vary for cancer that is in partial remission. Some of the factors doctors take into consideration are the type of cancer, how aggressive it is, how well the patient tolerated and responded to treatment, and her age and overall health.

There are no assurances with chronic cancer, which can make it difficult to cope with. Lean on your medical team to guide you on how to go forward. Ask your doctor to lay out a best- and worst-case scenario for you, so you understand your options and can manage your expectations. Ask her how she will monitor your health, which aches and pains you can anticipate and which symptoms require you to see her. Does she recommend any lifestyle changes? How often will I need follow-up tests? Do I see her for all ailments, or do I go to my general practitioner if I get a cold or the flu?

Living with cancer in partial remission is a different emotional, physical and financial hurdle than when you first learned you had cancer. It is not going to go away completely. Patients can, and do, live years with chronic cancer and still lead a full and productive life. It may require adjustments to your routine such as more frequent doctor visits, follow-up tests and treatment if the cancer begins to progress, but you can make plans and enjoy your life again.

Emotional support and guidance from others with chronic cancer can help you manage your expectations. They understand what it feels like to hear that status and set up a routine around it. There are women willing to help and support those who have the same diagnosis. They will share with you what they are doing to cope with it emotionally and how they are living with the uncertainty of it. A helpline or support group will connect you with someone who has chronic cancer and understands what you are experiencing. (See Badass Cancer Resources, Online Communities, page 253; Patient Support—Helplines, Peer-to-Peer, Live Chats, page 254.)

Recurrence

A cancer recurrence means it has returned after not being detectable for a period of time. When cancer returns, it is referred to as a local recurrence, when the cancer comes back in the treated breast or near the mastectomy scar; a regional recurrence, when the cancer has come back in nearby lymph nodes; or as a metastasis, or distant recurrence, when the cancer has left the original site and traveled to other organs of the body.

Most recurrences happen in the first five years after breast cancer treatment, but cancer can recur anytime. The larger the tumor, and the more lymph nodes with cancer at the initial diagnosis, the higher the chances of a recurrence. The increased possibility of a recurrence does not mean it will happen.

Local recurrences are typically found in a physical exam by a physician, or through a mammogram, ultrasound or MRI. If you experience any of the symptoms below, contact your doctor right away. The symptoms for a local recurrence are as follows:

- Breast or nipple pain
- A discharge from the nipple other than breast milk
- New lump or irregular area of firmness
- Dimpling of the skin. It sometimes looks like an orange peel
- Red, swollen or hot breast
- Inverted nipple (if this is not normal for you)
- Skin irritation or rash
- Swelling under your arms where lymph nodes are located
- Change in size or shape of the breast

Symptoms for a regional occurrence may include:

- Lump or swelling of the lymph nodes: under your arm, near your collarbone, in your neck
- Swelling in the arm on the same side as the initial diagnosis
- Pain or loss of feeling in the arm and shoulder
- Persistent pain in the chest
- Trouble swallowing

A metastasis is usually found in a diagnostic exam when a patient reports the symptoms below during a follow-up office visit:

- Weight loss
- Shortness of breath

- Bone pain
- Extreme fatigue
- Headaches
- Decreased alertness

Someone can be metastatic and still be diagnosed as NED (no evidence of disease). It means the cancer spread beyond the original site, but currently no evidence of disease can be found in the body. It does not mean it will never return. The patient needs to stay on top of her health through regular screenings and follow-up visits to her doctor.

Treatment for a recurrence varies depending on the type of protocol used for the initial diagnosis, whether it is local or if the cancer has metastasized. It also depends on the age and health of the patient. It could involve surgery, chemotherapy, targeted therapy, radiation and/or hormone therapy. If the cancer appears in the opposite breast than the one that initially had cancer, it may be considered a new cancer and treated the same way the initial cancer was.

Discuss with your doctor your prognosis and what to anticipate when cancer recurs, so you can manage your expectations. Talk to her about clinical trials and if she thinks you would be a good candidate. Ask her how much time you have to make a decision about the next steps.

How to handle treatment at this phase of your illness is up to you. Drugs, therapies, new discoveries and breakthroughs keep people with metastatic cancer alive longer and allow them to live a full productive life. Some people choose to continue treatment until their quality of life becomes too compromised to enjoy; others decide to stay on it permanently.

There is no right or wrong way to manage this phase of the disease. Discuss all your options with your doctor and ask for her advice. Have her lay out the pros and cons of each point she offers. Talk to your family about your choices so they can help you figure out the next steps.

Information and support are critical when handling the challenges of a metastatic breast cancer diagnosis. These are several websites and organizations that offer help on living with and managing the disease. (See Badass Cancer Resources, Advanced Breast Cancer, page 243; Clinical Trials, page 245; Metastatic Breast Cancer, page 252; Financial Assistance, page 247; Hospice and Palliative Care, page 248; Patient Support—Helplines, Peer-to-Peer, Live Chats, page 254.)

Always keep in mind that there is no absolute timeline for life expectancy or a road map with cancer. A doctor can give a patient her best guess, but that is all it is, an estimate based on what she knows at that moment. Medicine and therapies for cancer advance every day. People are living longer with metastatic cancer. There is one thing to know about cancer: A prognosis is a best guess, not etched in stone. Never give up hope.

Living with cancer

My mother's first recurrence was fourteen years after her initial diagnosis. Her cancer was determined to be metastatic, and she was told to get her affairs in order. She underwent chemotherapy for a second time, even though we were advised it usually was not as effective as the first time around. When she finished the treatment, we were told her cancer was in remission. We took the good news in stride but now understood her life with cancer would never end.

When we heard her cancer was back, it was more frightening than learning about her initial diagnosis. It took all thoughts of a future without the disease off the table. The uncertainty that came with her recurrence felt more unsettling. Now that it had returned, we knew it always could.

Her next recurrence was five years later. She went through chemotherapy a third time, and her doctor warned us not to get our hopes up. Once again, her cancer went into remission. He said, "It may not appear that she has cancer now, but make no mistake: It is the cancer that will take her life." Seven years later, and twenty-six years after her initial diagnosis, she had her third recurrence and was undergoing chemotherapy for the fourth time when a pulmonary embolism ended her life.

The first time my mother was diagnosed, I was nine and did not understand what was happening. When she had her first recurrence, I was twenty-three and understood very well what her diagnosis meant. It was shocking and hugely disappointing to us when her cancer returned. After so many years, we had put her illness behind us and went on with our life.

Her recurrence took away any ease in our existence. Every phone call I received from her or my sister, I readied myself for cancer to come up. The disease put my mother, sister and me in a tenuous place. It was hard to make plans, short- or long-term, when she was in treatment. When she was in remission, we lived from blood test to mammogram to bone scan and back again. It was difficult to think of the future. When she bought a new car. I thought, *Really? Well, I guess that's a good sign you'll be around for a while.* She always told my sister and me she just wanted to live long enough to see us get married. My sister and I jokingly agreed we would not get married—the idea being that we could postpone her death by postponing our marriage. Neither of my parents was alive for our weddings.

The emotional toll the first and all subsequent recurrences had on her must have been extremely difficult. I think helping other patients was a way for her to deal with her own feelings. I do not know; she would not talk to me about her cancer. She would always say, "Don't you worry about me, I'm fine," when I asked her about it. I did not push her to talk about it because part of me wanted to believe everything was fine, and I feared she would tell me something I could not do anything about.

My mom lived with chronic cancer for twelve years. She worked around her treatments and lived her life as she did before her diagnosis. She was hysterically funny and continued to play practical jokes on my sister and me. She tended to her roses, registered people to vote and went camping. After her initial diagnosis, she volunteered and drove women to their appointments and stayed with them through their treatments. Her doctors, other patients, loved ones and friends all told her, "Slow down. Take it easy. You are doing too much." Her response was always the same: "What am I going to do? Just sit and wait for cancer to kill me? No, thank you."

She was in the hospital the last five days of her life. My sister and I took turns sleeping in her room with her. It was Saturday night, two nights before she passed, and she and I were watching the television show *Twin Peaks*. We thought she would be home in time for Thanksgiving in five days. During a commercial break, we began talking about family coming for the holiday, and she said, "You know, Theresa, we both know I am living on borrowed time. But I could die next week and still outlive you. It is better to realize life can be that short on your own before something forces you to."

Loving someone who had cancer was frightening and sad and made me angry. I could not imagine the terror she must have been feeling. There are no directions to living with cancer or loving someone who has the disease. Creating a life around such uncertainty means accepting disorder as routine. Even with that doubt, you can create a space for yourself to experience life without thoughts of disease and illness. Appreciate the moment you are living right now, and continue to find meaning in your life. Remember what made you happy before cancer disrupted your world, and engage in it again, the best you can. Make memories with family and friends. Be patient and kind to yourself as you find your place in this new world.

Survivor

A lot of emotional weight is put on the word "survivor." It implies there is a happy ending. The patient has triumphed. Everyone diagnosed with the disease strives to be classified as a cancer survivor.

Some assign the word to those who no longer have cancer, not ones who will live with it forever. Others associate it with winners and losers of a battle. I believed once I was done with treatment, I would consider myself a survivor and all thoughts of the disease would be behind me and I could relax about it.

Many are proud to say they are a cancer survivor and find solace in it. As they should—cancer is hard. I do not discount the word or how difficult it is to get through a diagnosis. I do not take lightly the euphoria you feel when you have struggled for months or years and can finally say you do not have cancer anymore. Being classified a survivor is intoxicating and liberating. But, contrary to the medical definition, it is not reserved for those who show no evidence of disease. It is for anyone who has been diagnosed with cancer and gets up every day, regardless of her status, and gives life her best shot.

When people find out I am a cancer survivor, they say, "Congratulations! What a fighter you must have been" and "I am not surprised—you are one tough cookie." I am grateful to be classified that way, but I did not do anything special or different or fight any harder than someone who is in partial remission or metastatic. Women living with the disease did not miss a key piece of information or make a bad decision or not try enough when going through it than I did. A survivor is not more resilient and does not have any special powers or a magical elixir that afforded her that status. The only difference between someone who has chronic cancer and me is I am a breast cancer statistic who has not had a recurrence. Being classified a survivor does not mean I now have a pass on the disease for life. Cancer is unpredictable; it can come back at any time.

The National Coalition for Cancer Survivorship defines "survivorship" this way: "From the time of diagnosis and for the balance of life." Dictionary.com defines the term "survivor" as "a person who continues to function or prosper in spite of opposition, hardships or setbacks."

It is up to you how you want to describe yourself. Some women do not want a label; they just want to be known as someone who has been treated for cancer, or they simply want to be identified as who they were before their diagnosis: math teacher, financial analyst, chef, dog walker, cabaret singer.

You get to define what "survivor" or "living with cancer" means to you. "Cancer survivor" is a description, not a last act. Do not let one word define or categorize you or your experience. You are more than a label. Congratulate yourself for everything you have done to get where you are. It is an achievement.

Survivor's guilt

"Well, you didn't have *real* cancer then!" one woman yelled when I told her I had radiation and tamoxifen but not chemotherapy. "Only people who go through chemotherapy have real cancer!" I told her I would get a peer whose experience was similar to hers to call her. "Yes, I want to talk to someone else. Because you have *no idea* what it feels like to really have cancer!"

She was halfway through her chemo treatment and having a difficult time with it. I understood her anger, but her comment shut me down for years: I felt incredibly fortunate that I did not have to have chemotherapy but also guilty that I was spared when so many must suffer through it. I had not felt shame about my survival until that phone call.

I told a friend my story, and she told me how she had endometrial cancer, cancer on the lining of the uterus, which was caught early. She was able to have it surgically removed without need for further treatment. When she began to tell friends, their question was the same: "What kind of chemo are you having?"

"I had surgery and don't need additional treatment," she told them.

"Oh, you're fine then," they said. "You didn't really have cancer."

She stopped telling anybody about her diagnosis and never spoke about it again until I shared my story with her. She was so surprised and relieved to know someone else had a similar experience. She also

> **Tip**
>
> *"Cancer survivor" is a description, not a last act. Do not let one word define or categorize you or your experience. You are more than a label. Congratulate yourself for everything you have done to get where you are. It is an achievement.*

felt guilty that she "got away" with something because she did not have chemotherapy or suffer more.

Survivor's guilt is when someone feels remorse for having survived after a traumatic event when others did not. It usually happens to people after a horrible experience such as war, a plane crash or an act of violence. The survivor feels at fault because they did not suffer the same fate as others.

It does not have to be a large-scale disaster for someone to have intense feelings of guilt. Many women in support groups feel it when they are still alive after a fellow patient in their group passed. Owning the only home still standing when a natural disaster leveled a neighborhood or being spared from layoffs at work when an equally qualified colleague lost her job can have someone feeling survivor's guilt and questioning why it was not them.

It took me years to accept there was nothing to apologize for or feel bad about because I did not have chemotherapy. I continually questioned my ability to help and support others through their diagnosis. I did not talk about the details of my treatment unless specifically asked. I feared I would not be taken seriously.

There is no such thing as "cancer light," as I have heard it referred to when someone does not have chemotherapy, a double mastectomy or awful side effects from treatment. The fear, trauma, pain, depression and isolation that are part of a diagnosis are the same no matter the stage or treatment. It is all terrifying.

You did not "get away" with anything, and there is nothing to feel guilty about if you were diagnosed at an early stage or had a different form of treatment. There is also no reason to apologize to anyone or feel bad if you survived when someone else did not given the same diagnosis, or if someone's cancer was more advanced than yours when diagnosed. It is hard, I know, but there is nothing she did wrong or you did right that caused the different outcomes. It is just what happened. Your survival did not cost someone else her life.

Survivor's guilt is distressing and can cause depression, nightmares, loss of sleep and withdrawal from others. Some women question their worthiness or what they did to deserve their favorable outcome. It is tempting to ignore these deep, painful feelings; that is why it is so important to address them. The psychological impact and loneliness they cause can add another dimension to the emotional upheaval you are left with after a diagnosis.

Below are some ways to help you work through the emotion of survivor's guilt:

- Recognize you have no control over another patient's outcome.
- Acknowledge your feelings. Accept that they are a normal reaction to an unusual situation.
- Think about the people who love you and how they would feel if you did not survive.
- Believe that your survival did not cost someone else her life.
- Help others. Volunteer for something that makes you feel as if you are giving back.
- Become a cancer advocate. Lobby for policy changes, speak to community audiences and fundraise for research.
- Talk about it. Contact support through a chat line or call a helpline to get matched to another survivor. (See Badass Cancer Resources, Patient Support—Helplines, Peer-to-Peer, Live Chats, page 254.)

I feel less guilt over my experience with cancer and can talk about it more easily. I do not apologize for my experience anymore or shy away from telling someone about it. I have learned to accept that everyone has their own path, which I cannot change. But I can help them through this difficult time in their life, and that gives me purpose.

None of us know what our end will be until we are there. A person's diagnosis may predict that cancer will cause her passing, but no one knows for sure that the disease is what will end her life. Stay engaged and address the future with everything you have to make it the best it can be. The whole reason you are standing up to cancer, after all, is so you can have your life.

CHAPTER 19

The New Normal

It is a big mental and emotional leap to go from your precancer life to one after a diagnosis. There is no set path or one way back to something normal. Finding a new routine takes time. The way it happens and how long it takes are different for everyone.

My last day of radiation was at 9 o'clock on a Friday morning. The nurses and technicians congratulated me and wished me well as I left the hospital. Michael and I went out to dinner that evening with friends and celebrated. We popped Champagne, ate cake and cheered that I was done with cancer. It was awesome.

Unfortunately, it did not take long for me to recognize the reality of survival was not that simple. The mental and emotional evolution to cancer survivor takes much longer than I ever imagined. The first year after treatment was the most difficult, and my feelings of fear and anxiousness about cancer lingered for several years.

I was eager to move on and put cancer behind me, but I was not prepared for how challenging it was to go back to a "normal" life. It was all too daunting: the long-lasting side effects of surgery, treatment and medication; the fear that the cancer could return; the bills that kept coming. Family and friends watched me pick up a routine and assumed I was okay. They too were ready to put my disease behind us and go back to the way things were before my diagnosis. They moved away from my cancer long before I did.

I felt isolated and depressed after treatment when I had counted on feeling relieved and normal again. I thought I could move on the way my loved ones had. But instead I felt like that one person standing still in the middle of a rapidly moving crowd, completely out of sorts. I no longer had the patience or tolerance for behavior I found acceptable prior to my diagnosis. The thoughts and opinions that were of the upmost importance before, I now found trivial. It was difficult to relate to people and activities around me.

My family and friends were relieved and delighted for me and would say, "You should be happy. You survived it. Just be grateful and move on. Stop thinking about it." I *was* extremely grateful to be alive, but I could not get comfortable being a survivor. I could not move on.

I became fearful of what *could* happen. Prior to my diagnosis, I felt great. I thought I was healthy. But then it scared me that I felt perfectly fine yet had a deadly disease growing inside me. It was disconcerting that I did not even have a lump in my breast that gave me any indication something might be wrong.

Prior to my diagnosis, little white dots that appeared in my breasts—as seen in mammogram results—were not that concerning. When a cluster of them proved to be cancerous, every white dot necessitated a biopsy followed by more mammograms, MRIs or ultrasounds to confirm nothing else was present. This went on for several years until eventually the dots appeared stable and no new ones showed up.

I thought that when I was done with treatment, my life would pick up where it left off. Cancer would be behind me, and I would get back to building my business and living again. I did not anticipate or imagine I would still be undergoing biopsies, tests and scans or have multiple doctor appointments long after I was done. I had not planned on writing letters, sending documents and making follow-up calls with insurance companies years after my diagnosis. I did not expect all the lingering doubts, paranoia and sleepless nights after I was done with treatment. I missed my old, comfortable and familiar life, and I wanted it back.

How to move on after a diagnosis

To truly move on to a new life, you must first mourn the one you lost. You lived it for too long not to concede that it had passed. Recognize the impact cancer had on your relationships, security, financial stability, self-confidence and identity. Acknowledge the changes, and express the sadness and anger you have about them. The painful feelings you are left with after a diagnosis do not go away if you do not deal with them. They just go deeper inside and come out in other ways such as depression, indifference or aggression. Until you grieve for what is gone, you will not be able to let go and embrace your new life.

Progress also takes self-examination of what you truly want for yourself now. You sidelined or put areas of your life on hold because of your diagnosis. You might feel differently about them after what you have been through. Some things will fall by the wayside right away or be replaced, and other shifts will come over months or years. It is a process of figuring out what works for you now and what does not. Take your time, and think about your routines and relationships and if you want them to be the same as they were before you were diagnosed. You may decide you want projects you work on to be more simple, engaging or altruistic, or the people you are around to be positive and inspiring. A new normal happens in small steps and over time.

"Motion is lotion," my physical therapist once said to me. That advice applies not only to your physical health but to your mental and emotional health as well. Activities that stimulate your brain and mobilize your body are motivating. It is important to engage and connect with others.

There are several ways to ease yourself into becoming active:

- Share your story on a cancer blog or in a community room. (See Badass Cancer Resources, Online Communities, page 253.)
- Join a Meetup group for survivors or one that centers on a hobby or interest of yours. In the search bar of a search engine— for example, Google or Yahoo!—type in your city and *breast cancer meetups* or *breast cancer survivors,* or *movie meetups* or *pet lovers meetups.* Some examples: Portland meetups breast cancer survivors, young breast cancer meetups San Francisco, metastatic breast cancer meetups Dallas, or Brooklyn pet lovers meetups,

Philadelphia movie meetups. You will find a list of what is available in your area.

- Write your story, and share it in a writing group.
- Consider attending a camp or retreat for survivors. Different nonprofit organizations host weekend or weeklong getaways designed exclusively for those affected by cancer. Some camps offer adventures as ambitious as kayaking; others are more restful, with activities such as swimming or crafts. They are in various locations across the country. The camps are free, but you are responsible for your transportation to and from the location. (See Badass Cancer Resources, Camps and Retreats, page 243.)

Additional activities:

- Volunteer at a favorite organization: local soup kitchen, Red Cross, ASPCA.
- Pick a new hobby, and take a class for it: gardening, photography, writing, bird watching.
- Update your vision board or create a new one. (See Badass Cancer Resources, Vision Board, page 258.)
- Set realistic weekly and monthly goals, and recognize the progress you have made.

Advocacy is another way many people get active again. Advocates support breast cancer organizations, speak to people who were recently diagnosed or get involved with activities, such as cancer walks or runs. Others volunteer at hospitals, visit patients, fundraise for a cure and raise awareness. They feel useful in a way that is related to their experience and, in doing so, find healing. Some volunteer for one event, whereas others make advocacy a lifelong passion. You do not have to be involved forever, just until you feel better.

I had to break a routine I was afraid to let go of to truly move on. I had become physically active, but mentally I stayed a patient. Long after I was done with treatment, I still approached everything in my life as if I were sick. Prior to my diagnosis, I paid little attention to my health; now I was neurotic about it. I diligently read the labels on everything I purchased, whether apple juice, pasta, deodorant or lipstick. I continued with the thirty supplements, two immune-boosting drinks and three tinctures I took every day while I was in treatment. It was good for my body but overwhelming and exhausting to maintain. The rigidity I had created around this protocol became stressful and counterproductive to my overall well-being.

It took me letting go of my belief that the only thing between my good health and a cancer recurrence were the supplements, drinks and tinctures I took. I put faith in myself to find other ways to maintain my good health. I dropped the drinks and tinctures and reduced the number of supplements. I began to eat well, exercise and get more sleep—three improvements I did not do prior to my diagnosis. It was a new routine that allowed me to relax and still preserve my health and enjoy life.

There is not a set timeline on how long it will take or what will have to happen to make you feel as if your life is routine again. I did not wake up one day and feel better, as I hoped I would. I had to let go of how I thought my road back should go and focus my energy on projects and activities that were engaging and productive. Once I did, I saw my days go from lost and depressed to motivated and energized, and eventually my life felt right again.

If you are having a difficult time picking up and moving on from cancer, speak with your doctor. It is not uncommon for patients to feel invigorated after treatment then, eight months or a year later, find they are having a difficult time returning to their life. Tell your doctor if you are having issues with depression, appetite, sleep, sex or concentration. Let her know if you are concerned about a recurrence or worried about the future.

Many cancer patients call a helpline or go to a support group years after their diagnosis because they are still struggling. Consider seeking medical help if you are having difficulty. Ask your doctor to recommend a therapist for you, or search online for one who meets your needs. (See Badass Cancer Resources, Find a Doctor, page 248.)

Let go of *how* you are going to get yourself on a path to living fully. Simply focus on doing something toward achieving your goal every day. If you worry about how you will do it, chances are you will get stuck there. Keep putting one foot in front of the other and pushing ahead. How it happens will take care of itself once you become engaged in moving forward.

The transition from your pre-cancer life to a new normal is a process of letting go, beginning anew and being open to change. Focus on what you do have, not on what you do not, and build from there. In time you will see you can build and award yourself a life that is enjoyable and fulfilling.

Switching your care back to your primary doctor

The timing of this changeover is a decision you will make with your oncologist. When you are ready, the two of you can have a conversation in which you ask her any questions you may have. It would be helpful if she could summarize in writing your diagnosis and treatment protocol as well as give you an outline of her recommendations for follow-up care.

Her recap should cover the following:

- Type of cancer
- Date of diagnosis
- Pathology results: stage, grade, hormonal status, tumor marker information
- Treatment protocol: type and site of surgery, amount of radiation, names and doses of chemotherapy and any other medication she prescribed for you
- Results of treatment, blood tests, X-rays and scans

Tip

Let go of how you are going to get yourself on a path to living fully. Simply focus on doing something toward achieving your goal every day.

When the time is right to transition, ask her the following:

- Whom should I see for my follow-up care?
- Is there any point at which I need to see her again for follow-up care?
- What kind of follow-up tests should I have?
- How often should I have them?

Be sure to discuss the following at follow-up appointments:

- Anything new and different for you: a pain, a symptom or something out of the ordinary that has gone on for two weeks or more
- Any changes in your daily life: fatigue, loss of appetite, inability to sleep
- Something that makes you think you have cancer again
- Pain anywhere on your body
- Feelings of depression or anxiety
- Rapid changes in weight
- Limitations in movement
- Difficulty with concentration or memory

Also review the following:

- Medications you are taking
- Supplements, herbs and over-the-counter medicines you are taking
- Integrative or alternative therapies you are following

For optimal health, it is important to maintain a regular schedule for the following appointments and tests and share the results with your other physicians:

- Physical
- GYN exam
- Mammogram
- Colonoscopy
- Bone density

Once, when I went for a routine annual follow-up with my breast surgeon, I declared I was done with all my doctor appointments for the year.

"You are my last doctor's appointment for the year," I said. I used my fingers to count out who I had seen as I continued, "Over the last two weeks, I saw my GYN, dentist, ophthalmologist and primary doctor for a physical. I am so happy to be done!"

She smiled and said, "Well, that may be the most efficient way to do it, but it's not necessarily the healthiest. You should stagger your appointments, especially with cancer doctors who will be examining your breasts. By seeing all your doctors over a short period of time, a full year can go by between checkups. A better plan is to schedule your appointments throughout the year. That way, someone is always examining your body and more likely to catch something early."

It is important to keep a routine schedule with your doctor and not see her only when you do not feel well. Waiting long periods of time between checkups, or going only when you are sick, does not give her a timeline for any abnormalities that might appear in test results. She will not know if something that is worrisome started recently or if it has been developing much longer. Seeing her for regular visits will help her detect something early and keep both of you on top of your health.

I am often asked how long I continued to see my cancer doctors after I was done with radiation. I saw my radiation oncologist twice a year for five years and my medical oncologist twice a year for five years until I finished tamoxifen. I still see my surgical oncologist, or breast surgeon, after my annual breast cancer screenings. Over the years, atypical cells that have required biopsies and benign lumps show up. Those things, combined with my mother's three recurrences, have kept me on the alert. Some women continue to see their oncologist for years after they have completed treatment, and others choose to go back to their primary care physician as soon as they reach the five-year mark, when the chance of recurrence is considered reduced. Have a conversation with your oncologist or surgeon to discuss what protocol you feel comfortable with.

If you are uninsured, underinsured or have other financial limitations to maintaining annual health checkups, there are resources that can help you find health centers in your area. These centers deliver primary health care and charge on a sliding fee scale. (See Badass Cancer Resources, Financial Assistance, page 247.)

Health and wellness

I took for granted that my health would be there for me whether I took care of it or not. It was not until I was diagnosed with breast cancer that I began to pay attention to what was on my dinner plate. It was also when I concluded that taking the elevator downstairs and walking a hundred feet to the deli for Cokes and cheese sticks was not a healthy exercise routine or diet. After forty-three years of giving my health a passing glance, I was scared: Cancer made me take it seriously. I felt that if I continued to neglect my body, I was telling cancer I did not care; it had my permission to come back.

Michael is good about taking care of his health and eating well. He tried to get me to do the same, but I had no interest in food or exercise. My attention was on my job. I snacked when I got hungry during the day and ate whatever he put in front of me, if at all, when I got home late from the office. I knew very little about food and even less about nutrition and exercise.

After my diagnosis, I cleaned all junk food out of our kitchen, then found I did not have a next step. I struggled with my commitment to living a healthy life. I ran out of excuses to avoid a change when I accepted it was not about time or money, my go-to reasons, or access to fresh food, which is everywhere in Manhattan; it is about education. Without an understanding of what constitutes good, nutritious food or what is meant by exercise or activity, I could not incorporate these concepts into my life. I had to educate myself.

I began by picking up a few food magazines and reading about the fundamentals of food and cooking. I looked for articles on the nutritional value of ingredients and the different ways to prepare food, what to look for when shopping and what to avoid on restaurant menus. I took Michael up on his offer to teach me the basics of cooking and listened to his tips on how to buy and store food. Friends sent me simple recipes, and I made a point of sitting down to eat a meal instead of standing over the kitchen counter.

My exercise routine began the first time I took the stairs to get up to our fifth-floor apartment instead of the elevator. After that I got out a subway stop before mine and walked the rest of the way home. I eventually joined a gym and developed a workout routine of swimming and land exercises. I stopped and started numerous times before I stuck to living healthfully. I was diligent right after my diagnosis and for the year or so after I was done with radiation. The further away I got from my diagnosis, the easier it was to slip into old habits.

My downfall was trying to do everything at once each time I attempted a change. Here is what I eventually learned: Start with what is easiest for you, and build from there. Congratulate yourself on your progress, and each time you slide back, start again—do not get stuck there.

To successfully manage a transition to something new, it takes education and commitment. There are several websites focused on health and wellness specifically for cancer patients. They have tips, suggestions, recipes and ideas to inform and guide you. Education is your fastest route to living healthfully. (See Badass Cancer Resources, Nutrition and Lifestyle, page 253.)

Managing stress

Stress is part of living. There are ways to manage stress so you benefit from it instead of having it wear you down.

There are two types of stress: good stress, or eustress; and bad stress, also called distress.

Eustress is short-term. It is motivating and exciting and will push you to meet a goal. Good stress is what you feel when you work to finish a presentation, give a speech or accomplish a health goal. You have the skill to do it, and you have control over the outcome of your efforts. It has a beneficial effect on your motivation and performance.

Bad stress can be short- or long-term. When you are suffering from bad stress, you do not feel as if you have control over the situation. It is draining, and there is no reprieve or time to recover from the cause of your tension. It has a negative effect on your physical, mental and emotional well-being and causes constant inflammation in the body, which, studies show, is an underlying factor in all disease. You may not be able to eliminate the cause of your anxiety or distress, but there are ways you can manage and reduce the cause.

A helpful tool to manage daily pressures is to write a stress diary. It is a simple and effective activity to gain insight to your stressors, so you can begin to address them. Write down what is causing your worry, and at the end of the week, analyze your writings. This exercise allows you to clarify your stressors and identify what prompted them.

By analyzing your behavior, you will be able to find areas where you can better manage the energy or channel it to something beneficial. You will also be able to determine if your reaction was appropriate to the incident and, if not, change it in the future. Overreacting to something or acting inappropriately can fuel the anxiety, anger and other emotions you are feeling.

Below are simple tips for keeping a stress diary:

- Write in it every day.
- At the top of the page, write the day and date.
- Note the time of each entry.
- The first entry should be the level of pressure you feel as you start the day. Measure it on a scale of 1 (low) to 10 (high).
- Throughout the day, jot down every time you feel strained.
- Write what you think started your anxiety: The car would not start, a disturbing phone call, an email with bad news, meeting with your boss, equipment at work malfunctioned, you opened a bill.
- Put down what was happening before you felt the stress.
- Note who was around you when you felt your tension level rise.
- Describe in detail how you behaved: I yelled at the kids for spilling milk, then locked myself in our

Tip

To successfully manage a transition to something new, it takes education and commitment.

bedroom. I ate a box of cereal and a package of cookies. I shut down and would not speak to anyone. I started crying.

- Note how you felt physically: I felt my heart start to race and a burning sensation throughout my body. I got a headache, and my palms got sweaty. I felt anxious, nauseous and light-headed.
- Explore how you felt emotionally: I felt defeated and helpless. I felt anger and panic.
- How long did the episode last?
- Rate the stressor on a scale of 1 (not intense) to 10 (very intense); compare your reaction using the same scale. Was the cause a 4 and your reaction to it an 8?

At the end of the week, review all your entries.

- Examine your patterns of stress, what caused them and how you reacted.
- Go through the list, and note which ones brought you the most and least amount of anxiety.
- Note the episodes you rated as very intense.
- Take notice if there was something that regularly caused them.
- Determine if your reaction was in alignment with the difficulty.

Be honest with yourself when noting and analyzing what causes your suffering. No one will see your list. Cancer is a huge contributor to stress, but it is not the only source.

Once you have reviewed everything, pick an event or a trigger that caused high stress. The goal is to better understand your emotions around the stressor and put a plan together to lessen the effect it has on you. Think of ways to reduce your stress. Do not limit your options to what you have done in the past to address this stress. Write down all possibilities before you judge them. It may mean a change in routine at home or responsibility at work or replacing a draining activity with one that is inspirational and engaging. A plan to address what is causing you the most anguish will give you some control over the situation, and your anxiety will begin to lessen.

Start by keeping a stress diary for a month. Write in it daily, and review it at the end of every week. Doing this will give you insight to patterns and coping mechanisms you have established over time. It will allow you to see what has worked for you and what has not—and make changes accordingly. You can continue to write in the diary after a month or use it as needed. Make it your safe place to let go of your emotions and get perspective on your circumstances.

Several websites offer stress diary templates or worksheets you can print and follow. In a search engine—for example, Google or Yahoo!—type in *stress diary template* or *stress diary worksheet.*

There are additional ways to reduce bad stress. Below are more options:

- Get involved in a group activity: community garden, reading group, a local sports team.
- Practice mindful meditation: *Little Book of Mindfulness: 10 Minutes a Day to Less Stress, More Peace,* by Patricia Collard; *Mindfulness in Plain English,* by Bhante Gunaratana. (See Recommended Books, page 399.)
- Exercise.
- Take a yoga or t'ai chi class.
- Practice breathing exercises. (See Breathing Exercises, page 149.)
- Get restful sleep.
- Maintain a routine.
- Talk with a therapist.
- Avoid caffeine, alcohol and nicotine.

Stress does not go away on its own. It builds, festers and influences your health, relationships and behavior. You do not have to accept stress as a way of living. A method to reduce it and an active effort to keep it in check will help you manage stress so it does not mange you.

Life after a diagnosis starts as a crawl. Next you will stand, then you will walk. What comes after is up to you. Some women want to slow down their life; others want to take on more. Some have a bucket list of desires to accomplish, and still others pursue their lifelong passions. There are those who become immersed in advocacy and fight for a cause, and women who just want things to be normal again.

Lean on women who have been through cancer to guide you. They know the roller coaster of emotion this part of the experience brings, as well as the surprise of how hard it is to pick up your life after a diagnosis. They understand how tough it is to let go of the life or body you had and regain your identity and purpose. Let them be a good listener as you work it all out.

Learn and get ideas from others, but do not compare your life with theirs. You will never know their full story, only what they want you to see. Think about what matters to you now and what makes you happy. Let that guide you to what you want as you reclaim your life.

It is in our nature to want to know how things will turn out. It feels safer when we think we can control where our life will go and what will happen. But that thinking limits what is possible to what you already know. To find out how big your life can be, you have to let go of expectations and be flexible, then see where it takes you. You were thrown into the unknown in a jarring way with cancer, and you figured it out and righted yourself again. Have faith that you will know what to do with the opportunities that come your way too.

CHAPTER 20

Prelude to a Postscript

When one of my dearest friends suggested I include a chapter on end-of-life planning, I balked at the idea, but she persisted.

"Cancer is not a death sentence," she said. "Whether or not someone is diagnosed with a terminal illness, the fact remains, everyone's life will come to an end someday. It would be helpful for people to understand what they need to take care of and that they have a say in their life up to the end."

She was right. We do have choices and a say in our life until the moment we are gone. But who wants to talk about it before we have to?

When I was initially diagnosed and uncertain of my fate, my first thought was, *If it is going to be painful, please just let it be quick.* My next thoughts were about how unorganized my life was and how unprepared I was to go. I had two very close friends who passed away from AIDS. They handled their death very differently and showed me what I did—and did not—want for myself.

Not long after he found out his illness was terminal, one friend managed every part of his exit. He took care of his memorial and funeral, completed arrangements with his favorite charity for his belongings and orchestrated the paperwork for his apartment to be sold after he passed. He made sure his dog would be well taken care of, organized home care for himself and wrote down how to maintain his apartment if his mind slipped. Then he relaxed into the last two years of his life knowing his wants and needs would be met and his wishes would prevail. He spent the time traveling and enjoying loved ones and his dog. He passed away at home surrounded by family, friends and his dog. He was at peace when he died.

My other friend was in denial about his death up to the end. He refused to complete a will or express his desires of how he wanted to be cared for or where he wanted to die. His mother came to visit and decided he should go back with her to the town in which she lived. He died 2,500 miles away from all his friends, alone in a hospital bed. By default, his mother had legal authority over everything in his life. She was overwhelmed and at a loss. She did not know how to deal with all of it, so she did what she could and walked away from the rest. His estranged and abusive father, with whom he had not spoken in more than twenty-five years, found out his son had passed away. Because there was no paperwork in place to stop him, he claimed—and received—half his estate. That result certainly would have been my friend's demise if he had not already passed.

My wishes aligned with my friend who went peacefully, but my life was more in the position of my friend who did not. My family and friends knew what I wanted, but that is very different from having it documented, legally or otherwise. I knew that, but I did not know what to do or where to begin. My first friend was right. Information on end-of-life planning would be helpful.

Americans as a whole, do not readily talk about death and dying until we have to. It was not always that way. In the 18th and 19th centuries, death and grieving were a way of life. It was so common, people routinely planned their funeral when they learned they were dying. Funerals were a public affair instead of a private matter. There were particular clothes for grieving men, women and children and specified lengths of time for how to long to wear them. People offered condolences whenever they came across someone in mourning. Some graves were designed to be planters, and the family plot was tended to as a garden space. The living family gathered together at the cemetery and had picnics like a reunion with deceased family members. To people then, death was part of life and addressing it was a form of moving on.

Today, generally speaking, most of us dodge any conversation about death. We do so for various reasons: We are not prepared; it brings to our attention what we have not accomplished; we fear a family dispute over end-of-life planning and estate distribution. Also, how we die is disconcerting. It is often equated with pain and suffering, and that is frightening. For others, it is not dying or death that is hard; it is the family members they leave behind and their worry about how they will cope. In addition, what we know about death is scary and unnerving. It happens to everyone, we do not know when it will happen, no one alive has done it before and there is no concrete evidence of what really happens.

But more people are beginning to understand the benefits of choreographing their end-of-life arrangements before it is a necessity. Doing so affords them the most options when choosing their care. They have time to deliberate over their estate and put plans in place to ensure their comfort. It awakens some to the limited time they have to fulfill their dreams and live the life they want.

Planning end-of-life care is not about dying; it is about living. Preparing for your last days does not hasten your death or extend your life. It also does not mean you are ready to go or that you are giving up. It is a compassionate and significant way to take care of yourself and your loved ones. When you put the appropriate documents in place and communicate how and where you want to be cared for, you live fully with the knowledge that the ones you care about have a road map to follow to help them through this complicated time. The alternative is to leave your end-of-life decisions to others to figure out.

Most of us tend to think we still have time to take care of the important things that matter to us. When the timeline of departure is suddenly moved from *unknown* to *four months,* you need to move quickly. End-of-life decisions should not be made in a panic or when you are distraught. It is better if they are not talked about in bits and pieces or mentioned in passing to someone. Such important decisions require thought, honesty

> **Tip**
>
> *Planning end-of-life care is not about dying; it is about living. Preparing for your last days does not hasten your death or extend your life. It also does not mean you are ready to go or you are giving up.*

and information to determine what is realistic, and you need to document them. Below will help you understand what goes into end-of-life planning. (See Badass Cancer Resources, End-of-Life Planning, page 246.)

Estate planning

An estate is the entirety of what you own at the time of your death. It is more than wealth and investments. It includes your home, car, insurance policies and all your personal possessions. Regardless of the size, everyone has an estate.

A brief list of items to consider for your estate planning:

- Who will take care of my children and pets?
- How do I provide for my spouse or partner and children after I am gone?
- How shall I direct my loved ones to deal with my end-of-life health issues?
- How should they dispose of my possessions?
- How can I pass as much of my estate as possible to my spouse or partner, children, grandchildren and charities dear to my heart?

Documenting how and to whom you want your estate distributed is something everybody needs to figure out, not only those who are wealthy. If you do not do it, the courts, the government and other family members will do it for you. If you knew their choices and decisions ahead of time, you probably might not be happy—as evidenced by my friend who did not plan.

Paperwork

The first step in planning for your estate is writing a will. This document dictates in writing how all your money and possessions will be distributed, including who will take care of your children and be the executor of your estate, among other things. If you die without one, it means you have died "intestate." The intestacy laws of your state will determine how your estate is distributed. This includes all your personal possessions and assets at the time of death—bank accounts, properties, investments. Having a last will and testament in place can help your family avoid possible conflicts and legal issues after your death.

Estate planners agree that everyone needs a will, but increasingly they are saying people could also benefit from a living trust. A difference between a will and living trust: A will goes into effect after you die; a living trust goes into effect as soon as you create it. A few of the reasons people include a living trust in their estate planning: Assets are dispensed more quickly; you avoid the cost and time delays of probate court; you can protect government benefits for a person with disabilities; you can better protect inheritances from creditors and lawsuits; it does not go through probate, therefore personal information about property and other assets does not become public record. (See Badass Cancer Resources, End-of-Life Planning, page 246; Legal Information and Documents, page 251.)

In addition to a will, Kiplinger (https://www.kiplinger.com) advises everyone to have these four key documents in place:

- Durable power of attorney: This document will give your loved ones the authority to manage your finances and legal matters if you become incapacitated or need their help
- Advance directive, or living will: This document allows you to provide written guidance on what actions should be taken for your health if you are no longer able to make decisions for yourself. This includes measures to keep you alive as well as matters such as pain management and organ donation.
- Health-care proxy, also known as a health-care surrogate or medical power of attorney: Through this document, you appoint an agent to make health-care decisions on your behalf should you lose the ability to make decisions for yourself. A health-care proxy works in conjunction with an advance directive. The difference between them: In a living will, you provide written guidance for actions to be taken regarding your health care; with a health-care proxy, you give someone else the power to decide what actions are taken. It is advised to have both.

- Medical-information release: This is written authorization to give your doctors permission to share your medical information with your family

Additional paperwork to set up:

- Guardianship designations: This document allows the parents of a minor to legally designate another person or other people to be the guardian of the child. This matter is usually covered in a will but not always.
- Beneficiary designations: These are investments such as 401(k)s, IRAs or Roth IRAs, trusts and life insurance policies that you can pass on to your heirs without documenting them in your will. A financial adviser, certified public accountant (CPA) or life insurance agent can help you properly set up these important designations. If you do not name a beneficiary, or the one you have named has become incapable or has died, the courts could get involved, and delays will follow.
- Do not resuscitate (DNR): This legal directive allows someone to die naturally without the intervention of cardiopulmonary resuscitation (CPR) or advanced cardiac life support to maintain a heartbeat.

You can acquire this paperwork, as well as other valuable forms such as diminishing capacity letters and organ donor letters, through an estate planner, or you can download it from websites. It is prudent to periodically review and update all your end-of-life paperwork to ensure all the documents reflect your current wishes. A good standard practice is to review your estate planning documents for each major life event: birth of children or grandchildren, marriage, divorce, children become adults or a major disability brought on by illness or an accident.

When documenting instructions for your estate, remember to include information for any services you have set up electronically. The two areas to consider:

- Digital items: online accounts, passwords
- Physical items: advisers, account statements, insurance policies, safety box keys

Write down everything that requires confidential information to get into—such as your computer, email, web addresses and electronic accounts—along with access information: login ID, password, secret answers. It may be difficult, or impossible, for your family to get into important online accounts and electronic records without your security codes and passwords. Access to bank accounts and safety deposit boxes will require your loved ones to provide an original death certificate if they do not have your information. Obtaining multiple death certificates will cost money and cause time delays.

Below is a list of digital accounts to think about when documenting your estate:

- Computer
- Email
- Electronic devices: cell phones, tablets, PDAs
- Bank account: account number, type of account
- Financial investment accounts: account numbers
- Online accounts: bills, digital records, pictures, medical portals, social media accounts

Additional items to document:

- Codes: safety deposit box, storage unit, safes
- Addresses: bank, financial investment institutions, storage unit
- Contact information: accountant, broker, banker, employer
- Documents: assets, contracts, business agreements

Make sure the location of keys needed to open safes, vaults and storage units is included in the documents. Keep this information in a secure place along with your will, living will, durable power of attorney and other important documents. Be sure to communicate to the executor of your estate where everything is located. If you choose to keep the information in a safe, make sure the executor knows the lock combination to open it.

Several legal websites provide comprehensive details on planning an estate. Many provide legal paperwork you can download for free and do it yourself. If you choose this option, it is advisable to have an estate planner or lawyer review the completed documents. You may prefer to hire an estate planner or an attorney to assist you with the paperwork. If that is the case, ask family and friends for recommendations. Remember to ask for references before selecting one to assist you. In addition, online directories allow you to search for a planner by city, state and ZIP code, or by name. (See Badass Cancer Resources, Legal Information and Documents, page 251; End-of-Life Planning, page 246.)

Care options

Estate planning is more than communicating in what way you want your money and possessions distributed. It also expresses how and where you want to spend your final days. Paperwork will cover your legal and medical wishes, but there are other important questions to consider: Who do you want to take care of you? Where do you want to be when you die—in a hospital, at home, out in nature or at a different location? Do you want all life-prolonging measures performed, or do you just want to be kept comfortable?

Many people have no idea what their loved ones want for their final days. When asked, most people will say they want to die at home or at a favorite location surrounded by the people they love. Very few say they want to die in a hospital or nursing home. But that is where the majority of people pass away. You have options. Before you start making decisions or assumptions about your care, learn about what is available.

Below will help you understand the definitions of treatments:

- Active treatment: Health-care practices that aim to cure patients, not only reduce pain or stress. Chemotherapy would be considered active treatment for someone with cancer.
- Passive treatment: When the patient no longer seeks active or curative treatment but moves to pain management and comfort.

Below will help you understand the choices for care:

Home care

Home care is a wide array of services that allows you, as an ill or injured person, to receive care in your home.

It can include, but is not limited to, personal care—for example, helping you bathe, wash your hair and get dressed. It can involve cleaning, cooking, delivering meals, laundry and yard work. It might mean physical therapy or occupational therapy (or both) to improve mobility and complete simple household activities. It also can include monitoring blood pressure, temperature, breathing and pain levels and communicating your status and condition with your doctor. It may require managing and administering medication. Home health-care services can be arranged and administered, but family and friends will handle much of the day-to-day care.

Online care calendars can help organize support from the community for routine tasks such as preparing meals, transportation, helping with housework and picking up a prescription. (See Badass Cancer Resources, Care Calendars, page 244.)

Assistance can also be found through organizations such as the American Cancer Society (https://www.cancer.org/). It has set up community programs across the country to help and support those with cancer. In addition, online directories provide lists of home health-care agencies if a patient needs or prefers to hire a home health-care aid. (See Badass Cancer Resources, End-of-Life Planning, page 246.)

Palliative care

Palliative is a term for medical treatment that concentrates on reducing symptoms and managing pain for a serious illness whether it is terminal or not. It can be given to you at any time or stage of illness, from diagnosis on.

A palliative care team includes, but is not limited to, specially trained doctors and nurses as well as psychologists, nutritionists and physical therapists. Everyone works together to improve the quality of

> **Tip**
>
> *Estate planning is more than communicating in what way you want your money and possessions distributed. It also expresses how and where you want to spend your final days.*

life for you and your family. You can continue this care as you pursue a cure. You can also get care on an as-needed basis for a chronic or long-term illness. Palliative care can be administered at home or received in a hospital, a nursing home or another extended care facility.

If you are diagnosed with metastatic cancer, you may choose palliative care early after your diagnosis to help you and your family manage your illness. Hospice care at the end of life includes palliative care.

Hospice care

Hospice care is a service, not a location. It is for patients considered terminally ill or those who have less than six months to live. The caregiver team includes trained hospice physicians as well as nurses, psychologists, social workers, volunteers and clergy.

Caregivers concentrate on comfort, support and the emotional aspect of dying rather than extensive life-prolonging treatment. The team helps you and your family members cope with illness and approaching death together. Hospice care offers psychological support, pain management and symptom control. You can receive it in a hospital, a hospice center, a skilled nursing facility or at home.

The difference between palliative and hospice care: Palliative care can begin at the time of diagnosis; hospice care begins once treatment for the disease has stopped. Most private health-care plans cover palliative and hospice care. Always check your insurance policy for any limits. Medicare and Medicaid cover most programs. (See Badass Cancer Resources, Hospice and Palliative Care, page 248; End-of-Life Planning, page 246.)

In-patient care

In-patient care is when you are admitted to a hospital or long-term care facility. Some people prefer or require the continuous care those environments provide. Hospice and palliative care can be administered there as well.

If your prognosis demands that you address your care now, discuss your situation with your health-care team or a social worker to understand what will be involved in your case. These professionals can guide you to the right service. They can also get support teams to assist you and your family. Lean on the pros, and let them guide you to what is achievable.

Additional sources of information about arrangements:

- Hospital care managers
- Hospital discharge planners
- Online directories for providers: In the search bar of a search engine—for example, Google or Yahoo!—type in your location and *hospice care* for details about services in your area. Some examples: New Orleans hospice care, New York City hospice care, hospice care Denver.
- The Department of Human Services website for your state: On the home page of your state's website—for example, www.iowa.gov, www.myflorida.com, www.maine.gov—type in *Department of Human Services* in the search bar for information on hospice care services available in your area.
- National hospice and palliative care organizations such as Hospice Foundation of America (https://hospicefoundation.org/) and the National Association for Home Care and Hospice (https://www.nahc.org/) (See Badass Cancer Resources, End-of-Life Planning, page 246; Hospice and Palliative Care, page 248.)
- Patient advocates (See Badass Cancer Resources, Patient Advocates, page 254.)
- Friends who have used hospice services in the past for loved ones

When deciding on care, take into consideration how much support and help your loved ones are capable of. Have an honest and open conversation with family members about your wants, desires and expectations, and ask them to be frank about what they are willing and able to do. Once you know what you have to work with, you can put together an achievable plan for your care.

When you understand your options and prepare in advance, you eliminate the pressure on your loved ones to make these decisions for you. It guides them in what manner you want to be taken care of, where you want your final days to be and how they can best support you.

Talk about it

Death is hard to think about, but talking about it helps. A conversation about dying and end-of-life planning does not have to be morbid. It can be fact-finding and informative. Talk with family and friends to find out their thoughts on death and dying. Ask what they have done to plan for their end of life. Discussing it with others helps reduce the anxiety about it.

Having a belief or philosophy about death and dying can help you feel less fearful about it. It does not matter if you are religious or not or if your thoughts about death and the afterlife now conflict with your ideas in the past. What is important is that you find peace with your beliefs today.

If your prognosis is terminal and you are facing the end of your life, speak with your doctor or a nurse, a social worker or a counselor to help you cope with your thoughts and anxiety. If you are so inclined, speak to a respected religious person about this stage of your life. Spend time having conversations with family and friends who are willing to talk and who accept your situation. Do not be afraid to be honest and vulnerable. To shut down or internalize these emotions is isolating and will increase your fears. Accept that there will be loved ones who will not talk to you about it. You can assist them by providing information and guiding them to support. (See Badass Cancer Resources, Grief, page 248.)

It is helpful to connect with patients who know what you are facing. Ask your doctor if the hospital has a support group for people with a terminal illness. A local religious organization may have or know of groups. Write about your experience, and share your story with others through online communities. They can help ease your anxiety, answer questions or give you tips on how to cope or communicate with family. (See Badass Cancer Resources, Online Communities, page 253.)

Myth
Most women die of breast cancer.

Truth
Women fear cancer in general and breast cancer in particular more than any other disease. And because breast cancer now gets so much attention, many people believe most women die of breast cancer. But that is not the case. In the United States, breast cancer is the fifth leading cause of death in women. Heart disease is first.

—DR. SUSAN LOVE RESEARCH FOUNDATION

The more you can remain mentally stimulated, the less stress and depression you will feel. Stay active and engaged with people as much as possible for as long as possible. Continue to work, write the novel, plant the garden, take the vacation, sign up for an art class. Carry on with your social life, and stay involved with friends. Maintain as much of your routine as possible, and direct your energy toward what you love.

Patients who are terminal have found solace in leaving letters for loved ones to read after they are gone. Project yourself into the future, and compose letters or write cards for your spouse, significant other and children to open on anniversaries, birthdays and other special occasions. If you have children, consider a video log for your son or daughter for their graduation, wedding or birth of their first child. A few minutes of your telling them how much you loved them and your hopes and dreams for them as they celebrate a birthday, achieve a milestone or cheer a new beginning will make you a part of their special day.

Some patients get involved in planning a celebration of their life. It helps them relieve their anxiety regarding death and feel as if they have some control over what is happening to them. Some want a say over the remembrance they leave. Others take care of it to keep their family members from having to do such an emotional task while they are in mourning. Some plan ahead for financial reasons; some funeral homes offer discounts for preplanned funerals. Your loved ones will have to take care of the arrangements if you do not get involved. But they will appreciate your input and be relieved and grateful for whatever you do.

I visited a friend in the hospital who had advanced lung cancer. She was thin and frail, and her skin was pallid. She had an IV in her arm, oxygen tubes in her nose and machines monitoring all her vitals. Three days prior, she had had back surgery to help reduce the pain in her spine. When I got there, she was in an upbeat mood. She had sung in a cabaret four weeks earlier, despite her frail lungs, and was excited about new music for her next show, which she planned on performing the following month. She was not delusional or in denial about her health; she chose to put her attention on what she loved—singing in cabarets—not her circumstances. She died three days later and worked on new songs until her end. It made her happy.

She told her friends that when the time came, she wanted a cabaret to celebrate her life. She gave big-picture ideas of a perfect song and dance memorial, and let her fellow actors put together the show. She found comfort in knowing she would be remembered for what she loved: music and performing.

One year for Christmas, Michael and I gave our dear friend Aunt Dee a bottle of wine with her name engraved on it. She was thrilled but refused to drink it.

"I'm going to be buried with it," she said. "I want it lying in my arms in the casket. It is a lovely chardonnay with my name on it. I don't know what they are serving on the other side, so I'm going prepared."

It was a simple request and one that captured what a funny character she was.

Death, dying and end-of-life planning are not easy subjects to tackle. Not talking about them, though, does not delay or circumvent the inevitable. It is better to speak about them and work out the details before you are forced to. No one knows if her death is imminent or years away. Having all your affairs in order gives you the freedom to live without worrying about dying. Several websites offer information on how to plan a celebration of life as well as checklists, ideas and funeral customs and etiquette. (See Badass Cancer Resources, End-of-Life Planning, page 246.)

Putting our life to rest is a time for reflection on all we have loved, enjoyed and achieved while we were here. A memorial is a salute to who we are and the life we have lived. Death is a momentous occasion, and you have a say in the memory you leave with loved ones. It is the last time you will have a voice in your life. Why not take it?

The two biggest moments in your life are the one when you come into it and the one when you make your exit. Unlike your entrance, you have a say over the details of your departure. No matter when, where or how you go, you owe yourself peace and comfort at the end.

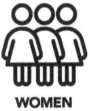

WOMEN

COVID-19

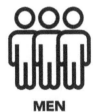

MEN

BADASS

CANCER RESOURCES®

Information and support are good medicine.

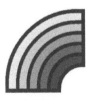

LGBTQ

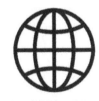

INTERNATIONAL

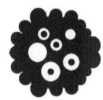

OTHER

There are more than 140 resources provided here to help you with your diagnosis. Each site has been reviewed for content and relevancy. You can quickly determine by the information provided below if it is the right resource for you without spending time going through each site.

These links and resources provided are for informational, educational and support purposes only and are not an endorsement. The material in the Badass Cancer Resources guide is not a substitute for medical or other professional services from a qualified health-care provider. Search results do not replace advice from your doctor.

The websites listed in the Badass Cancer Resources guide are from established organizations. I appreciate that website addresses and internal links can change or get updated. Many, not all, of the resources listed here are also on my website: www.theupsidetoeverything.com. Please check the online guide for current web addresses and new resources. Or a simple search using the name of the organization will take you to the website and you can navigate the pages from there. I regularly review and update the Badass Cancer Resources guide on my website. I welcome information on any resources you find helpful and will include them in the resource guide on my website. Cancer support is a community effort. Please note: The "Other" category in the Badass Cancer Resources logo is for resources other than breast cancer. Those resources are available only my website.

Arranged Alphabetically by Category

A

C

Cancer Information

All the resources provided have information on cancer. The organizations below offer clinical information and explanations on types, diagnosis, treatment and studies of the disease.

Care Calendars

Caregiver Support—Helplines, Peer-to-Peer, Live Chats

E

G

H

I

International

Many of the organizations listed here and the information they provide can be utilized from anywhere in the world through their websites; the organizations below provide services outside the United States.

L

Languages and Ethnic-Specific Resources and Support

N

Nutrition and Lifestyle

O

Online Communities

P

Podcasts, Radio Shows, Videos and Webinars

The following websites offer information in audiovisual formats.

Pregnant With Cancer

Prosthesis

S

Second Opinion

Self-care

Sex

V

Vision Board

W

Wigs

Y

Young Adult

In the world of cancer, young adult is generally considered ages 15 to 39.

Arranged Alphabetically by Name

C

W

Y

Badass Cancer Resources: A-to-Y

A

Air Care Alliance

https://www.aircarealliance.org/
mail@aircarealliance.org *Email*
(888) 260-9707
General information, Monday – Friday, 9:00 AM – 5:00 PM PT
Air Care Alliance is an umbrella organization that provides an online directory of more than sixty groups with volunteer pilots who will **fly patients** for care or provide other flight or aviation services to help those in need.

Submit a Request Online
http://www.aircarealliance.org/submit-request-for-assistance
Request a flight or information.
Service is free.

Air Charity Network

http://aircharitynetwork.org/
Air Charity Network comprises a network of member organizations with volunteer pilots who utilize their own aircraft, fuel and time to provide free air transportation to medical facilities for citizens who are financially distressed or otherwise unable to travel on public transportation.

Request a Flight
http://aircharitynetwork.org/request-a-flight/

Members also coordinate flights to fly organ transplant candidates and people involved in clinical trials, chemotherapy or other repetitive treatment.

Passenger Qualifications
http://aircharitynetwork.org/home/passengers/qualifications/
Passenger requirements are necessary to be transported.
Services are free.

AirMedCare Network

https://www.airmedcarenetwork.com/
https://www.airmedcarenetwork.com/contact *Contact form*
https://www.facebook.com/AirMedCareNetwork/
(855) 568-5984 / (800) 793-0010
Membership lines, Monday – Friday, 8:00 AM – 8:00 PM CT
AirMedCare Network is an **air ambulance** membership network. It owns a fleet of helicopters that will fly you to the closest facility. The membership covers the expense of the air ambulance fees not covered by your health insurance.
Membership fees apply.

Alliance for Fertility Preservation

https://www.allianceforfertilitypreservation.org/
https://www.facebook.com/search/top?q=alliance%20for%20fertility%20preservation
https://twitter.com/AllianceForFP
(925) 290-8950
Information; leave a voice mail and someone will get back to you.
Alliance for Fertility Preservation is a coalition of professionals with expertise in **oncology, reproductive endocrinology**, urology, psychology, oncology nursing, reproductive law and **fertility preservation** for cancer patients.

One-on-One Support
https://www.allianceforfertilitypreservation.org/resources/get-and-give-support

Alliance for Fertility Preservation has partnered with Imerman Angels to provide **free one-on-one support** to **previvors, patients, survivors** and **caregivers** who want to learn about fertility preservation.

Fertility Options for Women
https://www.allianceforfertilitypreservation.org/options-for-women/
Explanation and information on options, costs, potential risks and eligibility.

Fertility Options for Men
https://www.allianceforfertilitypreservation.org/options-for-men/
Explanation and information on options, costs, potential risks and eligibility.

Financial Assistance Programs
https://www.allianceforfertilitypreservation.org/financial-assistance-programs/
Information on programs to help offset some of the costs of fertility preservation.

Fertility Scout
https://www.allianceforfertilitypreservation.org/about-fertility-scout/
Fertility Scout helps oncology health-care providers and patients find fertility preservation **services around the world** quickly—before they start their treatment. Locate a fertility and reproductive health center in your area. *Online Fertility Scout is free.*

American Association of Sexuality Educators, Counselors and Therapists
https://www.aasect.org/
https://www.facebook.com/AASECT
https://twitter.com/TheAASECT
American Association of Sexuality Educators, Counselors and Therapists is professional organization devoted to the promotion of **sexual health** by the development and advancement of the fields of sexual therapy, counseling and education.

Directory of Therapists, Councilors and Educators
https://www.aasect.org/referral-directory
A list of **sexuality educators, sexuality counselors** and **sex therapists** in the United States and around the globe. AASECT is a membership organization for medical and health-care professionals, but anyone can access the map and list of professionals.
Directory is free.

American Breast Cancer Foundation

https://www.abcf.org/
website: *English and Spanish*
info@abcf.org *Email*
https://www.facebook.com/americanbreastcancerfoundation/
https://twitter.com/TweetABCF
(844) 219-2223 / (410) 730-5105
Breast Cancer Assistance Program, Monday – Thursday, 9:00 AM – 4:00 PM; Friday 9:00 AM – 11:45 AM ET
The American Breast Cancer Foundation provides access and **financial assistance** to aid in the **early detection, treatment** and **survival** of breast cancer for **underserved** and **uninsured individuals,** regardless of age or gender. In conjunction with its Breast Cancer Assistance Program, ABCF maintains a Community Partnership Program with medical clinics and health-care consortiums to provide **reduced-fee breast cancer screenings, diagnostic mammograms** and **ultrasounds**.

Breast Cancer Assistance Program
https://www.abcf.org/our-programs/breast-cancer-assistance-program/
Information on financial assistance for breast cancer screenings and diagnostic tests for uninsured and underserved individuals, regardless of age or gender.
Information and support are free.

American Cancer Society

https://www.cancer.org/

website: *English and 12 additional languages*

https://www.facebook.com/AmericanCancerSociety

https://twitter.com/americancancer

(800) 227-2345

Helpline/information: English 24/7. Live Spanish help, Monday – Friday, 7:00 AM – 7:00 PM CT; after hours, third-party translation. Third-party translation service for other languages.

Live chat available, Monday – Friday, 7:00 AM – 6:30 PM CT. English and Spanish

The American Cancer Society is a nationwide, community-based voluntary health organization dedicated to eliminating cancer as a major health problem. It provides **information, education, resources** and **support** for all types of cancer including alternative approaches, clinical trials and tips for living with cancer.

Understand and Manage Your Diagnosis

https://www.cancer.org/cancer/breast-cancer.html

Information on **managing, understanding** and **coping with cancer.**

Understand and Manage Advanced and Metastatic Cancer

https://www.cancer.org/treatment/understanding-your-diagnosis/advanced-cancer/what-is.html

Information on managing, understanding, and coping with **advanced** and **metastatic cancer.**

Treatment

https://www.cancer.org/treatment.html

Information on **side effects; finding** and **paying for treatment; understanding financial** and **legal matters**; helping children when a family member has cancer; staying healthy during and after treatments; managing a diagnosis during and after a natural disaster.

COVID and Cancer

https://www.cancer.org/about-us/what-we-do/coronavirus-covid-19-and-cancer.html

Routine medical care during the pandemic; preventing and managing infections. Tips for **managing stress** and **emotions** related to coronavirus; ways to **stay healthy** while stuck at home; steps for cancer caregiving during a pandemic; questions to ask your health-care team.

Videos on Clinical Trials

https://www.cancer.org/treatment/treatments-and-side-effects/clinical-trials/clinical-trials-videos.html

Better understand what is involved in a trial and if a trial is right for you.

About Clinical Trials

https://www.cancer.org/treatment/treatments-and-side-effects/clinical-trials/what-you-need-to-know/picking-a-clinical-trial.html

Information on understanding clinical trials: where they are done, how they work and who is eligible.

Personal Health Manager

https://www.cancer.org/treatment/treatments-and-side-effects/planning-managing/personal-health-manager.html

Information, tools and worksheets to **stay organized** and **prepared** for talking with your doctor.

Sex and the Woman With Cancer

https://www.cancer.org/treatment/treatments-and-side-effects/physical-side-effects/fertility-and-sexual-side-effects/sexuality-for-women-with-cancer/faqs.html

Sex and the female body; **surgery and sex; chemo and hormone treatment and sex; cancer, sex and the single woman.**

Cancer, Sex and the Male Body

https://www.cancer.org/treatment/treatments-and-side-effects/physical-side-effects/fertility-and-sexual-side-effects/sexuality-for-men-with-cancer/how-male-body-works-sexually.html
Sex and the male body; **surgery and sex; how testosterone works; how the male body works**; and **sex and cancer.**

Talking to Children

https://www.cancer.org/treatment/children-and-cancer/when-a-family-member-has-cancer/dealing-with-diagnosis/how-to-tell-children.html
Steps, advice and resources on how to tell children when a family member has cancer.

Caregiver Information and Support

https://www.cancer.org/treatment/caregivers/caregiver-support-videos.html
A video series and downloadable guide for understanding a **caregiver's role**: **patient nutrition; coping skills; dealing with money issues; living wills** and **facing end of life**; how to assist with the everyday needs of their loved one and self-care techniques to improve their own **quality of life.**

Healthy Eating, Active Living

https://www.cancer.org/healthy/eat-healthy-get-active/healthy-eating-active-living-videos.html
Two- to four-minute videos: Healthy choices can affect your risk; the truth behind cancer myths; incorporating healthy behaviors into your busy life. *Services are free.*

American College of Trust and Estate Counsel

https://www.actec.org/
https://www.actec.org/about-us/contact-us/ *Contact form*
https://www.facebook.com/ACTECFellow
https://twitter.com/ACTECNEWS
(202) 684-8460

Information, Monday – Friday, 9:30 AM – 5:30 PM ET
American College of Trust and Estate Counsel is a nonprofit association of peer-elected lawyers and law professors skilled and experienced in the preparation of **wills and trusts; estate planning;** and **probate procedure** and administration of trusts and estates of decedents, minors and incompetents.

Videos, Podcasts and Resources
https://www.actec.org/estate-planning/resources-for-families/
Estate planning resources for individuals, families and professionals. Find information related to estate planning and regulatory matters affected by the pandemic.

Directory of Trust and Estate Attorneys
https://www.actec.org/fellows/directory/
The directory assists consumers in identifying and locating trust and estate attorneys in their area.
Directory is free.

American Indian Cancer Foundation
https://www.americanindiancancer.org/
info@aicaf.org *Email*
https://www.facebook.com/AmericanIndianCancer
https://twitter.com/AICAF_Org
(612) 314-4848
Information; messages left are returned ASAP.
The American Indian Cancer Foundation is a nonprofit organization that was established to address the cancer inequities that American Indian and Alaska Native communities face.

COVID and Cancer
https://americanindiancancer.org/covid-19/
Services are free.

Ana Ono

https://www.anaono.com/
cs@anaono.com *Email*
https://www.anaono.com/pages/contact-us *Contact form*
anaonointimates (@AnaOnoIntimates) / Twitter
(866) 879-1744
Information and customer support
Ana Ono is an **intimate** and **lifestyle apparel** line for women with **two breasts, one breast, no breasts** or **new breasts**. The line includes pocketed bras as well as bras for radiation, for reconstruction and for women who have gone flat. It also offers support leisure bras, front-closure bras and robes with a drain-management belt.

Insurance Coverage

https://www.anaono.com/pages/insurance-faq
Many insurance companies cover mastectomy bras. With a qualifying prescription from your doctor, you may be eligible. Ana Ono will help you process your coverage and claims.
Prices available online.

Anti-Cancer Club

https://anticancerclub.com/
https://anticancerclub.com/contact-us/ *Contact form*
https://www.facebook.com/AntiCancerClub/
https://twitter.com/anticancerclub
Anti-Cancer Club provides **information, resources, weekly tips** and insights into the cancer experience and anti-cancer living. Information includes resources to help patients and survivors create a **healthy lifestyle mentally, physically** and **emotionally.**

Healthy Eating Recipes

https://anticancerclub.com/topic/recipes-and-eating-healthy/

Recipes and information on **healthy eating**. Each week the culinary experts offer one food, flavor or idea as it relates to an **anti-cancer diet**.

Online Cooking Classes
https://anticancerclub.com/?s=cancer+fighting+kitchen
The Cancer Fighting Kitchen
Fees apply.

Book Club
https://anticancerclub.com/club-activities/cancerbookclub/
The Anti-Cancer Book Club, #Bullseye, meets through a live video meeting. Check website for dates.
Free

Artful Parent
https://artfulparent.com/
The **Artful Parent** has a directory of more than 500 art and crafts projects for kids. Includes instructions for creating a vision board.

Vision Board in 10 Steps
https://artfulparent.com/make-vision-board-works-10-steps/
Free

Awesome Breastforms
www.awesomebreastforms.org
website: *More than 100 languages*
https://www.facebook.com/Awesome-Breastforms-Orders-1601722360097846/?fref=ts#
Awesome Breastforms are **prosthetic breast forms** handmade with **100% cotton fiber yarn**. They are created by a group of women who have come together for the single purpose of crocheting and knitting handmade prosthetic breast forms for women who have had breast surgery—including

mastectomy, lumpectomy and **explant surgery**—and for **women with developmental conditions**. Washable and easy to care for.

How to Order
https://awesomebreastforms.org/index.php/how-to-order-awesome-breastforms-2/
Breastforms are free

B

The Balance
https://www.thebalance.com
Contact@thebalance.com *Email*
https://www.facebook.com/thebalancecom/
https://twitter.com/thebalance/
The Balance is useful to patients dealing with medical bills. It explains the different types of debt and provides a state-by-state list of statutes of limitations by category. Experts from the financial industry post up-to-date industry information and trends.

Statute of Limitations on Debt
https://www.thebalance.com/state-by-state-list-of-statute-of-limitations-on-debt-960881
Explanation of categories of debt and information on statutes of limitation by state.
Free

Body Med Boutique
https://bodymedboutique.ca/
anne@bodymedboutique.com *Email*
admin@bodymedboutique.com *Info/book and appointment*
https://www.facebook.com/bodymedboutique/

(289) 337-1508

Information, Tuesday – Friday, 10:00 AM – 4:00 PM; Saturday 10:00 AM – 2:00 PM CT, Ontario, Canada. Messages left will be returned ASAP.

BodyMed Boutique fits products for women and men including a full line of mastectomy bras and breast forms, post-surgical bras and girdles, abdominal binders, medical shape wear, vascular compression socks, hosiery and sleeves.

Products

https://bodymedboutique.ca/product-category/postsurgical/
BodyMed has large selection of post-surgical **compression garments**, **mastectomy bras** and **prosthesis,** as well as hot-flash pajamas, head coverings and cancer treatment aids.

Shop Been-A-Boob

https://bodymedboutique.ca/shop/breast-forms/heart-ultralight-been-a-boob-by-janac/
Been-A-Boob **prosthesis** by Janac Mastectomy Wear is available through Body Bed Boutique. Been-A-Boob is a non-silicone prosthetic device made for sports, swimming and every day. Filled with little beads that mold to any shape of bra, it can be worn in a swimsuit and a regular mastectomy bra. *Prices available online.*

The Camisole Project

https://bodymedboutique.ca/camisole-project/
The Camisole Project provides a **free Because We Care package** to anyone diagnosed with breast cancer. The package includes a post-surgical camisole with drains that will make the days following surgery more comfortable, a heart-shaped pillow for under your arm to help with the discomfort of a lymph node surgery, a journal and pen for taking notes at doctor appointments, baby wipes to use after surgery when bathing or showering is not recommended, a pair of cozy socks, a pack of Kleenex, an all-natural lip balm and a chill-out aromatherapy roller to give you a lift.

Free

Breasthealth.org
http://www.breasthealth.org
breasthealth@breastcancer.org *Email*
https://www.facebook.com/breasthealth?ref=hl
https://twitter.com/GoBreastHealthy
(610) 642-6550
Information, Monday – Friday, 9:00 AM – 5:00 PM ET
Breasthealth.org has information on steps you can take today to affect your breast health tomorrow. Dr. Marisa C. Weiss, a globally recognized breast oncologist, founded Breasthealth.org.

Breasts: Facts and Fiction
http://www.breasthealth.org/category/breasts-101/
Information, tips and advice on breast health.

Healthy Eating
http://www.breasthealth.org/category/healthy-eating/
Information, tips and advice on **healthy eating**.

Healthy Habits
http://www.breasthealth.org/category/healthy-habits/
Information, tips, and advice on how to develop and maintain **healthy habits**.

Healthy Home
http://www.breasthealth.org/category/healthy-home/
Information on the greener way to clean; guide to maintaining a BPA-free life; DIY cleaning products that are safe and effective.
Free

Breastcancer.org

http://www.breastcancer.org

website: *English and Spanish*

https://www.facebook.com/breastcancerorg/

https://twitter.com/Breastcancerorg

Breastcancer.org is a nonprofit organization that provides information, resources and education on breast cancer. It has an extensive library of articles, slide shows, blogs, podcasts and videos.

Videos

http://www.breastcancer.org/treatment/surgery/reconstruction/videos.

Doctors and survivors discuss topics that include but are not limited to **understanding breast cancer;** breast **reconstruction; treatment;** breast cancer and **your job; sex** and **intimacy; hormone therapy; lymphedema; pain management; mastectomy** and **reconstruction.**

Podcasts

http://www.breastcancer.org/community/podcasts.

Topics include but are not limited to **recurrence; COVID and breast cancer; breast cancer risk and race; inflammatory breast cancer; immunotherapy; mastectomy and reconstruction; sexual side effects of cancer treatment.**

Men With Breast Cancer

https://www.breastcancer.org/symptoms/types/male_bc

Information on **risks, symptoms, diagnosis,** what to expect from a **pathology report** and the **treatment** of male breast cancer.

Talking to Older Children and Teens

http://www.breastcancer.org/tips/telling_family/older_kids

Seven-step guideline with tips on talking to young and older children when a family member has cancer.

Free

BreastFree.org

http://breastfree.org/

info@breastfree.org *Email*

https://breastfree.blogspot.com/

BreastFree.org offers advice and support for women who want to learn more about **living breast-free**. It has information on how to select breast forms, bras and swimsuits and provides a resource list for purchasing. It also recommends creative ways to look good and feel good.

Free

C

Camp Erin—Eluna Network

https://elunanetwork.org/

https://elunanetwork.org/contact-us/ *Contact form*

https://www.facebook.com/elunanetwork

https://twitter.com/elunanetwork

(267) 687-7724

Information; messages will be returned ASAP.

Camp Erin is a national **bereavement program** managed by Eluna Network **for youth, ages 6 to 17,** who are grieving the death of a significant person in their life. **Eluna Network** offers weekend camps that combine traditional, fun camp activities with grief education and emotional support.

Camp Dates, Location and Contact Information

https://elunanetwork.org/camps-programs/camp-erin/

Camps are offered in every Major League Baseball city as well as additional locations across the U. S. and Canada. To register for a camp, go to the map at the bottom of the page and click on the camp you are interested in.

Resource Center

https://elunanetwork.org/resources/

Parents can find help and support for their children. Categories include **activities, art therapy, counseling, depression, parenting, peer support, self-esteem, grief** and **substance abuse**.

Camps are free of charge for all families.

Camp Kesem

http://campkesem.org

Contact Us (campkesem.org) *Contact form*

https://www.facebook.com/CampKesem

https://twitter.com/campkesem

(260) 225-3736

Information; messages will be returned ASAP.

Camp Kesem is a nationwide community, driven by passionate college student leaders, that supports **children, 6 to 16 years of age,** through and beyond their parent's cancer. Kesem is the largest national organization dedicated to supporting children affected by a parent's cancer, at no cost to families. The innovative and fun-filled programs connect children with peers who understand their unique needs.

Camp Kesem Locations

https://www.campkesem.org/find-a-camp

Camps are free.

Camp Widow

http://www.campwidow.org/

contact@soaringspirits.org *Email*

https://www.facebook.com/CampWidow

https://twitter.com/soaringspirits

Information and phone numbers for each camp available online under locations.

Camp Widow is an innovative program that provides practical tools and research-informed resources for **widowed people of any gender, race, religion, age or sexual orientation**. Any person who has experienced the death of a spouse or partner is welcomed. The organization brings together widowed people from around the world to celebrate the healing power of community. Camp Widow has in-person, virtual and pop-up camps.

Regional Social Groups

https://soaringspirits.org/programs/regional-social-groups/
Meetings are focused on assisting widowed people in rebuilding their social structure post-loss.

Camp Widow Weekend

https://campwidow.org/camperships/request/
Information on registering for weekend camps that offer hope and healing. *Travel and lodging fees apply. Financial help and support available.*

Camp-Mak-A-Dream

http://www.campdream.org/
http://www.campdream.org/about-us/contact-us/ *Contact form*
https://www.facebook.com/Camp-Mak-A-Dream-37094882711/
https://twitter.com/campdream
(406) 549-5987
Program information, Monday – Friday, 8:00 AM – 5:00 PM MT
Camp-Mak-A-Dream offers **weeklong camps** in Montana for **children, teens, young adults, women** and **families** affected by cancer, as well as programs for children who have a sibling or a parent with cancer. Campers of all ages are welcome. People up to the age of 80 have attended. Young adult retreats are for ages 18 to 35. There are four sessions specifically for women older than 21. The camp provides medically supervised cost-free Montana experiences.

Apply for a Camp

https://www.campdream.org/apply/

Information on how to apply for a camp. Participants are asked to cover the cost of travel to Montana.

Camp is free.

Cancer + Careers

www.cancerandcareers.org

website: *English and Spanish*

https://www.cancerandcareers.org/en/about-us/contact *Contact form*

https://www.facebook.com/CancerandCareers

https://twitter.com/cancerandcareer

(646) 929-8032

Information only, Monday – Friday, 9:00 AM – 5:00 PM ET

Cancer + Careers empowers and educates people with cancer to thrive in their workplace, by providing expert advice, interactive tools and educational events for **employees** with **cancer**. Includes information on insurance, résumé writing, legal and financial matters, self-employment, networking and getting back to work after cancer.

Ask a Career Coach

https://www.cancerandcareers.org/career-coach

Submit questions to experts in their field about **career change, career management, image and professionalism, workplace politics** and more.

Résumé Review

https://www.cancerandcareers.org/resume_reviews/new

Receive free, personalized feedback on your résumé from a professional career coach.

Guide Your Conversations

https://www.cancerandcareers.org/en/resource/charts-and-checklists

Questions to help you gather information and guide your conversations with your employer and health-care team.

Webinars

https://www.cancerandcareers.org/en/community/videos/bwc
A series of 60-minute webinars on balancing work and cancer. Topics include **job search; working through treatment; managing long-term stress** and **body confidence; self-confidence** in the **workplace;** and strategies for eating well on the job.

Library

https://www.cancerandcareers.org/en/community/videos
Videos on balancing work and cancer.
Services are free.

Cancer Be Glammed

http://www.cancerbeglammed.com/
http://www.cancerbeglammed.com/contact *Contact form*
https://www.facebook.com/CancerBeGlammed
https://twitter.com/CancerBeGlammed
Cancer Be Glammed helps women diagnosed with all forms of cancer address the nonmedical, appearance-related side effects of surgery and treatment. The site provides **fashionable products** and **lifestyle solutions** to help women recover with dignity, self-esteem and style.

Cancer Be Glammed: The Guide

https://cancerbeglammed.com/recover-in-style-book
A guide that prepares women, facing all forms of cancer, for the most common **appearance-related questions** and **concerns.**

Recovery Boutique

https://cancerbeglammed.com/shop-cancer-be-glammed-for-recovery-clothing-and-essentials
Clothing, accessories and lifestyle solutions to help you recover in comfort and style.

Gifts for Cancer Patients

https://cancerbeglammed.com/shop/gift-her
Gifts for the cancer patient curated by the women of the Cancer Be Glammed community.
Prices available online.

Cancer Cactus Society

https://cactuscancer.org/
https://cactuscancer.org/contact/ *Contact form*
https://www.facebook.com/CactusCancer
Cancer Cactus Society is an online organization that encourages, empowers and connects young adult cancer survivors and caregivers throughout the globe, 24/7. It provides support and resources to young adults, ages **18 to 45,** dealing with cancer as **patients, survivors** or **caregivers** in the form of wellness resources, lifestyle encouragement and a peer support community.

Young Adult Cancer (YAC) Hangout

https://cactuscancer.org/programs/young-adult-cancer-hangout/
Brings together young adult cancer survivors and caregivers each month in an informal video hangout where they can chat about anything they would like.

Awkward Auntie

https://cactuscancer.org/programs/awkward-auntie/
A question-and-answer section in which a **doctor answers questions about sex and relationships** that patients are too uncomfortable to ask their oncologist.

Programs

https://cactuscancer.org/programs/
Programs include **game night, journaling, drawing workshop, watercolor notecard workshop, book club** and **blogging**. It also has a webinar on how to turn your cancer story into comedy.

Yoga & Mindfulness Workshops

https://cactuscancer.org/programs/grief-to-gratitude-a-yoga-mindfulness-workshop/

A **six-week program** that will normalize grief and help you tune in and connect to your body, mind and soul through yoga, breathwork, meditation and other contemplative practices.

Creative Writing Group

https://cactuscancer.org/programs/unspoken-ink-creative-writing-workshop/

Unspoken Ink: Creative Writing Workshop is designed to take you on a journey through your cancer diagnosis and into your survivorship with a small group of your young adult cancer patient and survivor peers. Each **eight-week writing workshop** consists of a weekly writing night attended via online video chat in an intimate, 18-person setting. It addresses issues that transport you from initial diagnosis into the new normal and survivorship.

Guys Discussion Group

https://cactuscancer.org/programs/guys-discussion-group/
Guys-only program led by LCSW Dennis Heffern. Each month, different community members offer up a certain topic with a chance for open discussion at the end. For men of all young adult cancer experiences. *Services are free.*

Cancer Council Victoria

https://www.cancervic.org.au/
https://www.cancervic.org.au/about/contact_us *Contact*
https://www.facebook.com/cancervic
https://twitter.com/CancerVic

Cancer Council Victoria is an organization in Australia that started more than 80 years ago to reduce the deaths and improve the quality of life for people living with cancer while empowering the community by leading and integrating research through prevention, support and advocacy.

Cancer Types

https://www.cancervic.org.au/cancer-information/types-of-cancer
Information on **diagnosis, treatment** and **living** with cancer-by-cancer type.

Managing Daily Life

https://www.cancervic.org.au/living-with-cancer
Information and advice on managing life after a cancer diagnosis. Topics include **side effects, emotions, life after treatment, nutrition,** and **sexuality** and **intimacy.**

Talking to Kids About Cancer

https://www.cancervic.org.au/cancer-information/children-teens-and-young-adults/talking-to-kids-about-cancer/overview.html
A comprehensive booklet with advice on **telling children** and **family about cancer.**
Free

Cancer Fighters Thrive

http://www.cancerfightersthrive.com
info@cfthrive.com *Email*
Cancer Fighters Thrive is an online magazine to inform, inspire and empower cancer patients, their friends and families with **healthy recipes, helpful tips** and **information on nutrition, health and wellness.**

Cancer Support Organizations

https://www.cancerfighters.com/s/cancer-support-organizations
Information on **support organizations.**
Free

Cancer Financial Assistance Coalition

https://www.cancerfac.org/

Cancer Financial Assistance Coalition is an alliance of financial assistance organizations joining forces to help cancer patients manage their financial challenges. Find assistance from **organizations providing financial** or **practical help.** Categories include co-pays, financial assistance, food, genetic testing, home care, meal delivery, wigs and prosthesis. You can search by diagnosis, ZIP code, type of assistance and specific population.

Free

Cancer Hope Network

http://www.cancerhopenetwork.org/

info@cancerhopenetwork.org *Email*

https://www.facebook.com/CancerHopeNet/

https://twitter.com/CancerHopeNet

(877) 467-3638 (877-HOPENET)

Helpline, Monday – Friday, 9:00 AM – 5:30 PM ET. Support available in 15 languages.

Cancer Hope Network offers free **one-on-one phone support** to **adult cancer patients** and their **loved ones, 18 years** and **older,** at any stage of cancer. It provides trained individuals who have recovered from cancer, or cared for someone who has recovered from cancer, and matches them with cancer patients currently undergoing a similar experience.

Patient Support

https://www.cancerhopenetwork.org/get-support/support/

Information for a cancer patient to request support from a peer.

Caregiver Support

https://www.cancerhopenetwork.org/get-support/support/caregiver-support.html

Information for a caregiver to request support from a peer.

Support After Treatment
https://www.cancerhopenetwork.org/get-support/support/survivor-support.html
Connect with a volunteer after treatment.
Services are free.

Cancer Legal Resource Center

https://thedrlc.org/cancer/
website: *English and Spanish*
CLRC@drlcenter.org *Email*
https://www.facebook.com/CancerLegalResourceCenter/
https://twitter.com/cancerlegalhelp
(866) 843-2572
Information, Monday – Friday, 9:00 AM – 5:00 PM PT. English and Spanish
Cancer Legal Resource Center is a program of the Disability Rights Legal Center, a nonprofit public interest advocacy organization that champions the civil rights of people with disabilities as well as those affected by cancer. CLRC's national telephone assistance line, outreach programs and community activities **educate** and **support cancer patients, their families,** health-care professionals and advocates on matters such as **maintaining employment through treatment, accessing health care** and **government benefits, taking medical leave** and **estate planning.**

Request for Assistance
https://thedrlc.org/cancer/clrc-intake-form/ Contact form, English and Spanish

Webinars
https://thedrlc.org/cancer/publications-webinars/
Webinars and recorded presentations for cancer patients and their families, survivors, caregivers, health-care professionals and others coping with cancer. People can participate by phone or online.
Service is free.

Cancer Support Community

https://www.cancersupportcommunity.org

help@cancersupportcommunity.org *Email*

https://www.facebook.com/CancerSupportCommunity

https://twitter.com/CancerSupportHQ

(888) 793-9355

Helpline, answered by licensed oncology mental-health care providers; English and Spanish

Monday – Friday, 9:00 AM – 9:00 PM ET; Saturday – Sunday, 9:00 AM – 5:00 PM ET

Live web chat, Monday – Friday, 9:00 AM – 9:00 PM ET; Saturday – Sunday, 9:00 AM – 5:00 PM ET

Cancer Support Community organization offer social and emotional support for people affected by cancer. It offers **support groups, educational sessions, health** and **wellness programs** as well as hope and a community. The programs are free of charge to anyone affected by cancer, including **patients, caregivers, loved ones** and **children**.

Cancer Support Community Locations

https://www.cancersupportcommunity.org/find-location-near-you

The Cancer Support Community has 175 locations worldwide, including 52 licenses affiliates and health-care partnerships.

MyLifeLine

https://www.cancersupportcommunity.org/mylifeline

Connect to others through a **private community website**. Create a personal webpage with a support calendar that allows for updates, guest messages, financial support, and inspirational quotes and photos.

Radio Shows

https://www.cancersupportcommunity.org/RadioShow

Medical experts, opinion leaders, authors, caregivers and survivors share information and advice on how to live a better life with cancer.

Services are free.

Cancer.Net—American Society of Clinical Oncology

https://www.cancer.net

website: *English and Spanish*

contactus@cancer.net *Email*

https://www.facebook.com/CancerDotNet

https://twitter.com/cancerdotnet

(888) 651-3038

Information, Monday – Friday, 9:00 AM – 5:00 PM ET. Other times, leave a message; your call will be returned within 24 hours.

Cancer.Net provides timely, comprehensive, **oncologist-approved information** and resources from the American Society of Clinical Oncology with support from the Conquer Cancer Foundation. With almost 45,000 members who are leaders in advancing cancer care, the American Society of Clinical Oncology is the voice of the world's cancer physicians.

Information Guides—Breast Cancer

https://www.cancer.net/cancer-types.

Guides with comprehensive, oncologist-approved information and illustrations.

Information Guides—Metastatic Breast Cancer

https://www.cancer.net/cancer-types/breast-cancer-metastatic

Guides with comprehensive, oncologist-approved information and illustrations.

Navigating Cancer

https://www.cancer.net/navigating-cancer-care

Learn about cancer, its causes and its treatment. Topics include **financial considerations; dating, sex** and **reproduction; coping** with cancer; **telling children**; and resources for teens, young adults and older adults.

Navigating Cancer Videos

https://www.cancer.net/navigating-cancer-care/videos
Information covering various aspects of cancer. Topics include cancer basics; after treatment and **survivorship**; treatment, tests, and procedures; and **quality of life**.

Choose an Oncologist

https://www.cancer.net/navigating-cancer-care/cancer-basics/cancer-care-team/choosing-doctor-your-cancer-care
Information on how to find and choose a cancer doctor.

Oncologist Database

https://www.cancer.net/find-cancer-doctor
Database includes the names of **physicians** and other **health professionals** searchable by ZIP code.

COVID and Cancer

https://www.cancer.net/blog/2021-02/common-questions-about-covid-19-and-cancer-answers-patients-and-survivors
Resources and commonly asked questions about COVID and cancer.

Cancer Care and Costs

https://www.cancer.net/navigating-cancer-care/financial-considerations
Questions to ask your medical team and how to calculate your **out-of-pocket costs**.

PRE-ACT (Preparatory Education About Clinical Trials)

https://www.cancer.net/research-and-advocacy/clinical-trials/welcome-pre-act
Educational program that provides general information on **clinical trials**.

Clinical Trial Video Library

https://www.cancer.net/research-and-advocacy/clinical-trials
Forty-second to two-minute recordings with information.
Free

Men With Breast Cancer

https://www.cancer.net/cancer-types/breast-cancer-men
Information specific to men with breast cancer.

Advanced Cancer Care Planning Guide

https://www.cancer.net/sites/cancer.net/files/advanced_cancer_care_
planning.pdf
Comprehensive decision-making guide to help patients and families
facing serious illness. Topics include options for **advanced cancer,** making
decisions about your care and finding support near the **end of life.**
Free

Cancer*Care*

https://www.cancercare.org/
website: *English and Spanish*
info@cancercare.org *Email*
https://www.facebook.com/cancercare
https://twitter.com/cancercare
(800) 813-4673
*Helpline, Monday – Thursday, 10:00 AM – 6:00 PM; Friday 10:00 AM –
5:00 PM ET. This number is for all services except chemotherapy co-pay assistance.
English and Spanish*
(877) 880-TNBC / (877-880-8622)
*Triple Negative Breast Cancer Helpline, Monday – Thursday, 10:00 AM –
6:00 PM; Friday, 10:00 AM – 5:00 PM ET. English and Spanish*
(800) 813-4673
*Pet Assistance & Wellness Program (PAW) Hopeline, Monday – Thursday,
10:00 AM – 6:00 PM; Friday, 10:00 AM – 5:00 PM ET*
(866) 552-6729
*CancerCare Co-pay Assistance Foundation Line, Monday – Thursday,
9:00 AM – 7:00 PM; Friday, 9:00 AM – 5:00 PM ET. This number is for
help with chemotherapy assistance only. English and Spanish*

CancerCare is a national organization that provides professional **support** services with information to help people manage the **emotional, practical** and **financial challenges** of cancer. Cancer*Care* oncology social workers are licensed professionals who offer individual counseling, locate services that help with practical needs (home care, transportation), and guide people through the process of applying for Social Security disability or other forms of assistance.

COVID and Cancer
https://www.cancercare.org/coronavirus
Up-to-date coronavirus guidelines and a list of **informational** and **financial resources**.

Educational Workshops
https://www.cancercare.org/connect_workshops
Phone, online or as podcasts. **One-hour workshops** with leading experts in oncology. Registration required. Extensive library of podcasts include **coping** with cancer; **children; clinical trials; doctor-patient communication; end-of-life** care; **immunotherapy; pain; diagnostic technologies; nutrition**.

PAW Program
https://www.cancercare.org/paw
Assistance with **cats** and **dogs** for people living with cancer in active treatment and their loved ones during the emotional, physical and financial challenges of cancer treatment.

Young Adult Survivorship: Fertility, Sexuality and Intimacy
https://www.cancercare.org/connect_workshops/359-young_adult_survivorship_fertility_sexuality_intimacy_2013-06-28
Topics covered include but are not limited to **fertility, sexuality** and **intimacy, desire,** tips on **vaginal dryness** and **premature menopause; sexual self-esteem;** and **pregnancy**.

Employment and Career Workshops

https://www.cancercare.org/tagged/workplace_issues
Available over the telephone, online or on podcasts. Understand your **legal rights** and **legal protections; workplace transitions; living** and **working with cancer.**

Co-pay Assistance

http://portal.cancercarecopay.org/Funds-Available/Diagnoses
Assistance for **pharmaceutical products** to insured individuals who are covered by private insurance, employer-sponsored health plan or have Medicare Part D or Medicare Advantage. Check the portal for **funds currently available** for each type of type of cancer. Check back regularly for the co-pay funding status if availability for the specific fund is currently closed.

Limited Financial Assistance

http://portal.cancercarecopay.org/Enroll-Now
Financial assistance for cancer-related costs such as **co-pays** for **chemotherapy** and **cancer medications**. Downloadable forms to enroll or reenroll in a program.

Additional Resources for Financial Assistance

https://www.cancercare.org/copayfoundation
The professional oncology social workers can help you find other resources.

Directory for Financial and Practical Help

https://www.cancercare.org/helpinghand
Directory of assistance from organizations providing financial and practical help.
Services are free.

Care Calendar

https://www.carecalendar.org
admin@carecalendar.org *Email*

Care Calendar is a **personalized online care calendar** that allows you to post requests for members of your community to find ways to help and support you. Update family and friends on your health or other topics and post photos. The site provides a setup worksheet to help you gather all the information you will need prior to developing your calendar.
Free

CaringBridge

https://www.caringbridge.org/

https://www.facebook.com/CaringBridge/

CaringBridge offers **personal websites** to help people communicate with and support loved ones during a critical illness, treatment or recovery. The website allows you to share news and updates with your community, communicate in private, post your needs, coordinate tasks, and activate your community for help and support, receive emotional support and strength, send email and text updates and post a personal fundraiser.
Free

Centers for Disease Control and Prevention

https://www.cdc.gov/

website: *17 languages*

https://wwwn.cdc.gov/dcs/ContactUs/Form *Contact form*

(800) 232-4636

Information, Monday – Friday, 8:00 AM – 8:00 PM ET. English and Spanish

The **Centers for Disease Control and Prevention** is a federal agency that conducts and supports health promotion, prevention and preparedness activities in the United States, with the goal of improving overall public health.

National Breast and Cervical Cancer Early Detection Program

https://www.cdc.gov/cancer/nbccedp/

Provides breast and cervical **cancer screenings** and **diagnostic services** to **low-income, uninsured** and **underinsured** women across the United States.

Find a Screening Program Near You
https://www.cdc.gov/cancer/nbccedp/screenings.htm
Interactive map to locate **free** and **low-cost** breast and cervical cancer **screenings** by state, tribe or territory.

COVID
https://www.cdc.gov/coronavirus/2019-ncov/index.html
Information and what you need to know about COVID.
Free

CenterWatch

https://www.centerwatch.com/
CenterWatch provides patients and their advocates information on **clinical trials, specific drugs** and other essential **health** and **educational resources**. CenterWatch has a database searchable by medical condition and geographic location; medical specialty and geographic location; FDA drug information; and new drugs in research.

Find a Trial
https://www.centerwatch.com/clinical-trials/pns/

COVID and Participation in Clinical Trials
https://www.wcgclinical.com/covid-19/covid-19-patient-resources/
Information and patient concerns and insights on clinical trials in the time of COVID.
Free

Chemocare.com

www.chemocare.com
website: *English and Spanish*
Chemocare.com is a comprehensive resource for cancer patients and their caregivers that provides chemotherapy drug and **side effect information,**

cancer wellness information, and links to additional reliable resources and organizations.

Drug Information

https://chemocare.com/chemotherapy/drug-info/default.aspx
Information on chemotherapy drugs and drugs most often used during chemotherapy. What they are used for, how they are given and possible side effects.

Managing Side Effects of Chemotherapy

https://chemocare.com/chemotherapy/side-effects/default.aspx
A list of chemotherapy side effects categories, symptoms within each category and links to additional side effects information.

Complementary Medicine

https://www.chemocare.com/complementary-medicine.aspx#cognitive
Information on complementary medicine in five categories: sensory, cognitive, expressive, physical and medical systems.

4th Angel Mentoring Program—Support

https://4thangel.ccf.org/
Patients and caregivers are matched with trained volunteer mentors with similar age and cancer experiences. The program is a national, free service that emphasizes one-on-one contact to best empower caregivers and patients with knowledge, awareness, hope and a helping hand.
Free

The Children's Treehouse Foundation

https://childrenstreehousefdn.org/
info@childrenstreehousefdn.org *Email*
https://childrenstreehousefdn.org/contact-us *Contact form*
https://www.facebook.com/The-Childrens-Treehouse-Foundation
-314365928577957/

(303) 322-1202
Information, Monday – Friday, 10:00 AM – 5:00 PM MT
The **Children's Treehouse Foundation** is an organization providing group-based, manualized psychosocial intervention developed specifically to support the **emotional needs of children** with a parent or caregiver who has cancer. Its CLIMB program—Children's Lives Include Moments of Bravery—is a six-week program designed specifically to support the emotional needs of children, 6 to 18 years of age, with a parent or caregiver who has cancer. CLIMB also helps parents understand what to expect from their children and improves communication involving their cancer diagnosis. CLIMB programs are available in cancer centers around the world.

Find a CLIMB Program
https://childrenstreehousefdn.org/climb-locations-worldwide
Map of CLIMB programs around the world.

Online CLIMB programs
https://childrenstreehousefdn.org/register-for-a-climb-group
Information on the program and how to register.
CLIMB services are free.

Chronic Sex
http://www.chronicsex.org/
https://www.facebook.com/ChronicallySexy/
https://twitter.com/chronicsexchat
Chronic Sex opens up frank discussions about how quality of life and **sex** are **affected** by **chronic illnesses** and **disabilities**. The information, discussions and articles focus on self-love, self-care, relationships, sexuality and sex itself. Under resources, find information and articles on dating, fertility, talking to doctors, abuse and violence, and illness and disabilities.

Podcast
https://www.chronicsex.org/podcast/
The podcast talks about how **self-love, relationships, sex** and **sexuality** are all affected by **chronic illness** and **disability**. It also touches on intersectionality, social justice, empathy, current events and more. Given the range of subject matter, this podcast is not suitable for those under the age of 18.

Resource Sex Toys
https://www.chronicsex.org/sex-toys/
Prices available online.

Cleaning for a Reason

http://cleaningforareason.org/
info@cleaningforareason.org *E-mail*
https://www.facebook.com/cleaningforareason
https://twitter.com/clean4areason
Cleaning for a Reason is a nonprofit organization that gives the gift of **free house cleaning** to women, over 19, actively undergoing treatment for any type of cancer. The service provides women with one general house cleaning per month for two consecutive months. The service is available in the United States and Canada.

Apply for Cleaning Service
https://cleaningforareason.org/patients/
Information on how to apply and to check the status of an application.

Find a Provider
https://cleaningforareason.org/service-provider/
Service is free.

Cleveland Clinic

https://my.clevelandclinic.org/

myconsult@ccf.org *Email*
https://www.facebook.com/ClevelandClinic
https://twitter.com/clevelandclinic
(216) 444-3223 / (800) 223-2273, ext. 43223
Information, Monday – Friday, 8:00 AM – 5:00 PM ET
Cleveland Clinic's MyConsult Online Medical Second Opinion program connects you to top Cleveland Clinic specialists for a **second opinion** without the time and expense of travel. The specialists review the patient's medical history, records, test results and images, and provide a comprehensive, personalized report and answers to individual questions.

Virtual Second Opinions
https://www.eclevelandclinic.org/myConsultHome
Information on how to get an online second opinion from a doctor at the Cleveland Clinic.

Online Second Opinions
https://myconsult2020.com/landing.htm
Fees apply. Does not accept insurance.

ClinicalTrials.gov
https://clinicaltrials.gov/
ClinicalTrials.gov is a **database** of privately and publicly funded **clinical trial studies** conducted around the world. ClinicalTrials.gov is part of the National Institutes of Health, U.S. National Library of Medicine.

Clinical Trail Locator
https://clinicaltrials.gov/
Find studies taking place by condition and country. Clinical study locations and specific contact information are listed to assist with enrollment. Each study record includes a summary of the study protocol, including the purpose, recruitment status and eligibility criteria.

Read a Study
https://clinicaltrials.gov/ct2/help/how-read-study

Medical Encyclopedia
https://medlineplus.gov/
Information on **drugs, supplements, genetics** and **medical tests**. Articles and images for diseases, symptoms, tests and treatments through MedlinePlus.
Service is free.

CONQUER: The Patient Voice

https://conquer-magazine.com/
https://www.facebook.com/conquermag/
https://twitter.com/conquermagazine
CONQUER: The Patient Voice is an **online magazine** that addresses issues facing cancer patients and survivors, their family members and caregivers for all types of cancer.

COVID and Cancer
https://conquer-magazine.com/web-exclusives/1498-covid-19-one-year-later-what-patients-with-cancer-need-to-know

Wellness and Nutrition
https://conquer-magazine.com/wellness-corner
Healthy recipes and information on nutrition, stress management, exercise and cancer.

Financial Support
https://conquer-magazine.com/financial-support
Articles, videos and directories with information on **financial support** available for cancer patients.

Cancer Center Locator

https://conquer-magazine.com/interactive-media/cancer-center-locator

Interactive map of cancer centers by state.

Free

Cook for Your Life

http://www.cookforyourlife.org/

website: *English and Spanish*

info@cfyl.org *Email*

https://www.facebook.com/CookForYourLife/

https://twitter.com/cookforyourlife

Cook for Your Life teaches **healthy cooking** for people touched by cancer. It provides nutritious recipes to **promote healthy survivorship** for people in **different stages of treatment**. Recipes can be searched by specific needs. Popular categories include healthy survivorship, in treatment, neutropenic diet, gluten-free, fatigue, low-calorie, bland diet, nausea, high-protein, high-fiber, low-fiber, easy-to-swallow and high-calorie. The blog has articles on how to cope with tastes changing during treatment as well as benefits of certain spices, probiotics during cancer, sugar alternatives and more.

Videos

https://www.cookforyourlife.org/videos/

Four- to six-minute videos with step-by-step instructions.

Free

Corporate Angel Network

www.corpangelnetwork.org

info@corpangelnetwork.org *Email*

https://www.corpangelnetwork.org/contact-us *Contact form*

https://www.facebook.com/corporateangelnetwork/

https://twitter.com/CorpAngelNet

(914) 328-1313

Information, Monday – Thursday, 9:00 AM – 5:00 PM; Friday 9:00 AM – 4:00 PM ET

Corporate Angel Network arranges **free travel** on **private planes** for **cancer patients**, bone marrow donors and recipients, and stem cell donors and recipients. CAN pairs empty seats on both private and corporate planes with qualified patients who need the rides—at no cost.

Patient Flights
https://www.corpangelnetwork.org/patient-flight-process
Information on how the process works, from registration to flight.

Request a Flight
https://www.corpangelnetwork.org/flight-request
Patient inquiry form.
Cancer patients fly free.

Creative Funeral Ideas
www.creative-funeral-ideas.com/
Creative Funeral Ideas offers access to tools to create a **personalized** and **individualized service** to reflect and highlight the personality and life of the deceased. The website provides information, resources and guidance for planning a memorial service.

Plan a Memorial
https://www.creative-funeral-ideas.com/planning-a-memorial-service.html
Step-by-step guide for planning a memorial service.
Information is free. Fees apply for e-books, custom poems, eulogies, etc.

CURE, Cancer Updates, Research & Education—Magazine
http://www.curetoday.com/
https://www.facebook.com/curemagazine
https://twitter.com/cure_magazine

CURE, Cancer Updates, Research & Education is an online magazine that provides **information, articles** and **educational videos** on cancer, treatment and clinical trials and includes stories by those diagnosed with cancer.

Breast Cancer

https://www.curetoday.com/tumor/breast

Information and articles on living with and managing a **breast cancer diagnosis.**

Psychosocial News

https://www.curetoday.com/news/psychosocial

Information and articles on the **social factors** and Individual thoughts and **behavior around cancer.**

Sexual Health

https://www.curetoday.com/news/sexual-health

Information and articles on **sexual health** and **quality of life.**

Managing Side Effects

https://www.curetoday.com/news/side-effect

Information and articles on managing the **physical, mental** and **emotional** side effects of cancer.

Magazine and newsletter are free.

CureDiva

https://www.curediva.com/

https://www.curediva.com/contacts/ *Contact form*

https://www.facebook.com/CureDiva/

(877) 596-9681

Information, Monday – Friday, 9:00 AM – 6:00 PM. Messages will be returned ASAP.

CureDiva is an **online store** that offers **stylish apparel, accessories, wigs, hair-loss solutions, compression** and **lymphedema products,**

and **personal-care** items for women coping with breast cancer and its aftereffects, including the side effects that treatments cause.

Prices available online.

D

Dana-Farber Cancer Institute

http://www.dana-farber.org

website: *More than 100 languages*

https://www.facebook.com/danafarbercancerinstitute

https://twitter.com/danafarber

(617) 632-3000

General information, English

(617) 632-3673

General information, Spanish

(617) 632-6366

General information, all other languages

(800) 941-9309

Patients located in the United States, the Grand Rounds care team initiates the online second opinion process by phone, Monday – Friday, 9:00 AM – 9:00 PM ET.

(775) 440-2559

Patients located outside the United States, the Grand Rounds care team initiates the online second opinion process by phone, Monday – Friday, 9:00 AM – 9:00 PM ET.

Dana-Farber Cancer Institute is a comprehensive cancer treatment and research center in Boston, Massachusetts. It is a principal teaching affiliate of Harvard Medical School and a federally designated Center for AIDS Research. The institute offers adult **cancer patients** from around the country and around the world a **remote second opinion** through its **Second Opinion Program**. The program is coordinated through Grand Rounds, a digital health-care company that connects patients with local and remote specialty care.

Remote Second Opinion
https://www.grandrounds.com/dana-farber
Information on how to get a **written online second opinion**. The website offers a sample consultation to show you what to expect in a report. Check with your medical insurance for coverage. Consult the website for additional information and details.
Fees apply.

Death Café
http://deathcafe.com/
website: *More than 100 languages*
http://deathcafe.com/contact/ *Contact form*
https://www.facebook.com/deathcafe
https://twitter.com/DeathCafe
Death Café is a group-directed **discussion of death** with no agenda, objectives or themes. It is a discussion group rather than a grief support or counseling session. Individuals, often strangers, come together in restaurants, coffee shops, bookstores and living rooms to talk about death and living well over tea and cake.

Search for a Death Café
https://deathcafe.com/deathcafes/
Information on Death Cafés taking place searchable by ZIP code or area code.

Worldwide Map
https://deathcafe.com/map/
Map of Death Café locations around the world.
Free

DoYou
https://www.doyou.com/
https://www.facebook.com/doyouyoga

DoYou is an **online yoga** and **fitness coach**. It offers **yoga, Pilates, meditation, fitness and detox programs.**

Free and fee-based

Dr. Susan Love Research Foundation

https://www.drsusanloveresearch.org/
website: *English and Spanish*
info@DrSusanLoveResearch.org *Email*
https://drsusanloveresearch.org/contact/ *Contact form*
https://www.facebook.com/DrSusanLoveFoundation
https://twitter.com/drloveresearch
(310) 828-0060
Information; messages left will be returned ASAP.

The **Dr. Susan Love Research Foundation** has a comprehensive website with information on breast **cancer basics, newly diagnosed, screening** and **testing, living with breast cancer, metastatic stage IV breast cancer, menopause** and women's health, and **treatment options.** Dr. Susan Love is a surgeon, a prominent advocate of preventive breast cancer research and an author and is regarded as one of the most respected women's health specialists in the United States. She helped establish the National Breast Cancer Coalition.

Breast Cancer Explained

https://drsusanloveresearch.org/breast-cancer-explained/
Information to educate and inform patients and their families and friends.

ImPatient Science Video Series

https://www.drsusanloveresearch.org/impatient-science
Two- to five-minute videos on the science of breast cancer. Topics include **metastatic breast cancer, breast cancer subtypes, understanding immunology, clinical research** and **collateral damage.** English and Spanish

Free

Dr. Susan Love Research Foundation's Love Research Army
https://www.armyofwomen.org/studies
An initiative that connects women and men of all ages, ethnicities and locations to researchers committed to encouraging and facilitating breast cancer research in all people. The goal is to forge partnerships between their members and the scientific community and teach members about the clinical research process and connect them with innovative research studies. You can sign up to receive periodic emails with information about breast cancer research studies that are recruiting volunteers. It lists **clinical studies** and projects that are currently open and enrolling volunteers.

E

EmergingMed Clinical Trial Navigation Service
https://app.emergingmed.com
https://app.emergingmed.com/emed/contactus *Contact form*
(877) 601-8601
Information, Monday – Friday, 8:00 AM – 6:00 PM ET. English and Spanish
EmergingMed Clinical Trial Navigation Service helps you **find clinical trials** that match your diagnosis and treatment history and update you on when new trials and sites open that match your profile. A drop-down menu allows you to view trials taking place. The clinical trial database includes all treatments trials from ClinicalTrials.gov along with updates reported directly by trial sponsors and sites.
Free

Epic Experience
http://www.epicexperience.org/
Info@epicexperience.org *Email*
https://www.facebook.com/EpicExperience/
https://twitter.com/epicxperience

(855) 650-9907
Program information, Monday – Friday, 9:00 AM – 5:00 PM MT; other times leave a message, and your call will be returned.
Epic Experience offers free camp adventures in Colorado for **adults, 18 years and older,** who have been **affected by cancer.** Camp adventures are for those who were diagnosed at any time in their life. Epic Experience offers six to eight **weeklong outdoor experiences** each year, which feature outdoor activities such as white-water adventures in the summer and snowshoeing and cross-country skiing in the winter. Camp is for **cancer patients and survivors** only; it does not include caregivers.

Register for an Epic Experience
https://www.epicexperience.org/apply/
Participants are asked to cover the cost of travel. Some financial assistance for travel may be available; call for details.
Camp is free.

Everplans
https://www.everplans.com
Everplans is an **online digital record-keeping service** for your important documents.

Information and legal documents
https://www.everplans.com/guides/state-by-state-guides
State-by-state health, legal and **end-of-life paperwork.**

Advanced Directives
https://www.everplans.com/articles/all-you-need-to-know-about-advance-directives
Information and explanation on the components of an **advanced directive.**

Advanced Directive Forms

https://www.everplans.com/articles/state-by-state-advance-directive-forms
Advanced directive **forms state-by-state.**

Checklists

https://www.everplans.com/checklists
Checklists to plan and stay organized in all areas of your life and death. *Downloadable forms are free. Fees apply for digital archiving services.*

F

First Descents

https://firstdescents.org/
Programs@firstdescents.org *Email, questions about the programs*
info@firstdescents.org *Email, general inquiries*
https://www.facebook.com/FirstDescents
https://twitter.com/FirstDescents
(303) 945-2490
Program information, Monday – Friday, 8:00 AM – 5:00 PM MT
First Descents provides life-changing **outdoor adventures** for **young adults, 18 to 39, affected by cancer** and other serious health conditions; also for frontline health-care workers. The one-week camp each year is for **caregivers,** and a two-week camp is for those **40 to 49** who have been **affected by cancer.**

Frequently Asked Questions

https://firstdescents.org/first-time-participant-faq/
Information on what participants were concerned about prior to their program and what they learned.

Find a Program

https://firstdescents.org/programs/

Programs include **multiday local weekend outdoor experiences** and **weeklong adventures** for **cancer survivors**.

All food, lodging, instruction, gear and activities throughout the week are included. Participants are asked to cover the cost of travel. Travel scholarships are available if costs are prohibitive.

FORCE: Facing Our Risk of Cancer Empowered

http://www.facingourrisk.org

website: *English and Spanish*

info@facingourrisk.org *Email*

https://www.facebook.com/facingourrisk

https://twitter.com/FacingOurRisk

(866) 288-7475

Helpline, general questions about genetics. Leave a message and your call will be returned within 24 to 48 hours. English and Spanish

FORCE: Facing Our Risk of Cancer Empowered provides information, resources and support for families and individuals affected by **hereditary breast**, **ovarian** and **related cancers**.

Support Programs

https://www.facingourrisk.org/support/local-groups

FORCE offers a **peer navigation program** that connects cancer survivors, people at high risk and their caregivers to support and resources personalized for their situation.

InformedDNA

https://informeddna.com/

Information and education on genetics and genetic testing. For general questions about genetics, call the phone number above.

Services are free.

Free Meditation Info

http://www.freemeditationinfo.com/

https://www.facebook.com/FreeMeditationInformation

Free Meditation Info shares information on the benefits of **mantras** and **meditation**. It provides **easy-to-understand techniques** and methods with instructions, both basic and detailed. The information provided is not specific to one particular meditation organization, philosophy or religion.

World Meditation Directory

http://www.freemeditationinfo.com/places-to-meditate/worldwide-meditation-directory.html

Fuck Cancer

https://www.letsfcancer.com/

info@letsfcancer.com *Email*

https://www.letsfcancer.com/contact-us/ *Contact form*

https://www.facebook.com/letsfcancer

https://twitter.com/letsfcancer

Fuck Cancer is dedicated to **cancer prevention** and **early detection**. It runs digital and on-the-ground programs and events that seek to change the way people think and talk about cancer, ultimately improving health outcomes.

Careline

https://www.letsfcancer.com/careline/

Provides **emotional support** and **guidance** to those affected by cancer administered through the Patient Advocate Foundation.

Prevention

https://www.letsfcancer.com/resources/prevention/

Information guides on **food, vaccinations, exercise** and **lifestyle** to promote health and wellness.

Early Detection

https://www.letsfcancer.com/resources/early-detection/

Information guides with **cancer facts**, clinical trials and guides to self-tests.

Life With Cancer

https://www.letsfcancer.com/resources/life-with-cancer/

Information guides with advice and tips on **self-care**, and communicating with **family**, **friends** and **co-workers**.

Resources

https://www.letsfcancer.com/resource/helpful-links/

Resources for information for different types of cancer, emotional support, financial assistance and more.

Free

G

Good Wishes

http://www.goodwishesscarves.org/

Info@goodwishesscarves.org *Email*

(888) 778-5998

Information; leave a message and your call will be returned ASAP.

Good Wishes provides a headscarf to anyone experiencing the **thinning or loss of hair** as a result of illness or treatment. The It's a Wrap or the Good Wishes scarf comes in a variety of fabric colors and prints to choose from.

Request a Wrap

http://www.goodwishesscarves.org/request-a-wrap/

Information on how to request a wrap. If you do not have internet access you can call the number above, and the staff will walk you through the options of patterns and colors.

Scarf is free.

Greatest

https://greatist.com/
https://www.facebook.com/greatist
https://twitter.com/greatist
Greatest has information and tips to **living healthfully**.

Food and Exercise

https://greatist.com/eat
Information and articles on food and how to live a healthy life.

Fitness and Stress Reduction

https://greatist.com/move
Information and articles on exercise, the benefits of specific workout routines and how to work out smarter not harder.

Beauty and Relaxation

https://greatist.com/beauty
Articles and tips on food, products and exercises that help promote beauty and relaxation.

Home and Hearth

https://greatist.com/home
Information, articles, tips and ideas to promote a healthy home environment.
Free

Grief Healing

http://www.griefhealingblog.com/
https://www.facebook.com/GriefHealing
https://twitter.com/GriefHealing
Grief Healing is blog with information, resources and reading material on **grief, healing, caregiving** and transition for anyone coping with loss.

Marty Tousley, a nationally certified grief counselor, facilitates and monitores the website.

Children, Teens & Grief
https://www.griefhealingblog.com/p/blog-page.html
Articles with information about grief in children and adolescents.

Coping With Special Days and Holidays
https://www.griefhealingblog.com/p/h.html
Articles, links and resources grouped according to season.

Pet Loss
https://www.griefhealingblog.com/p/pet-loss-articles.html
Articles and links with information on **coping** with the **grief** that accompanies the loss of an animal.

Discussion Groups
https://www.griefhealingblog.com/p/experience-teaches-us-that-when-facing.html
Free

H

Heal in Comfort
https://www.healincomfort.com/
healincomfort@ymail.com *Email*
https://www.facebook.com/healincomfort
https://twitter.com/healincomfort
Heal in Comfort offers **mastectomy recovery products** for **women** and **men after breast cancer surgery,** including mastectomy shirts with drain pockets, drain-management products, mastectomy recovery pillows, mastectomy recovery and reconstruction bras, post-surgery robes and camisoles.
Prices available online.

HealGrief.org—Actively Moving Forward

http://healgrief.org/actively-moving-forward/
https://healgrief.org/about-us/contact-us/ *Contact form*
https://healgrief.org/actively-moving-forward/general-inquiry/ *General inquiry contact form*
https://www.facebook.com/ActivelyMovingForward/
https://twitter.com/GoAMF

HealGrief.org—Actively Moving Forward is a national network that responds to the needs of grieving young adults. The website has **information, advice** and **support** for people at the particularly vulnerable ages of **18** to **30**.

College Student Grief

https://healgrief.org/actively-moving-forward/college-student-grief/

Young Adult Grief

https://healgrief.org/actively-moving-forward/young-adult-grief/
A network of **young adults,** 18 to 30, supporting young adults who are dealing with a death or their personal diagnosis of a terminal illness. *Services are free.*

Heart2Soul

http://heart2soul.com/
https://www.facebook.com/heart2soul
https://twitter.com/karenzinn

Heart2Soul provides information, tips and advice when **planning a funeral, memorial** or **end-of-life celebration**.

Before You Begin

http://heart2soul.com/funeral-plans
Decisions that need to be made **before planning a funeral**.

Funeral, Memorial and Celebrating a Life
http://heart2soul.com/funeral-plan
Resources and information on **planning a memorial.**

Funeral
http://heart2soul.com/funeral-arrangement
Advice and guidance on how to lay out your plans and make your desires known before you are on your deathbed.

Explaining Death to Children
http://heart2soul.com/explaining-death-to-children
Information on **how to speak to children about death,** what to say and what not to say.
Free

Help With Hope
https://helpwithhope.org/
info@helpwithhope.org *Email*
https://www.facebook.com/hotforhopeinc/
https://twitter.com/hotforhope
(310) 596-6168
Information; messages will be returned ASAP.
Help With Hope, previously Hot for Hope, is a website that offers support for **children,** 8 to 17, whose **parent** has been **affected by cancer.** Help With Hope moderates support groups with Hope director and registered nurse Jenny Yessaian.

Meditation Support
https://helpwithhope.org/support-group/
Focused on creating a personal practice of mindfulness meditation. Online groups for **young adults with cancer** and survivors, and **children of adults with cancer** and survivors.

Care Packages
https://helpwithhope.org/care-packages/
Bereavement care packages for **children** 4 to 17 and a care support package for parents.
Services and care packages are free.

HER2Support.org

http://her2support.org/
HER2Support is an **online community** of **newly diagnosed** and **long-term survivors**, caregivers, mothers, daughters, sons and husbands of breast cancer survivors who are **HER2 positive**. Newly diagnosed patients and long-term survivors share their experiences and knowledge.

Guide to HER2
https://her2support.org/her2-breast-cancer/her2-gene/guide-to-her2
Information, facts and glossary for HER2.

Chemotherapy Drugs
https://her2support.org/her2-breast-cancer/chemo-drugs
Information pertaining to chemotherapy drugs that are in use.
Free

High Top Coaching

www.hightopcoaching.com
john@hightopcoaching.com *Email*
https://www.facebook.com/hightopcoaching7/?ref=aymt_homepage_panel
(910) 200-7292
Information and appointments
High Top Coaching was founded by **leadership** and **consulting coach** John Alexander. John retired from a successful business career to dedicate his life to supporting individuals and corporations in achieving their goals. He is an avid student of life and studied human behavioral science at

Fordham University and the University of Bridgeport and completed the CTI Coaches Training program.

Contact for prices on coaching.

Hill-Burton Program—Health Resources and Services Administration (HRSA)

https://www.hrsa.gov
website: *14 languages*
https://www.facebook.com/HRSAgov/
https://twitter.com/HRSAgov
(877) 464-4772
Information, Monday – Friday, 7:00 AM to 8:00 PM ET (except federal holidays)
Hill-Burton Program provides free or low-cost medical care in select U.S. hospitals. The program is run by the Health Resources and Services Administration, an agency of the U.S. Department of Health and Human Services, the primary federal agency for improving health care to people who are geographically isolated and economically or medically vulnerable.

Hill-Burton Program

https://www.hrsa.gov/get-health-care/affordable/hill-burton/index.html
Information and guidelines for the Hill-Burton Program for **free** and **reduced-cost health care**.

Find a Hill-Burton Facility

https://findahealthcenter.hrsa.gov/

Frequently Asked Questions

https://www.hrsa.gov/get-health-care/affordable/hill-burton/FAQ/get-care-faq.html
Information and FAQs about the Hill-Burton program.

His Breast Cancer Awareness

https://www.hisbreastcancer.org
https://www.hisbreastcancer.org/contact *Email*
https://www.facebook.com/HISbreastcancer/
https://twitter.com/hisbreastcancer

His Breast Cancer Awareness was created to **assist men,** women, health-care professionals and anyone interested in learning about the **risk, treatments(s), emotional aspect** and **stigmatism** of men dealing with **breast cancer.**

Information About Male Breast Cancer

https://www.hisbreastcancer.org/information-about-male-breast-cancer
Information on **symptoms, risk factors, diagnosis, biopsy, screenings, hormone therapy** and **genetics.**

BRCA and Men

https://www.hisbreastcancer.org/genetics-of-male-breast-cancer
Information, facts and frequently asked questions about **BRCA1** and **BRCA2** and **men.**

Preventing Male Breast Cancer

https://www.hisbreastcancer.org/male-breast-cancer-prevention
Information, tips and advice on **health, wellness** and **cancer prevention.**
Free

Hope for Two—The Pregnant With Cancer Network

http://www.hopefortwo.org/
website: *More than 100 languages*
Info@hopefortwo.org *Email*
http://www.hopefortwo.org/contact-us/ *Contact form*
https://www.facebook.com/hopefortwo
https://twitter.com/HopeForTwoPWCN
(800) 743-4471

Information; messages will be returned ASAP.

Hope for Two—The Pregnant with Cancer Network is an international nonprofit online support organization for women diagnosed with **cancer during pregnancy.** Hope for Two connects women who are pregnant with other women who have been pregnant with the same type of cancer. The website also offers survival stories and a comprehensive glossary.

Get Support

https://hopefortwo.org/get-support/

Women lend support and share their experiences through phone and email conversation.

The Cancer and Pregnancy Registry

https://hopefortwo.org/dr-elyce-cardonick-obgyn-maternal-fetal-medicine-specialist/

Hope for Two—The Pregnant With Cancer Network board of advisors is collecting **information** on **pregnancies complicated by cancer.**

Cancer and Pregnancy

https://hopefortwo.org/news/

News and updates on cancer and pregnancy.

Services are free.

Hospice Foundation of America

https://hospicefoundation.org/

https://hospicefoundation.org/Contact-HFA *Contact info*

(800) 854-3402

Information, Monday – Friday, 9:00 AM – 5:00 PM ET. Messages are checked 24/7 and calls returned ASAP.

Hospice Foundation of America offers **information** and **resources** to educate the public and health-care professionals about **death, dying** and **grief.** It provides material on how to **access, choose, prepare** and **pay for**

care. The website has videos, tutorials and programs on understanding hospice care, starting the conversation and caregiving.

Explaining Hospice
https://hospicefoundation.org/Hospice-Care/Hospice-Services

Staring the Hospice Conversation
https://hospicefoundation.org/Hospice-Care/Starting-the-Conversation

How to Access Care
https://hospicefoundation.org/End-of-Life-Support-and-Resources/
Coping-with-Terminal-Illness/How-to-Access-Care
Steps to finding hospice care and when and how to proceed.

How to Choose a Provider
https://hospicefoundation.org/End-of-Life-Support-and-Resources/
Coping-with-Terminal-Illness/How-to-Choose
Questions to ask and what to look for when choosing care.

Paying for Hospice Care
https://hospicefoundation.org/End-of-Life-Support-and-Resources/
Coping-with-Terminal-Illness/Paying-for-Care
Explanation and information on paying for hospice care and extensions, discharge and revocation.

Hospice Directory
https://hospicefoundation.org/Hospice-Directory
Directory on hospice locations across the United States.

Support—Ask an Expert
https://hospicefoundation.org/Ask-HFA

Ask an Expert provides confidential guidance to patients, families and other interested parties regarding care at the end of life.

Free. A donation of $25 is requested but not required for Ask an Expert service.

I

Imerman Angels

https://imermanangels.org/

https://imermanangels.org/contact-us/ *Contact form*

https://www.facebook.com/ImermanAngels?ref=ts

https://twitter.com/imermanangels

(877) 274-5529

Helpline, Monday – Friday, 9:00 AM – 6:00 PM CT. English and Spanish

Imerman Angels is a **one-on-one cancer support community** that connects anyone seeking cancer support with a Mentor Angel, a cancer survivor or survivor's caregiver who is the same age and gender, and who faced the same type of cancer. The matching service is free and helps anyone touched by any type of cancer, at any cancer stage level, at any age, living anywhere in the world. Individuals 17 and younger will need parental consent; this situation typically involves connecting a parent or guardian.

Support

https://imermanangels.org/get-support/

Mentor Angels can lend **support** and empathy while helping those with **breast cancer** and their **caregivers** navigate the system, determine their options and create their own support team. Support is also provided to those who have lost someone to cancer and wants to speak to someone with the same experience. Forms are in English and Spanish. All other languages need to call the helpline to request a Mentor Angel.

Services are free.

J

Janac Mastectomy Wear

http://janacmastectomywear.com

Info@janacmastectomywear.com *Email*

https://www.facebook.com/Janac.Mastectomy.Wear/

(289) 337-1508

Information, Tuesday – Friday, 10:00 AM – 4:00 PM; Saturday 10:00 AM – 2:00 PM CT, Ontario, Canada. Messages left will be returned ASAP.

Janac Mastectomy Wear has a **non-silicone prosthetic device**, Been-A-Boob, made for sports, swimming, and every day. Been-A-Boob is made of soft fabric that simulates a natural breast. Filled with little beads that mold to any shape of bra, it can be worn by women with altered, removed or different-size breasts to balance their appearance.

Prices available online.

K

Knitted Knockers

www.knittedknockers.org

website: *Nine languages*

contact@knittedknockers.org *Contact form*

https://www.facebook.com/knittedknockers

Knitted Knockers are handmade **knitted breast prostheses** for women who have undergone mastectomies or other procedures to the breast. The website helps connect volunteer knitters with breast cancer survivors to offer **free** Knitted Knockers to any woman who wants them.

Request Knitted Knockers

https://www.knittedknockers.org/request-a-knocker/

Choose size, color and preferences on the online application.

International Locations
https://www.knittedknockers.org/international-groups/
Knitted Knockers are available in more than 25 countries.
Knitted Knockers are free.

Know Your Lemons

https://knowyourlemons.org/
website: *20 languages*
hello@knowyourlemons.com *Email*
https://knowyourlemons.org/contact *Contact form*
https://www.facebook.com/knowyourlemons
(801) 410-0231
Information; leave a message and your call will be returned. For immediate service, send a text.

Know Your Lemons is a charity focused on **early detection**. The site has comprehensive information on **breast health** and the **symptoms of breast cancer**. Presented in a friendly, accessible, and inclusive manner, it breaks down the barriers of taboo, fear and literacy that have slowed the progress of breast cancer awareness.

Symptoms
https://knowyourlemons.org/symptoms?rq=symptoms
Using lemons as the visual, find images of the **12 symptoms of breast cancer.**

Know Your Lemons App
https://knowyourlemons.org/self-exam-app
App that makes it easy to self-exam, report changes, calculate your risk and keep your regular screening appointments.
Free

L

Live by Living

http://livebyliving.org/

dsm@livebyliving.org *Email*

https://www.facebook.com/LiveByLiving/

(303) 808-2339

Information, Monday – Friday, 8:00 AM – 5:00 PM MT

Live by Living provides transformative **outdoor experiences** for **cancer survivors** and their **caregivers**. Day hikes, snowshoe outings and cancer survivor retreats are structured to help you build up your strength and stamina, find solace in the beauty of nature and make new friends with people who understand what you have been through.

Online Events

https://www.livebyliving.org/online-events.html

Information on programs and one-on-one counseling and mindfulness sessions.

Retreats

https://www.livebyliving.org/retreats.html

Information on when and where retreats take place and how to register for a day trip or a two-day retreat.

Day walks and retreats are free of charge.

Livestrong

https://www.livestrong.org/ *Cancer website*

https://www.livestrong.com/ *Health and wellness website*

https://www.facebook.com/livestrong

https://twitter.com/LIVESTRONG

(855) 220-7777

Cancer navigation services, Monday – Thursday, 12:00 PM – 4:00 PM CT. Someone will take your information and connect you with an appropriate navigator and cancer resources. English and Spanish
Livestrong provides information and **support** to **patients, caregivers** and anyone affected by cancer through **direct services** and **community programs.**

Livestrong Guidebook

https://www.livestrong.org/what-we-do/program/livestrong-guidebook
A two-book set that provides **information** and **resources** to address specific concerns that patients, loved ones and caregivers often have at the time of diagnosis, during treatment and post-treatment. Available in print and digital formats.

Fertility

https://www.livestrong.org/what-we-do/program/fertility
Information, resources and **financial support to survivors** whose cancer and its treatment present **risks to their fertility.**

Fitness and Nutrition

https://www.livestrong.com/challenges/
Monthly challenges designed to help you establish (and sustain) better **fitness** and **nutrition** habits all year long.

Livestrong at the YMCA

https://www.livestrong.org/what-we-do/program/livestrong-at-the-ymca.
Open to adults 18 and older in more than 750 YMCAs across the country. Survivors participate in exercise regimens catered to their individual needs from certified fitness instructors. The instructors are trained in cancer survivorship, post-rehabilitation exercise and supportive cancer care. *Programs are low-cost or free.*

Living Beyond Breast Cancer

www.lbbc.org
website: *English and Spanish*
mail@lbbc.org *Email*
https://www.facebook.com/livingbeyondbreastcancer
https://twitter.com/LivingBeyondBC
(888) 753-5222
Helpline—English, Monday – Friday, 9:00 AM – 9:00 PM ET
(844) 275-7427
Helpline—Spanish, Monday – Friday, 9:00 AM – 9:00 PM ET
Living Beyond Breast Cancer is an organization that provides information, support and educational programs for people with **all stages of breast cancer.**

Learn About Cancer

https://www.lbbc.org/learn
A library of **guides** to **understanding cancer; educational programs** and **webinars;** cancer blog of inspirational and empowering stories; tips for getting good support. Categories of information to further focus your search: **recently diagnosed; in treatment;** living with a history of breast cancer; living with **metastatic breast cancer; young woman.**

Let's Talk About It Video Series

http://www.lbbc.org/letstalk
The videos combine the perspectives of **young women** affected by breast cancer and their health-care providers. Topics include **early-stage** and **metastatic breast cancer.**
Services are free.

Look Good Feel Better

https://lookgoodfeelbetter.org/
website: *English and Spanish*

https://lookgoodfeelbetter.org/contact-us/ *Contact form*
https://www.facebook.com/lookgoodfeelbetter
https://twitter.com/LGFB

Look Good Feel Better is a nonmedical, brand-neutral public service program that teaches **beauty techniques** to women with cancer to help them **manage** the **appearance-related side effects** of cancer **treatment**. The program includes lessons on skin and nail care, cosmetics, wigs and turbans, accessories and styling.

At Home Beauty Guide

https://lookgoodfeelbetter.org/programs/beauty-guide/
Information and tips on makeup, new hair looks, nail care and styling.

Virtual Workshops

https://lookgoodfeelbetter.org/virtual-workshops/
Look Good Feel Better Live! Instructions and tips for dealing with the appearance-related side effects of cancer treatment during **one-hour online workshops**. Beauty professional volunteers guide a group of participants in **skin care** and **makeup application,** the use of **wigs** and other **head coverings,** or **body image** and **styling** to help manage appearance concerns. Participants can ask questions of the instructor and interact with other participants.

Global Programs

https://lookgoodfeelbetter.org/programs/around-the-world/#global-programs
The Look Good Feel Better Foundation oversees a **global network** of 26 licensed affiliates that deliver Look Good Feel Better support programs in countries across the globe.
Programs are free.

Look Good Feel Better for Men

http://www.lookgoodfeelbetterformen.org/
website: *English and Spanish*

https://lookgoodfeelbetter.org/contact-us/ *Contact form*
Look Good Feel Better for Men is a nonmedical, brand-neutral public service program that teaches self-care techniques to men with cancer to help them manage the **appearance-related side effects** of **cancer treatment** to look and feel confident and in control.

Video
https://lookgoodfeelbetter.org/programs/men/
A practical guide with **easy-to-follow tips** that deal with some of the side effects of treatment including **skin changes, hair loss, stress** and other issues. Information also available in a 15-page brochure.

Daily Routine Checklist
http://www.lookgoodfeelbetterformen.org/daily_routine.html
Simple steps to help you set up and keep a daily routine of personal care.

Additional Resources
http://www.lookgoodfeelbetterformen.org/resources.html
Information and support resources for men with cancer.
Programs are free.

Lotsa Helping Hands
http://lotsahelpinghands.com
info+contactus@lotsahelpinghands.com *Email*
Lotsa Helping Hands is a central place to coordinate meals and help for friends and family. An **online care calendar** allows cancer patients to post requests for members of their community to quickly find ways to get help and support. The service brings together caregivers and volunteers to help organize daily life during times of medical crisis or caregiver exhaustion in neighborhoods and communities worldwide. The information is private and accessible only to the people with the community ID.
Free

LympheDIVAs

https://lymphedivas.com/
https://lymphedivas.com/contact-us-1 *Contact form*
https://www.facebook.com/LympheDIVAs
https://twitter.com/LympheDIVAs
(866) 411-3482
Information, Monday – Thursday, 8:30 AM – 6:00 PM ET
LympheDIVAs provides medically correct and **fashionable compression sleeves, gauntlets** and gloves for the breast cancer survivor with lymphedema. Products feature moisture-wicking technology, which pulls sweat away from the body, and they dry quickly. They are completely seamless with 360-degree stretch, which allows for a full range of motion. Garments are infused with micro-encapsulated aloe vera to help moisturize and protect the skin. Shop a variety of pattern choices: fauna, flora, giving back, great artists, lace, paisley, tattoo, solid colors, crystals.

Size + Fit

https://lymphedivas.com/size-and-fit
LympheDIVAs has a **fitter's aid** to determine the approximate compression at any measuring point to make sure you are getting the compression you need to manage your swelling effectively. All the gauntlets and gloves are designed to have little to no compression at the wrist.
Prices available online.

M

Make a Vision Board

http://makeavisionboard.com/vision-board-apps/
Make a Vision Board offers information and links to seven digital vision board apps that allow you to create a vision board on your mobile device.
Free

Make Your Dialogue Count

https://makeyourdialoguecount.com/

website: *English and Spanish*

Make Your Dialogue Count provides information and tips for understanding and navigating the metastatic breast cancer care landscape and improving conversations with your friends, family and treatment team.

Discussion Guide

https://makeyourdialoguecount.com/physical-health/clinical-trials-and-treatment-options

Information on **clinical trials,** what the results mean and how they affect your care, so you can have a productive discussion with your doctor.

Personal Discussion Guide

https://makeyourdialoguecount.com/physical-health/make-your-dialogue-count-questionnaire

A questionnaire prompts you with six questions to create a **personal discussion guide** to help you speak with your doctor about treatment options.

Talking to Life Partner, Friends, Parents and Children

https://makeyourdialoguecount.com/mbc-and-relationships/sharing-news-with-friends-and-family

Tips and resources to help you prepare to talk to a life partner, friends and parents about metastatic breast cancer. The information on speaking to children is tailored to their age group.

Manage Emotional and Spiritual Health

https://makeyourdialoguecount.com/emotional-wellbeing

Downloadable PDFs with information on **navigating isolation** and managing **anxiety, depression** and **crisis of spirituality.**

Manage Your Physical Health
https://makeyourdialoguecount.com/physical-health
Information on **nutrition,** how to manage **pain** and understanding **fertility** options.

Evaluating Your Treatment Team
https://makeyourdialoguecount.com/mbc-and-relationships/your-potential-treatment-team
Information and guidance on selecting and evaluating your **treatment team.**

Planning Your Life Around MBC
https://makeyourdialoguecount.com/planning-your-life-around-mbc
How to have a **conversation** with your **employer** and **co-workers** as well as how to have conversation about end-of-life care.
Information and downloads are free.

MaleBC.org

http://malebc.org/
https://twitter.com/malefitness
MaleBC.org offers information and comprehensive resources specific to **men** with **breast cancer.** It provides material on understanding **risk, genetics, BRCA1 and BRCA2, sex** and **intimacy, diagnosis, treatment, surgery, reconstruction, metastasis, caregivers.** There are two- to three-minute videos on symptoms, treatment and overcoming the stigma.

Male Breast Cancer Report
https://paper.li/malefitness/1461822144#/
Informative, educational newsletter that features male breast cancer reports from all media.
Free

The Male Breast Cancer Coalition

http://malebreastcancercoalition.org/
http://malebreastcancercoalition.org/contact-us/ *Contact form*
https://www.facebook.com/MaleBreastCancerCoalition
https://twitter.com/MBCC_MHBT
The **Male Breast Cancer Coalition** is a **patient advocacy organization.** The website provides **information** and **resources for men** and their families.

Men Have Breasts Too—Videos

http://malebreastcancercoalition.org/men-have-breasts-too/
In this video series about breast cancer in men, you will meet men diagnosed with breast cancer and learn about male breast cancer and the impact genetic mutations have on them and their families.

Additional Resources

https://malebreastcancercoalition.org/category/resources/
Free

Medicaid

https://www.medicaid.gov
Medicaid.gov@cms.hhs.gov *Email*
https://www.medicaid.gov/about-us/contact-us/index.html *Contact*
https://twitter.com/cmsgov
(877) 267-2323
General prerecorded information, English and Spanish
(410) 786-3000
Information, Center for Medicaid and Medicare Services
(866) 226-1819
TTY General prerecorded information, English and Spanish
(410) 786-0727
TTY Center for Medicaid and Medicare Services

Medicaid is a **public-assistance program for Americans of all ages.** It provides **health coverage** to eligible low-income adults, children, pregnant women, elderly adults and people with disabilities. Medicaid is administered by states, according to federal requirements, and is offered in every state.

Contact Information by State
https://www.medicaid.gov/about-us/contact-us/contact-your-state-questions/index.html
You must contact your state Medicaid office for information. Here, find a list of offices by state and how to contact them.

Medicaid
https://www.medicaid.gov/medicaid/index.html
Information on **Medicaid programs** including outreach tools, eligibility, home and community-based services, quality of care, financial information, access to care, prescription drugs, and additional services and support.

Medicaid & You
https://www.medicaid.gov/medicaid-and-you/index.html
FAQs about guidelines, eligibility, coverage.

Medical Assistance Tool
https://www.mat.org/
website: *English and Spanish*
https://medicineassistancetool.org/Contact-Us *Contact form*
Medicine Assistance Tool is a search engine designed to help patients, caregivers and health-care providers learn more about the **resources available** through the various **biopharmaceutical industry programs.**
Service is free.

Assistance Tool

https://www.mat.org/My-Resources

Allows you to search by medication for available industry programs.

Find Free and Low-Cost Health Clinics

https://www.mat.org/find-a-clinic#find-a-clinic-results_e=0&find-a-clinic-results_distanceclinic=25

Map of free and low-cost health clinics.

Medicare

https://www.medicare.gov

website: *English and Spanish*

https://www.medicare.gov/forms-help-other-resources/contact-medicare

https://www.facebook.com/medicare

https://twitter.com/MedicareGov

Contact information

800-MEDICARE (1-800-633-4227)

877-486-2048 TTY

Information, 24/7

Medicare is a single-payer, **national social insurance program** administered by the U.S. federal government. It uses about 30 to 50 private insurance companies across the United States under contract for the administration. It provides health insurance for Americans age 65 and older who have worked and paid into the system through the payroll tax. Medicare is broken down into four categories: Part A: hospital insurance; Part B: medical insurance; Part C: Medicare advantage plus; Part D: prescription drug coverage. The comprehensive website provides information on how to find, apply and navigate these plans and get help with coverage.

Get Started With Medicare

https://www.medicare.gov/basics/get-started-with-medicare

Information on Medicare programs, how to sign up and how to use the benefits.

Live Chat 24/7
https://www.medicare.gov/talk-to-someone

Information in Other Languages
https://www.medicare.gov/about-us/information-in-other-languages
Information on Medicare available in more than 20 languages.

MedlinePlus
National Institutes of Health—U.S. National Library of Medicine
https://medlineplus.gov/
website: *English and Spanish*
https://www.facebook.com/mplus.gov/
https://twitter.com/medlineplus

MedlinePlus is the National Institute of Health's **consumer health website** for patients and their families and friends. Produced by the U.S. National Library of Medicine, it is the world's largest **medical library**. It provides information about diseases, conditions and wellness issues in easy-to-understand language. MedlinePlus health topics are regularly reviewed, and links are updated daily.

Health Topics
https://medlineplus.gov/healthtopics.html
Read about **symptoms, causes, treatment** and **prevention** for more than 1,000 diseases, illnesses, health conditions and wellness issues.

Drugs, Herbs and Supplements
https://medlineplus.gov/druginformation.html
Browse **dietary supplements** and **herbal remedies** to learn about their effectiveness, usual dosage and drug interactions.

Medical Tests
https://medlineplus.gov/lab-tests/

Learn about **medical tests**, including what the tests are used for, why a doctor may order a test, how a test will feel and what the results may mean.

Medical Encyclopedia

https://medlineplus.gov/encyclopedia.html

Medical Encyclopedia has more than 4,000 articles about diseases, tests, symptoms, injuries and surgeries. It also contains an extensive library of medical photographs and illustrations.

Healthy Recipes

https://medlineplus.gov/recipes/

Recipes show you how to prepare tasty, healthy meals that help you develop a healthy eating pattern.

Videos & Tools

https://medlineplus.gov/videosandcooltools.html

Health videos on topics such as anatomy, body systems and surgical procedures. Test your knowledge with interactive tutorials and games. Check your health with calculators and quizzes.

Free

Meetup

https://www.meetup.com/

https://www.facebook.com/meetup/

https://twitter.com/Meetup

Meetup is a **community of people who get together around shared interests**. A Meetup is created and set up by an individual or group. Browse categories to find an activity of interest. Each Meetup requires you to sign up to join.

Some groups are free; others have a fee.

Metastatic Breast Cancer Network

www.mbcn.org

mbcn@mbcn.org *Email*

https://www.facebook.com/MetastaticBreastCancerNetwork/

https://twitter.com/MBCNbuzz

(888) 500-0370

Information only

(844) 275-7427 (844-ASK-SHARE)

For helpline and peer-to-peer support, you will be referred to SHARE Cancer Support.

Metastatic Breast Cancer Network has a comprehensive website with information and resources to support people dealing with **metastatic breast cancer.**

Videos

http://mbcn.org/what-is-metastatic-breast-cancer/

Videos explain MBC in simple-to-understand terms. Information includes **MBC diagnosis,** info for those **newly diagnosed,** questions to ask your doctor, standard treatments for MBC, pain management and other side effects, **clinical trials** questions and answers, and **living with MBC.**

Brochures

http://mbcn.org/free-brochures/

The information on the website is also available in brochure form that can be downloaded or sent to you by mail.

Resources for Support

http://mbcn.org/peer-support-matches-telephone-hotline/

List of organizations that offer one-on-one and peer-to-peer breast cancer support.

Be Your Own Advocate

http://mbcn.org/be-your-own-best-advocate/

Information on **what questions to ask** your doctor and how to take charge of your cancer. Includes advice from patients living with MBC.

Clinical Trials
http://www.mbcn.org/clinical-trials-finder/
A **clinical trial search engine** to help people with metastatic breast cancer find trials.
Services are free.

METAvivor Research and Support
http://www.metavivor.org/
info@metavivor.org *Email general information*
support@metavivor.org *Email for support programs*
(818) 860-1226
Information and support, Monday – Friday, 8:00 AM – 7:00 PM ET
METAvivor is an organization dedicated to the specific fight of women and men living with **stage IV metastatic breast cancer**. Volunteer-led, it has trained metastatic breast cancer patients to create and lead peer-to-peer support groups across the country.

Support Programs
https://www.metavivor.org/support/finding-a-support-program/
An interactive map to find a list of support groups offered via the peer-to-peer program.

Clinical Trials
https://www.metavivor.org/mbc-prep/clinical-trial-search/
Information designed to help you better understand clinical trials. Clinical trial search and matching service.
Services are free.

COVID and Cancer

https://www.metavivor.org/support/covid-19-novel-coronavirus-resources/

Information, wellness tips and resources for COVID.

My Breast Cancer Coach

https://www.mybreastcancercoach.org/

My Breast Cancer Coach is an **online program** designed to help you better understand your type of breast cancer, so you can focus on the information that is most relevant to you. It provides information about personalized breast cancer treatment options to help manage your cancer care.

Personalized Treatment Guide

https://www.mybreastcancercoach.org/en-US/Your-Personalized-Treatment-Guide

By answering a few questions about your tumor type, the guide will present you with a report of treatment options that may be appropriate for patients with your diagnosis.

Prepare for Your Appointment

https://www.mybreastcancercoach.org/Prepare-for-Your-Appointment

Provides a list of questions you can download and print to take to a doctor's appointment.

My Cancer Coach Mobile App

https://www.mybreastcancercoach.org/breast-cancer-app

The mobile app provides information about **personalized cancer treatments** to help manage your cancer's progression. It also includes a personal guide, calendar, journal, glossary, resources and questions for your doctor.

Free

My Cancer Circle

http://mycancercircle.lotsahelpinghands.com

My Cancer Circle is an **online tool** for caregivers to coordinate family, friends and volunteers so they can help take care of all the tasks the patient faces every day. It directs their efforts by providing an online calendar to organize the community of helpers and caregiver resources to support you and your loved ones more efficiently.

Free

My Life Line

https://www.mylifeline.org

support@mylifeline.org *Support and general inquires*

https://www.facebook.com/MyLifeLine.orgCancerFoundation

https://twitter.com/mylifelineorg

My LifeLine offers cancer patients and caregivers a **free website** to **communicate** with **family** and **friends**. Create an online care calendar that allows you to post requests for members of your community to quickly find ways to help and support you.

Free

N

National Academy of Elder Care Lawyers

https://www.naela.org/

naela@naela.org *Email*

The **National Academy of Elder Law Attorneys** provides an **online directory** to assist consumers in identifying and locating elder and special needs law attorneys to provide legal services searchable by name or city, state and ZIP code. NAELA is a membership of attorneys who are trained in working with the legal problems of aging Americans and individuals of all ages with disabilities.

Online Directory

https://www.naela.org/findlawyer
Online directory with a list of lawyers by name or city, state and ZIP code.
Directory is free.

National Association for Home Care & Hospice

http://www.nahc.org
https://www.facebook.com/NAHC.org
https://twitter.com/OfficialNAHC
(202) 547-7424
Information, Monday – Friday, 9:00 AM – 6:00 PM ET
The **National Association for Home Care & Hospice** is a trade association that provides an online **Home Care/Hospice Agency Locator,** which contains a comprehensive database of more than 33,000 home care and hospice agencies. NAHC represents the interests of chronically ill, disabled and dying Americans of all ages and the caregivers who provide them with in-home health and hospice services.

Home Care and Hospice Basics

https://www.nahc.org/consumers-information/home-care-hospice-basics/
Information for those new to home care: selecting the right provider, accrediting agencies, standard billing and payment practices.

National Agency Location Service

https://agencylocator.nahc.org/
Use this resource to find all the agencies in any area of the country.
Free

National Breast Cancer Foundation

http://www.nationalbreastcancer.org/
http://www.nationalbreastcancer.org/contact-nbcf *Contact form*
https://www.facebook.com/nationalbreastcancer

https://twitter.com/NBCF

The National Breast Cancer Foundation website offers information, education, programs and resources for those affected with breast cancer. Patient services provide mammograms, diagnostic services and patient navigation for women in need.

Free Educational Guides

https://www.nationalbreastcancer.org/early-detection-of-breast-cancer/

Downloadable guides and e-books with information on **breast health, dense breasts, recurrence, abnormal mammograms,** what to do next, how to fit a bra, **early detection** and healthy-living tips.

Learn About Breast Cancer

https://www.nationalbreastcancer.org/about-breast-cancer/

Causes, breast anatomy, early detection, treatment, stages and **types.**

National Mammography Program

https://www.nationalbreastcancer.org/national-mammography-program

Free mammograms and **diagnostic services** for women in need.

Patient Navigator Program

https://www.nationalbreastcancer.org/breast-cancer-patient-navigator

Services to help women **navigate the complex cancer system.**
Services are free.

National Cancer Institute—U.S. Department of Health and Human Services

https://www.cancer.gov

website: *English and Spanish*

https://www.cancer.gov/contact/email-us *Email*

https://www.facebook.com/cancer.gov

https://twitter.com/thenci

(800) 422-6237

Information, Monday – Friday, 9:00 AM – 9:00 PM ET. English and Spanish
Chat line, Monday – Friday, 9:00 AM – 9:00 PM ET. English and Spanish

The **National Cancer Institute** provides a comprehensive website with **information, education, resources, advocacy** and **support** for all types and stages of cancer.

About Cancer

https://www.cancer.gov/about-cancer
Information on types of **cancer treatment, clinical trials, cancer drugs, complementary** and **alternative treatment, causes** and **prevention, advanced cancer, coping,** and **managing cancer care.**

Treatment Information

https://www.cancer.gov/types/breast/patient/breast-treatment-pdq
General information on breast cancer and treatment.

Self-Image and Sexuality

https://www.cancer.gov/about-cancer/coping/self-image#dating
Information on **self-image, sex** and **dating** during or after cancer.

Male Breast Cancer

https://www.cancer.gov/types/breast/patient/male-breast-treatment-pdq
General information for **men** with **breast cancer.**

Pregnancy and Cancer

https://www.cancer.gov/types/breast/patient/pregnancy-breast-treatment-pdq#_94
Information and options for **pregnant women** with **breast cancer.**

Dictionary of Cancer

https://www.cancer.gov/publications/dictionaries

Biomedical terms defined in nontechnical language. Contains definitions and synonyms for drugs and agents used to treat patients with cancer or conditions related to cancer. Each drug entry includes links to check for clinical trials listed in NCI's List of Cancer Clinical Trials.

Patient Education Publications
https://www.cancer.gov/publications
Free booklets with information on **clinical trials, screening, survivorship, support, types of cancer, treatment** and **side effects.**

Steps to Find a Clinical Trial
https://www.cancer.gov/about-cancer/treatment/clinical-trials/search/trial-guide

Clinical Trials
https://www.cancer.gov/about-cancer/treatment/clinical-trials/search
Services are free.

National Cancer Legal Services Network

www.nclsn.org
http://www.nclsn.org/contact-us/ *Contact form*
https://www.facebook.com/NCLSNetwork
https://twitter.com/NCLSNetwork

The **National Cancer Legal Services Network** promotes increased availability of **free legal service** programs so that **people affected by cancer** may focus on medical care and their quality of life. It supports the efforts of individuals and organizations intent on meeting the legal needs of the cancer-affected community. Pro bono legal services programs assist with insurance disputes, public benefits, housing, employment issues, future care and custody planning, immigration and advance directives.

Directory to Legal Services
http://www.nclsn.org/members-directory/
The directory helps patients find legal assistance and allows the NCLSN to identify locations where additional legal resources are needed to help low-income and at-risk populations dealing with cancer.
Directory is free.

National Center for Complementary and Integrative Health
https://nccih.nih.gov/
website: *English and Spanish*
info@nccih.nih.gov *Email*
https://www.facebook.com/nih.nccih
https://twitter.com/NIH_NCCIH
The **National Center for Complementary and Integrative Health** offers comprehensive information and resources for **complementary, alternative** or **integrative** health. The NCCIH is the federal government's lead agency for scientific research on complementary and integrative health approaches. It is one of the 27 institutes and centers that make up the National Institutes of Health within the U.S. Department of Health and Human Services.

Health Topics A-Z
https://nccih.nih.gov/health/atoz.htm
In-depth information on medication, conditions and supplements.

Herbs at a Glance
https://nccih.nih.gov/health/herbsataglance.htm
A series of brief fact sheets that provide basic information about specific herbs or botanicals—common names, what the science says, potential side effects and cautions.
Free

National Coalition for Cancer Survivorship

canceradvocacy.org

info@canceradvocacy.org *Email*

canceradvocacy.org *Contact form*

https://www.facebook.com/cancersurvivorship

https://twitter.com/canceradvocacy

(877) 622-7937 (NCCS-YES)

Information, Monday – Friday, 8:30 AM – 5:30 PM ET

National Coalition for Cancer Survivorship was founded by and for cancer survivors to help people develop skills to better meet and understand the challenges and navigate their illness.

The Cancer Survival Toolbox

https://canceradvocacy.org/resources/cancer-survivor-toolbox-english/

A **free audio program** created by leading cancer organizations with information on basic skills and special topics for people at any point in their care. Eleven downloadable audio tapes, 31 to 75 minutes in length, covering skills such as **communicating, making decisions** and **standing up for your rights,** as well as special topics that cover first steps for the newly diagnosed; dying well, the final stage of survivorship; and caring for caregivers.

The Cancer Survival Toolbox Spanish

https://canceradvocacy.org/resources/cancer-survival-toolbox/#tab-id-2

Resources

https://canceradvocacy.org/resources/

Resources and information on **care planning, advocating for yourself, employment rights** and **health insurance.**

Free

National Comprehensive Cancer Network

https://www.nccn.org/

https://www.nccn.org/patients/contact/default.aspx *Contact form*

https://www.facebook.com/NCCNorg

https://twitter.com/NCCN

(215) 690-0300

Information, Monday – Friday, 8:45 AM – 5:00 PM ET

National Comprehensive Cancer Network is an alliance of leading cancer centers devoted to patient care, research and education. The website provides cancer treatment information in easy-to-understand language.

The NCCN Guidelines

https://www.nccn.org/guidelines/patients

Step-by-step guides feature information on **cancer treatment**, with patient-friendly illustrations and glossaries of terms and acronyms.

COVID Resources

https://www.nccn.org/covid-19

Information, webinars and resources for COVID and cancer.

Webinars

https://www.nccn.org/patientresources/patient-resources/patient-webinars

NCCN provides free Know What Your Doctors Know webinars for people living with cancer and caregivers.

Map of NCCN Member Institutions

https://www.nccn.org/members/network.aspx

Locations of and information about the cancer centers that are a part of NCCN.

Patient and Payment Assistance

https://www.nccn.org/business-policy/business/virtual-reimbursement-resource-room-and-app

NCCN provides an extensive list of resources for financial support.

Free

National Hospice and Palliative Care Organization

https://www.nhpco.org/

Contact Us | NHPCO *Email*

https://www.facebook.com/NHPCO/

https://twitter.com/NHPCO_news

(800) 658-8898

Information, Monday – Friday, 9:00 AM – 5:00 PM ET

The **National Hospice and Palliative Care Organization** provides information, support and resources to help people make decisions about **end-of-life care** and **services** before a crisis.

Advance Directives

https://www.caringinfo.org/planning/advance-directives/creating-advance-directive/

Plan and Prepare

https://www.caringinfo.org/planning/

Information to help you make decisions about care and services before a crisis.

Palliative Care

https://www.nhpco.org/patients-and-caregivers/about-palliative-care/

Explanation and information on **palliative care, the goals, criteria, how** and **where it is delivered** and **who pays.**

Hospice Care

https://www.nhpco.org/patients-and-caregivers/about-hospice-care/

Explanation and information on **hospice care, the benefits, criteria, where hospice care is given** and **support for caretakers.**

Free

National LGBT Cancer Network

www.cancer-network.org

info@cancer-network.org *Email*

https://www.facebook.com/nationalLGBTcancerNetwork/

https://twitter.com/cancerLGBT

(212) 675-2633

Information, Monday – Friday, 9:00 AM – 5:00 PM ET

The **National LGBT Cancer Network** provides **education, support** and **information** for **LGBT** people affected by cancer and those at risk.

LGBT Cancer Information

https://cancer-network.org/cancer-information/

Current research data, with articles written in plain language, intended to be understandable to a broad audience.

LGBT-Friendly Cancer Screening Facilities

https://cancer-network.org/screening-providers/

Choose your state to find an LGBT-friendly cancer **screening facility** near you.

LGBT-Friendly Cancer Treatment Facilities

https://cancer-network.org/out-and-surviving/

The National LGBT Cancer Network has selected these resources and **treatment facilities** because of their commitment to offering safe, affordable, welcoming care to all LGBT people.

Cancer Resources

https://cancer-network.org/cancer-information/cancer-resources-for-the-lgbt-community/

Find a list of **cancer resources** for the LGBT community.

Support Resources

https://cancer-network.org/programs/support-groups-for-survivors/

Support for lesbian, gay, bisexual and transgender cancer survivors.

Free

National LGBT Cancer Project

www.lgbtcancer.com

darryl@lgbtcancer.org *Email*

https://www.facebook.com/LGBTCancerProject

https://twitter.com/lgbtcancer

(212) 673-4920

Information, Monday – Friday, 9:00 AM – 5:00 PM ET

The **National LGBT Cancer Project** is a lesbian, gay, bisexual and transgender **cancer survivor support** and **advocacy** nonprofit organization. The online support group community provides survivors with **peer-to-peer support, patient navigation, education** and **advocacy**. Volunteers include oncologists, social workers and psychologists.

LGBT Cancer Community

https://healthunlocked.com/lgbt-cancer

Write a post or pose a question to the LGBT cancer community.

Cancer Treatment Centers

https://lgbtcancer.org/cancer-treatment-center/

The **National LGBT Cancer Project** has compiled a list of cancer treatment centers across the country.

Clinical Trials
https://www.antidote.me/lgbtcancer-find-a-clinical-trial
A simple questionnaire will help you locate trials.
Free

National Widowers' Organization
https://nationalwidowers.org/
info@nationalwidowers.org *Email*
https://nationalwidowers.org/contact/ *Contact form*
(800) 309-3658
Information; messages are returned ASAP.
The **National Widowers' Organization** offers information, resources, books, blogs and articles to help men cope with loss. Through the site, you can connect with support groups in your area or with a peer through the **widower-to-widower support programs.** This organization was established in 2011 by a man who lost his wife to cancer and found it difficult to share in mixed-gender bereavement groups, so he started an organization only for grieving men.

Support Programs
https://nationalwidowers.org/widower-to-widower-peer-support-program/
Widower to widower: peer support programs.

Frequently Asked Questions
https://nationalwidowers.org/faqs/
FAQs about **how men grieve.** Topics include what to expect, anger, difference between grief and depression, how to handle household matters, how to find support, and dating again.
Free

Native American Cancer Initiatives
http://NatAmCancer.org/

mailto:nacr@natamcancer.org *Email*

https://natamcancer.org/contact *Contact*

(303) 838-9359

Information; voicemail messages will be returned ASAP.

The **Native American Cancer Initiatives** is an American Indian–operated, community-based site that offers **Native-specific cancer education information** and **resources** that address the continuum of cancer care.

The Quality of Life Tree

https://natamcancer.org/Quality-of-Life-Tree

Information on spirituality, communication, treatment, clinical trials, health information and side effects.

Survivor Support

https://natamcancer.org/Survivorship-Support

Information on ways you can help your loved one through cancer diagnosis, treatment recovery, care and healing.

Free

Necessity Bags

https://www.necessitybag.com/

Support@NecessityBag.com *Email*

(201) 830-7668

Information; messages will be returned ASAP.

Necessity Bags are lightweight, colorful, water-resistant bags filled with useful nonmedical items for patients to take with them to treatment: a blanket, headphones, a rubbing stone, an aluminum water bottle, a journal, sick bags, a head wrap, essential oils, cooling and cleansing wipes, throat lozenges, organic mint candies, organic lip balm and lotion, and ice packs–hot packs.

Check website for prices.

Needy Meds

https://www.needymeds.org/
website: *English and Spanish*
info@needymeds.org *Email*
https://www.facebook.com/needymeds
https://twitter.com/NeedyMeds
(800) 503-6987
Helpline, Monday – Friday, 9:00 AM – 5:00 PM ET. English and Spanish
NeedyMeds directs you to programs that may be able to **assist in paying** or your **medication**. The home page has a drug search and drug-pricing calculator.

Prescription Assistance

https://www.needymeds.org/pap
Prescription assistance can be offered in the way of patient assistance programs, which are created by pharmaceutical companies to provide **free or discounted medicines** to people who are unable to afford them. Each program has its own qualifying criteria.

Patient Assistance Program

https://www.needymeds.org/papus-home
Receive daily or weekly email reports for the most up-to-date **changes** in **patient assistance programs**. Information includes contact information; changes; new, closed or merged programs; drug additions and removals; new or changed applications and eligibility criteria; changes to programs.

Education

https://www.needymeds.org/advocates-education
An array of relevant health-care-related webinars, newsletters and videos. *Service is free.*

O

Oncofertility Consortium—Michigan State University

https://oncofertility.msu.edu/

oncofert@msu.edu *Email*

https://www.facebook.com/oncofertilityconsortium/

https://twitter.com/oncofertility

The **Oncofertility Consortium** is an international, interdisciplinary initiative designed to explore the **reproductive future** of **cancer survivors**. Oncofertility is a subfield that bridges oncology and reproductive research.

Save My Fertility

https://www.savemyfertility.org/

Save My Fertility is a resource for adult cancer patients and the parents of children with cancer who want to learn more about **preserving** their **fertility before and during cancer treatment** and protecting their **hormonal health after treatment.**

Patient Navigator

https://preservefertility.obgyn.msu.edu/

Medical professionals who provide female and male cancer patients with information about their fertility preservation options and help them coordinate their care.

Find a Clinic

https://oncofertility.msu.edu/find-a-clinic-or-center

Find fertility clinics around the world.

P

Patient Access Network Foundation

www.Panfoundation.org

info@panfoundation.org *Email*

https://panfoundation.org/index.php/en/contact *Contact form*

https://www.facebook.com/PANfoundation

https://twitter.com/PAN_Foundation

(866) 316-7263

Customer service, Monday – Friday, 9:00 AM – 7:00 PM ET. English and Spanish. Translation service available for languages other than English.

The **Patient Access Network Foundation** provides **financial assistance** for **prescription drug co-payments** to people with chronic or life-threatening illnesses for whom cost limits access to breakthrough medical treatments. PAN Foundation assistance is available **only for metastatic breast cancer**.

PAN Foundation Assistance

https://www.panfoundation.org/disease-funds/metastatic-breast-cancer/

For metastatic breast cancer only. The patient must have Medicare health insurance that covers his or her qualifying medication or product.

Apply for Assistance

https://www.panfoundation.org/get-help

Information on how to enroll and application information. You can apply online through the web portals 24/7. Or call the customer service line above during office hours.

Services are free.

Patient Advocate Foundation

www.patientadvocate.org

website: *English and Spanish*

https://www.facebook.com/patientadvocatefoundation/?ref=ts

(800) 532-5274

Information, Monday – Thursday, 8:30 AM – 5:00 PM; Friday, 9:00 AM – 4:00 PM ET. English and Spanish

(866) 512-3861

Co-pay relief assistance line, Monday – Thursday, 8:30 AM – 5:00 PM; Friday, 9:00 AM – 4:00 PM ET. English and Spanish

(877) 236–6626

DONNA CareLine for individualized case management assistance for breast cancer patients. Monday – Thursday, 8:30 AM – 5:00 PM; Friday, 9:00 AM – 4:00 PM ET. English and Spanish

Patient Advocate Foundation is a national nonprofit organization that serves as an **active liaison** between **patients and their insurer, employer** and/or **creditors to resolve insurance, job retention** and/or **debt crisis matters** relative to their diagnosis through case managers, doctors and attorneys. PAF patient services offers **one-on-one assistance** from a **professional case manager** to help patients, caregivers or providers **resolve health-care access** and **financial issues**. Case managers are available to assist patients who have a diagnosis of a chronic, debilitating or life-threatening disease.

COVID Care Resource Center

https://www.patientadvocate.org/covidcare/

Case managers provide patients diagnosed with a **chronic, debilitating** or **life-threatening disease** who are affected by COVID, and those hospitalized for COVID, with timely and relevant information. They answer questions that **patients** and **caregivers** have about accessing and **paying for care, managing basic cost-of-living needs** such as food, rent or mortgage, utilities, insurance and transportation costs—all of which have become difficult to manage because of the pandemic.

COVID Webinars

https://www.patientadvocate.org/covidcare/webinars/

Weekly webinars with timely information regarding the coronavirus pandemic.

DONNA CareLine Specialty Case Manager Program

https://donna.pafcareline.org/

Individualized case management assistance to patients who have been diagnosed with **breast cancer** and are seeking education, support and assistance in overcoming **insurance coverage** and **financial burdens** that affect their access to care. Case managers also assist patients who are experiencing **financial challenges** that are affecting their ability to **pay for care** and **basic cost-of-living expenses** by researching and linking them to available financial support programs that may meet some of these needs.

Resource Library

https://www.patientadvocate.org/explore-our-resources/education-resource-library/

A nine-module course to walk you through the process of **appealing a health insurance denial.** In each module, there is a short quiz and helpful resources that you can reference later. This training will help you identify a denial, **write an effective appeal letter** and gain valuable skills to pave the way to an easy health insurance approval.

National Financial Resource Directory

https://www.patientadvocate.org/explore-our-resources/national-financial-resource-directory/

Resources for **uninsured patients** and **underinsured patients** for a **broad range of needs** including **housing, utilities, food, transportation to medical treatment, home health care, medical devices** and **pharmaceutical agents**. Searchable by age, state, medical diagnosis and assistance needed.

Co-Pay Relief Program

https://www.patientadvocate.org/connect-with-services/copay-relief/

Financial assistance to qualified patients, assisting them with prescription **drug co-payments.** Counselors work directly with the patient as well as with the provider of care to obtain necessary medical, insurance and income information. Upon approval, payments are made directly to the doctor, the pharmacy or the patient.

All services are free.

Patient Resource

http://www.patientresource.com
prp@patientresource.com *Email*
https://www.facebook.com/PatientResource
https://twitter.com/PRPCancerGuide
(800) 497-7530 / (913) 725-1600
Information, Monday – Friday, 8:30 AM – 5:30 PM CT
Patient Resource is an online resource directory for people affected by any type of cancer.

Cancer Guides

http://www.patientresource.com/Cancer_Guides.aspx
Free guides that cover many of the major cancer types and include information about treatment options and side effects.

Breast Cancer Treatment Centers by State

https://www.patientresource.com/Breast_Cancer_Treatment_Facilities.aspx

National Cancer Institute–Designated Cancer Centers

https://www.patientresource.com/NCI_Designated_Cancer_Centers.aspx
Map of NCI cancer treatment centers.

Explaining Cancer

https://www.patientresource.com/Understanding_Cancer.aspx
Information on understanding cancer and cancer types. Topics include 10 things you should know, understanding your prescriptions, causes of cancer, cancer treatment, understanding immunotherapy, understanding radiation therapy, finding your medical team, clinical trials, basic cancer terms.

Treatment Centers and Financial Assistance Organizations in the United States
https://www.patientresource.com/Financial_Resources.aspx
Names and web address of **organizations** that offer **financial assistance** to
people affected by cancer.
Free

Psychology.com

http://www.psychology.com/
Psychology.com has a directory of licensed therapists across the country.
The website has an extensive self-help library with topics on depression,
anxiety and coping with chronic illness. Mental health topics are provided
courtesy of the National Institute of Mental Health.

Directory

http://www.psychology.com/therapist/
Directory of therapists searchable by state, ZIP code and specialty.
Free

Planned Parenthood

https://www.plannedparenthood.org/
website: *English and Spanish*
https://www.facebook.com/PlannedParenthood/
https://twitter.com/@PPFA
(800) 230-7526 / (800) 230-PLAN
Connects you to a Planned Parenthood in your area. English and Spanish
Planned Parenthood is one of the nation's leading providers of **high-
quality, affordable health care,** and it is the nation's largest provider
of sex education. More than 97% of Planned Parenthood's services are
primary and preventive health care, including lifesaving **cancer screenings,**
birth control, testing and treatment of STDs, annual exams and health
counseling. It provides **free or low-cost clinical breast exams,** checking
for changes or lumps in women's breasts. If the doctor finds something

abnormal or worth checking out, she refers the patient for a mammogram at a licensed facility. Planned Parenthood affiliates host free mammography mobile vans for low-income and uninsured women.

Find a Health Center
https://www.plannedparenthood.org/health-center.
Search for a facility near you. You can make an appointment online or by calling the number above.

Insurance
https://www.plannedparenthood.org/get-care/health-insurance.
Information on health coverage: how to sign up, what is covered and when to apply for insurance.

R

Resolve: The National Infertility Association
https://resolve.org
info@resolve.org *Email*
https://www.facebook.com/resolveinfertilityorg
https://twitter.com/resolveorg
(866) 668-2566
Helpline; messages will be returned within 48 to 72 hours.
Resolve: The National Infertility Association connects people challenged with building their family to information, resources and support.

HelpLine
https://resolve.org/support/helpful-resources/helpline/
Connect with a trained volunteer who has experience with infertility and can help you navigate the resources available to you.

Support Services
https://resolve.org/support/helpful-resources/online-support-resources/
Resolve has partnered with Inspire to connect you with people across the country to have real conversations about reproductive health and bring you support whenever, wherever, online.

Support Groups
https://resolve.org/support/find-a-support-group/
A map with locations of peer-led support groups across the country.

Coping With Infertility
https://resolve.org/support/managing-infertility-stress/coping-techniques/
Tips and information on **coping with infertility**. Learn how to get support for you and your partner.

Professional Services Directory
https://resolve.org/support/professional-services-directory/
A map with the locations of more than 600 professionals including **reproductive endocrinologists, urologists, mental health therapists** and other **family-building professionals**. Searchable by name, location and ZIP code.
Free

RxAssist.org

http://www.rxassist.org/
info@rxassist.org *Email*

RxAssist is a **resource center** with information on **patient assistance programs**. PAPs are run by pharmaceutical companies to provide **free medications** to people who cannot afford to buy their medicines. RxAssist does not operate any medication programs. RxAssist provides a PAP directory with names and phone numbers of providers that offer assistance with various services.

Medication Database Search Help

http://www.rxassist.org/help

The database can help you find out whether a drug is available, which pharmaceutical company program offers the drug and how to apply for the medication.

Patient Center

http://www.rxassist.org/patients

Patient Center provides a database to find current application forms and information on patient assistance programs.

Pharmaceutical Company Contact Information

http://www.rxassist.org/pap-info

The patient assistance program directory provides contact information for pharmaceutical companies. Patients can call them directly with questions and concerns.

Frequently Asked Questions About Patient Assistance Programs

https://www.rxassist.org/faqs

Information on patient assistance programs: who is eligible and how to apply.

RxHope

www.rxhope.com

RxHope is a **resource center** with information on **Patient Assistance Programs**. PAPs are run by pharmaceutical companies to provide **free medications** to people who cannot afford to buy their medicines. RxHope does not operate any medication programs. The site allows you to search for medication by brand name, PAP or pharmaceutical company.

Medication Search

http://www.rxassist.org/patients

Search for medication by name, patient assistance program or pharmaceutical company.

S

Save My Fertility—Michigan State University

http://www.savemyfertility.org/

https://www.facebook.com/oncofertilityconsortium/

https://twitter.com/oncofertility

(517) 884-8848

Information; voicemails will be returned typically in 24 to 48 hours.

Save My Fertility is an authoritative resource for adult cancer patients and the parents of children with cancer who want to learn more about **preserving** their **fertility before** and **during cancer treatment** and **protecting** their **hormonal health after treatment**. SaveMyFertility.org also offers information and guidance to oncologists, endocrinologists and other health-care providers concerned with the reproductive health of cancer patients and survivors.

Patient Navigator

http://preservefertility.northwestern.edu/

Provides information on options and offers tutorials on topics that include **family building, egg and embryo banking, ovarian tissue cryopreservation, normal female fertility,** and **normal male fertility.**

Downloadable Pocket Guides—Women with Cancer

http://www.savemyfertility.org/pocket-guides/patients/fertility-preservation-women-diagnosed-cancer

Understanding fertility preservation options available. The brochures are available for download at the end of each page. Guides available in English, Spanish, Chinese and Thai.

Downloadable Pocket Guides—Men With Cancer

http://www.savemyfertility.org/pocket-guides/providers/fertility-preservation-men-diagnosed-cancer

Understanding fertility preservation options available. The brochures are available for download at the end of each page. Guides available in English, Spanish, Chinese and Thai.

Global Map of Fertility Preservation Centers
https://oncofertility.msu.edu/find-a-clinic-or-center
Clinic and center finder has information to find fertility preservation centers around the world. Searchable by country and services.
Information and downloadable guides are free.

Savor Health
http://savorhealth.com/
http://savorhealth.com/about-us/contact/ *Contact form*
https://www.facebook.com/SavorHealth1
https://twitter.com/savor_health
Savor Health is **patient-specific**, evidence-based personalized **nutrition solutions** for **cancer patients** and **caregivers**.

The Heal Well: A Cancer Nutrition Guide
http://savor.static.assets.s3.amazonaws.com/pdfs/Heal_Well_Cancer%20 Guide_2015-web.pdf
General information on **nutrition** and **cancer**. Addresses common questions people have about diet, nutrition and physical activity during and after cancer treatment, and offers suggestions for common cancer or cancer treatment–related symptom management.

Curated Information
http://savorhealth.com/consumer/curatedinformationandresources/
The oncology **nutrition** experts sort through the overwhelming amount of data about cancer and nutrition and help you turn that information into action. They share ideas on **dining out**; healthy meals and snacks with minimal preparation; key studies on nutrition, cancer and fitness.

Nutritional Counseling

https://savorhealth.com/product-category/counseling/
Registered oncology dietitians who are board-certified specialists in oncology nutrition guide you through cancer treatment to ensure you get the nutrition your body needs, and they help you manage the nutrition-related side effects of your treatment.
Fees apply.

SHARE Cancer Support

www.sharecancersupport.org
website: *English, Spanish and Japanese*
info@sharecancersupport.org *Email*
helpline@sharecancersupport.org *Email helpline*
https://www.sharecancersupport.org/metastatic-breast-cancer/helpline/
Contact form – metastatic breast cancer
https://www.facebook.com/SHARECancerSupport
https://twitter.com/SHAREing
(844) 275-7427 (844-ASK-SHARE)
Helpline, Monday – Friday, 9:00 AM – 9:00 PM; Saturday – Sunday 9:00 AM – 5:00 PM ET. English and Spanish; ten additional languages available. Messages left are returned within 24 hours.
SHARE Cancer Support provides dedicated, experienced **support** for women facing **breast, ovarian** and **uterine or endometrial cancer.** The organization offers a **helpline, support groups, webinars, seminars** and lectures for newly diagnosed and young women with breast cancer, as well as women with advanced or metastatic breast cancer and caregivers and LGBT patients. It also has a support network that connects women diagnosed with breast or ovarian cancer with others who share similar diagnoses and experiences.

Dial-In and Videoconference Support Groups

https://www.sharecancersupport.org/calendar/support-groups/

Patients are part of a group without having to leave the comfort of their home. Call the helpline number above to register.

Online Support Communities

https://healthunlocked.com/login/share1

SHARE partnered with HealthUnlocked to create three **online support communities: breast cancer, metastatic breast cancer, ovarian cancer.**

Online Educational Programs

https://www.sharecancersupport.org/calendar/online-educational-programs/

Topics include **triple negative breast cancer, telehealth and breast cancer, stress reduction** and **exercise, pain, new developments in treatment, cannabis for medical disorders** and **preparing for loss.** Extensive library of programs; topics include but are not limited to **vaccines** and the future of cancer treatment, **age bias** in cancer care, **communities of color** and participation in breast cancer research, **sexuality** after cancer, persistent and intermittent **pain after breast cancer treatment** and tumor dormancy.

Publications

https://www.sharecancersupport.org/toolsresources/share-publications/

Free downloadable novellas, brochures and booklets with information on breast cancer.

Metastatic Trial Search

https://www.sharecancersupport.org/metastatic-breast-cancer/clinical-trial-matching-service/

Searchable by demographic, breast cancer type and the area of the body with current evidence of disease.

Services are free.

Sharsheret

http://sharsheret.org/

https://sharsheret.org/who-we-are/contact-us/ *Contact form*

https://www.facebook.com/sharsheret.org/

https://twitter.com/sharsheret

(866) 474-2774

Helpline, Monday – Thursday, 9:00 AM – 5:00 PM; Friday 9:00 AM – 1:30 PM ET

LiveChat 24/7

Pop-up window on the website.

Sharsheret supports **young Jewish women** and families facing **breast** and **ovarian cancer.**

Peer Support

https://sharsheret.org/resource/connect-with-a-peer-supporter/

Peer-to-peer support network that connects women newly diagnosed or at high risk of developing breast or ovarian cancer with others who share similar diagnoses and experiences.

Genetic Councilors

https://sharsheret.org/resource/speak-with-our-genetic-counselor/

Clinical team of trained skilled **mental health professionals** and **genetic counselors** are available to speak privately with you at any point in your cancer experience.

Hereditary Risk Family Support

https://sharsheret.org/resource/family-conference-call/

Confidential, **psychosocial support** and information to empower women and their families to better **understand** their **individual circumstances, cope with unique challenges** and **make informed decisions.**

Family, Friends and Caregivers Support

https://sharsheret.org/what-we-do/support-family-friends-and-caregivers/
Speak directly and confidentially with skilled social workers and learn about other cancer organizations to help you understand the diagnosis and treatment of breast cancer and the support options available to you.

Brochures and Booklets

https://sharsheret.org/resource/brochures-booklets/
Culturally relevant brochures and booklets.

The Best Face Forward

https://sharsheret.org/resource/best-face-forward/
A kit designed for women who are diagnosed with breast cancer and ovarian cancer, and who are currently undergoing chemotherapy or radiation therapy. The kit includes **makeup products** for all skin tones, easy-to-follow **makeup application instructions**, and **tips** for those facing **hair loss** and **changes in skin tone**.

Busy Box

https://sharsheret.org/resource/communicating-with-young-children/
Resource materials to **educate parents** about the **affect of breast** and **ovarian cancer on children**. Also included is a starter kit of games and activities for children.
Services, brochures, booklets and kits are free.

Social Security Administration

https://www.ssa.gov/
website: *English and Spanish*
Information found on the website is available in 12 languages including sign language.
https://www.facebook.com/socialsecurity/
https://twitter.com/socialsecurity/
(800) 772-1213

Information, Monday through Friday, 7:00 AM – 7:00 PM ET. English and Spanish. Free translation services for additional languages.

(800) 325-0778 TTY

The **Social Security Administration** is a **federal insurance program** that pays benefits to people who cannot work because of a medical condition that is expected to last at least a year or result in death. Social Security is not available for partial or short-term disability.

Information

https://www.ssa.gov/onlineservices/

Apply for retirement, disability and Medicare benefits online; check the status of an application or appeal; request a replacement Social Security card (in most areas); print a benefit verification letter; and more.

Online Booklet—Disability Benefits

https://www.ssa.gov/pubs/EN-05-10029.pdf

Information on who is eligible, how to apply and what you need to know about the benefits.

Soul Source Therapeutic Devices

https://www.soulsource.com/

https://www.soulsource.com/pages/contact-us *Contact form*

https://www.facebook.com/soulsourcedilators

https://twitter.com/SoulSourceTD

(888) 325-5870

Messages left will be returned ASAP.

Soul Source Therapeutic Devices specializes in **vaginal dilators**. A sex therapist and gynecologist created the dilators to help women undergoing progressive vaginal dilation therapy. All products are manufactured in the United States.

Check website for prices.

Stupid Cancer

http://www.stupidcancer.org

https://www.facebook.com/stupidcancer

https://twitter.com/stupidcancer

Stupid Cancer makes young adult cancer suck less for people **ages 15** to **39.** The organization addresses young adult cancer through advocacy, research, support, outreach, awareness, mobile health and social media.

CancerCon

http://cancercon.org/

Annual gathering for the young adult cancer movement. CancerCon has gone digital in 2021 and will return to live events in 2022.

Webinars

https://stupidcancer.org/webinars

Sessions include but are not limited to **body image, talking to your children, health, wellness, mental health, living with cancer, stress, getting active, sexual health, meditation** and **trauma.**

Stupid Cancer Show

https://www.youtube.com/user/stupidcancer

An award-winning talk radio podcast that gave voice to the nascent young adult cancer movement and elevated the cause.

Free

Susan G. Komen

https://www.komen.org/

helpline@komen.org *Email*

clinicaltrialinfo@komen.org *Email; specially trained oncology social workers*

https://www.facebook.com/SusanGKomen

https://twitter.com/SusanGKomen

(877) 465-6636

Helpline, Monday – Friday, 9:00 AM – 10:00 PM ET; 6:00 AM – 7:00 PM PT. English and Spanish

Susan G. Komen provides **information, resources, education** and **support** services to anyone with breast health and breast cancer concerns, including **breast cancer patients** and their **families.** The helpline provides information, **psychosocial support** and information about national and local organizations and **resources** that may provide **financial assistance** and other support services, including **low-cost mammography** and **support groups**.

Breast Cancer Information

https://www.komen.org/breast-cancer/
Information on breast cancer risk factors, screening, diagnosis, treatment, metastatic breast cancer and survivorship.

Tools and Resources

https://www.komen.org/support-resources/tools/
This section has information about the Komen Breast Care Helpline, as well as educational materials, toolkits, interactive resources and more.

Treatment Assistance Program

https://www.komen.org/treatment-assistance-program/
Information on eligibility, program overview and applying for assistance.

Men With Breast Cancer

https://www.komen.org/breast-cancer/facts-statistics/male-breast-cancer/
Information for **men** with **breast cancer** including types, genetic testing, treatment, surgery and radiation, hormone therapy and clinical trials.

Support for Men With Breast Cancer

Susan G. Komen offers **free six-week telephone support groups for men with breast cancer.** To learn more, call the helpline number above or email helpline@komen.org.

Videos

https://www.komen.org/support-resources/tools/komen-education-materials/videos/

Information on breast cancer screening, diagnosis, treatment, living with metastatic breast cancer and survivorship through **short** informative **videos**.

Translated Videos

https://www.komen.org/support-resources/tools/translations/

Videos translated into more than **40 languages including sign language**. *Services are free.*

T

Telling Kids About Cancer

http://www.tellingkidsaboutcancer.com/

Telling Kids About Cancer is an **online tool** to help parents tell their children they have cancer. It provides age-appropriate advice and information on talking with children, a **step-by-step tool** to create your own **conversation guide** and advice on how to prepare, when to talk and how to follow up. The tool includes stories and audiotapes from other parents on their experience. *Free*

Tender Loving Care

http://www.tlcdirect.org/

customerservice@tlcdirect.org *Email*

(800) 850-9445

Customer care line, seven days a week, 8:00 AM – 11:00 PM CT

Tender Loving Care is an online catalog of the American Cancer Society with **wigs, bras, clothing** and **accessories** for breast cancer patients. The guide will give you an idea of what most patients consider essential when they are setting out on their cancer journey.

Check website for prices.

Triage Cancer

https://triagecancer.org/
Info@triagecancer.org *Email*
https://www.facebook.com/TriageCancer
https://twitter.com/TriageCancer
(424) 258-4628
Messages will be returned ASAP.
Triage Cancer is a national nonprofit organization that provides education on the **practical and legal issues** that may affect individuals diagnosed with cancer and their caregivers.

Quick Guides

https://triagecancer.org/cancer-resources-and-educational-information/quickguides
Quick guides and checklists that offer legal and practical information about **health insurance, finances and financial toxicity, estate planning and medical decision-making, employment and work, and disability insurance.**

Resources and Webinars

https://triagecancer.org/resources-by-topic
Information on **navigating health care, stress management, psychosocial care, legal issues, caregiving, exercise, clinical trials** and **employment.**

Triple Negative Breast Cancer Foundation—Cancer*Care*.org

www.tnbcfoundation.org
https://www.cancercare.org
TNBCHelpline@cancercare.org *Contact form*
https://www.facebook.com/TNBCFoundation
https://twitter.com/TNBCFoundation
(800) 813-4673 / (877) 880-8622
Helpline, English and Spanish, Monday – Thursday 10:00 AM – 6:00 PM, Friday, 10:00 AM – 5:00 PM ET

The Triple Negative Breast Cancer Foundation (TNBC) partnered with Cancer*Care* to provide **information, support** and **resources** for patients and families coping with a diagnosis of **triple negative breast cancer.**

Living with TNBC
https://tnbcfoundation.org/living-with-tnbc
News and information about **living with TNBC,** treatment options and survivorship through articles and downloadable **guidebooks.**

Webinars
https://tnbcfoundation.org/living-with-tnbc/webinars
Information on **coping, clinical trials, advancements, fear of recurrence, standard of care,** precision medicine, updates on TNBC and more.

Caregivers
https://tnbcfoundation.org/living-with-tnbc/caregivers
Information to help the caregiver support the patient and themselves. *Services are free.*

U

Ulman Cancer Fund for Young Adults
http://ulmanfund.org
info@ulmanfund.org *Email*
https://www.facebook.com/ulmanfoundation
https://twitter.com/ulmanfoundation
(888) 393-3863, extension 105 / (410) 964-0202, extension 125
Information, Monday – Friday, 9:00 AM –5:00 PM ET. English and Spanish
The **Ulman Cancer Fund for Young Adults** is a patient navigation service for **young adult cancer patients** and **survivors.** It provides **information, resources** and **support** addressing various needs of young adults who face a cancer diagnosis, treatment and life with cancer.

No Way, It Can't Be Guidebook

http://ulmanfund.org/ucfguidebook/

Information on how young adults affected by cancer and their family and friends can face what lies ahead. Practical information about **medical care, education, relationships, emotional challenges, health and wellness, survivorship** and other topics relevant to the young adult cancer experience. The **guidebook** has usable and **practical tools** to help young adults and their families keep detailed records and documentation of their cancer treatment. *Services and guidebook are free.*

U.S. Department of Labor

Family Leave and Medical Act

https://www.dol.gov

https://blog.dol.gov/

(866) 487-2365

Information and referral service, Monday – Friday, 8:00 AM – 8:00 PM ET. Teletypewriter (TTY), English and Spanish

The Department of Labor's Wage and Hour Division administers the wage, hour and child labor laws of the **Fair Labor Standards Act.** The Family Leave and Medical Act was established for eligible employees of covered employers to take unpaid, job-protected leave for specified family and medical reasons with continuation of group health insurance coverage under the same terms and conditions as if the employee had not taken leave.

Family Leave and Medical Act

https://www.dol.gov/general/topic/benefits-leave/fmla

Education and information on FMLA.

Fact Sheets

https://www.dol.gov/agencies/whd/fmla

Information and **general guidance, fact sheets, e-tools, forms, interpretive guides, applicable laws** and **regulations** on FLMA.

Continuation of Health Coverage, COBRA
https://www.dol.gov/agencies/ebsa/laws-and-regulations/laws/cobra
Information on the **Consolidated Omnibus Budget Reconciliation Act,** which gives workers and their families who lose their health benefits the right to choose to continue group health benefits provided by their group health plan for limited periods of time under certain circumstances such as voluntary or involuntary job loss, reduction in the hours worked, transition between jobs, death, divorce and other life events.

U.S. Equal Employment Opportunity Commission

https://www.eeoc.gov
info@eeoc.gov *Email*
www.facebook.com/USEEOC
https://twitter.com/useeoc/
(800) 669-4000
Information line
(800) 669-6820
TTY for deaf and hard-of-hearing callers only.
(844) 234-5122
ASL video phone for deaf and hard-of-hearing callers only
The **U.S. Equal Employment Opportunity Commission** is responsible for enforcing federal laws that make it **illegal to discriminate** against a job applicant or an employee because of the **person's race, color, religion, sex** (including pregnancy, gender identity and sexual orientation), **national origin, age** (40 or older), **disability** or genetic information. The laws apply to all types of work situations, including hiring, firing, promotions, harassment, training, wages and benefit.

How to File a Charge

https://www.eeoc.gov/how-file-charge-employment-discrimination
Free

U.S. Food and Drug Administration

www.fda.gov

website: *English and Spanish*

https://www.facebook.com/FDA

https://twitter.com/US_FDA

(888) 463-6332

Information; messages left will be returned ASAP.

The **U.S. Food and Drug Administration** is a federal agency of the U.S. Department of Health and Human Services. The FDA is responsible for protecting the public health by ensuring the safety, efficacy and security of human and veterinary drugs, biological products and medical devices, and by ensuring the safety of our nation's food supply, cosmetics and products that emit radiation. The FDA advances public health by helping to speed innovations that make medical products more effective, safer and more affordable and by helping the public get the accurate, science-based information they need to use medical products and foods to maintain and improve their health.

Certified Mammography Facilities

https://www.accessdata.fda.gov/scripts/cdrh/cfdocs/cfMQSA/mqsa.cfm. Directory of **mammogram facilities** certified by the FDA, or certifying state, as meeting baseline quality standards for equipment, personnel, and practices under the Mammography Quality Standards Act of 1992 and subsequent Mammography Quality Standards Reauthorization Act amendments.

University of California San Francisco Medical Center

https://www.ucsfhealth.org/secondopinion

https://www.facebook.com/UCSFMedicalCenter

https://twitter.com/UCSFHospitals

(800) 941-1383

Information; Grand Rounds Digital Health Care Company, partners of the University of California San Francisco Medical Center on the second opinion program. Monday – Friday, 6:00 AM – 6:00 PM PT

(775) 440-2557

International Information; Grand Rounds Digital Health Care Company, partners of the University of California San Francisco Medical Center on the second opinion program.

University of California San Francisco Medical Center provides an **online second opinion** program that offers patients access to leading specialists at UCSF Medical Center, no matter where they live. The program is coordinated through Grand Rounds, a digital health-care company that connects patients with local and remote specialty care.

Getting Started

https://www.grandrounds.com/ucsfhealth.

A patient begins by creating an online account then submits her medical records and information. Grand Rounds Digital Health collects all the medical records and chooses the most appropriate doctor from UCSF Medical Center to review the patient's case. The physician reviews the documents then provides a written second opinion for the patient. You will be assigned a personal care coordinator and staff physician from Grand Rounds to assist you throughout the process. Does not accept insurance. Check with insurance company for coverage. *Fees apply.*

The Upside to Everything Life Coaching

www.theupsidetoeverything.com

theresa@theupsidetoeverything.com Email

https://www.facebook.com/theupsidetoeverything/

https://twitter.com/upsidetoeveryt1

https://www.instagram.com/theupsidetoeverything/

https://www.linkedin.com/in/theresadrescher/

(917) 545-0630

Information and appointments

Theresa Drescher is a **life coach,** founder of The Upside to Everything Coaching and author of *The Upside to Everything, Even Breast Cancer.*

Life Coaching

https://theupsidetoeverything.com/coaching-overview

For 15 years, **Theresa Drescher** coached people who were dealing with the terror of cancer, helping them **find** their **purpose, organize** their **chaos, persevere through painful obstacles** and **strategize about life changes.** She supported them as they made difficult decisions and were challenged by outside forces, and she helped them recognize their strengths. It is that experience, knowledge and empathy she offers in her coaching.

Contact for prices.

The US Oncology Network

https://www.usoncology.com

The US Oncology Network is an association of oncologists who provide medical care in cancer centers in the United States. The website provides a **listing of oncology centers** searchable by ZIP code, city or state, and a database of current and ongoing clinical trials.

Find a Location

https://www.usoncology.com/patients/find-a-location

Directory of oncology centers across the United States.

Find a Clinical Trial

https://www.usoncology.com/patients/clinical-trial-search

Clinical trials taking place by state and by disease. It provides information on the trial and the oncology practice conducting the trial.

Free

W

Walgreens Heart Beat Program

https://www.walgreens.com/topic/pharmacy/specialty-pharmacy/fertility-services.jsp

(800) 424-9002
Information and support from pharmacists and nurses 24/7
(888) 347-3415
Information, Heart Beat Program
Walgreens Heart Beat Program, along with Ferring Pharmaceuticals, provides you with **select fertility products** for your fertility preservation treatment at **no cost**. The fertility services provide support from pharmacists and nurses 24/7 including holidays. Additional services include same-day emergency service, insurance verification, overnight shipping and interactive educational tools. *Terms and conditions apply.*

Well Spouse Association

http://www.wellspouse.org
info@wellspouse.org *Email*
https://www.facebook.com/WellSpouseAssociation
https://twitter.com/WellspouseOrg
(732) 577-8899
Information, referral line, Monday – Thursday, 9:00 AM – 2:00 PM ET
Well Spouse Association is a membership organization that advocates for and addresses the needs of individuals caring for a **chronically ill** or **disabled spouse or partner**. The website provides resources for coping and survival skills, including an online chat forum for spousal caregivers. Coordinates a national network of support groups and facilitates a mentor program. WSA is only for spousal caregivers.
Membership fee applies. Assistance for membership fee available.

Support Groups
https://wellspouse.org/support-groups/telephone-support-groups.html
Peer-to-peer support for the special challenges and unique issues "well" spouses face every day. Support is directed for those who are in an ongoing caregiving situation, not for people in crisis.

Wikihow—Make-a-Vision-Board

http://www.wikihow.com/Make-a-Vision-Board

Step-by-step how to make a vision board.

Free

Wigs & Wishes

http://www.wigsandwishes.org

info@wigsandwishes.org *Email*

https://wigsandwishes.org/contact-us.php *Contact form*

https://www.facebook.com/WIGSandWISHES/

https://twitter.com/wigsandwishes

(856) 582-6600

Information, Monday – Friday, 9:00 AM – 5:00 PM ET

Wigs & Wishes provides **free wigs** to individuals battling cancer. A network of participating salons and stylists throughout the world donate wigs and **styling services to women** undergoing treatment for cancer. Wishes are granted to children battling cancer.

Request a Wig

https://wigsandwishes.org/request-a-wig.php

Information on how to request a wig.

Services are free.

Y

Young Survivors Coalition

www.youngsurvival.org

info@youngsurvival.org *Email*

https://www.youngsurvival.org/forms/contact-us *Contact form*

https://www.facebook.com/youngsurvivalcoalition

https://twitter.com/YSCBUZZ

(877) 972-1011

Information, Monday – Friday, 9:00 AM – 5:00 PM ET

Young Survivors Coalition provides **information, resources** and support for **young women** diagnosed in their **20s** with all stages of **breast cancer**. It offers **one-on-one support** by connecting young women with a peer diagnosed with breast cancer in their early 20s.

About Breast Cancer

https://www.youngsurvival.org/learn/about-breast-cancer
Information on breast cancer in young women. Download a guide to learn the **basics of breast cancer,** including the **signs** and **symptoms, risk factors** and what to do if you notice any changes in your own breasts.

Living With Breast Cancer

https://www.youngsurvival.org/learn/living-with-breast-cancer
Learn about your options, **understanding treatment, living with metastatic breast cancer, quality of life, fertility** and **family planning,** and tips for working with your health-care team.

Educational Materials and Resource Guides

https://www.youngsurvival.org/learn/resources-and-tools/educational-materials
Download breast cancer educational resources or order print copies.

One-on-One Support

https://www.youngsurvival.org/talk-one-on-one
Talk **one-on-one** with trained peer **mentors** who are young adults from all backgrounds and who volunteer as an empathetic listener.

Online Support

https://www.youngsurvival.org/connect
Find online support through virtual hangouts and Facebook.

Newly Diagnosed

https://www.youngsurvival.org/forms/newly-diagnosed-navigator

A cancer navigator guide that provides extensive practical information on diagnosis, decisions, treatment, daily living and quality of life for young women diagnosed with breast cancer.

Audio-Video Library

https://www.youngsurvival.org/learn/resources-and-tools/audio-video-library-

Extensive **audio-video library** that includes the following topics: breast cancer and young women; breast cancer by type; treatment, surgery, and reconstruction; clinical trials; emotional wellness; family, dating and relationships; all of you: sex, intimacy and body image; family planning and pregnancy; navigating end-of-life issues.

Resources

https://www.youngsurvival.org/directory

Directory of guides and resources for the **young cancer patient**.

COVID and Breast Cancer

https://www.youngsurvival.org/covid

Resources, information and community support for young adults diagnosed with breast cancer in the midst of the ongoing pandemic.

Services are free.

Afterword: Breast Health

I realize that by the time many of you get to this section, you will already know—or have lived through—what is written here. I have included this information to make it easy for you to share it with others.

There is no foolproof way to prevent a breast cancer diagnosis, but there are five simple steps you can take to help detect it earlier:

1. Know what your healthy breasts look like
2. Understand what factors increase your risk
3. Recognize the symptoms
4. Get annual breast exams
5. Have routine mammograms

Early detection is not a cure, but it can give you more treatment options and may make the outcome more successful.

Know your breasts

Everyone has breasts. They come in different sizes, shapes and colors. When we are young, they are round and plump, the skin is smooth, and they are sensitive. Like the rest of our body, they change as we age. They lose their firmness and sensitivity and can decrease in size. Their elasticity diminishes, which causes them to sag and the nipples to point downward. Fat replaces dense breast tissue as our ovaries produce less estrogen, which may cause soft, benign lumps to appear in areas that were once smooth.

These changes are normal. What is important is to know when something is not. The best way to do that is to know what your breasts normally look and feel like. What may be typical for one woman, such as an inverted nipple, may be atypical for another. Some women get cysts in their breasts before their period that then disappear when their cycle ends. There are women whose breasts ache and are sensitive to touch during their period but feel fine the rest of the month. When you know what is usual for you, something different or abnormal will stand out.

To be knowledgeable about your breasts takes more than a quick glance when getting dressed or swift feel when bathing. Our breasts are multifaceted and are made up of milk ducts, lobes, lobules, fibrous connective tissue, fatty tissue, nerves, lymph vessels, lymph nodes and blood vessels. They need your undivided attention if you are really going to know them. Once you establish a baseline of what they look and feel like, your routine breast checks will be more productive. If something new or different appears, keep an eye on it. If it persists for two or more weeks, make an appointment with your breast doctor if you have one. If not, see your gynecologist or general physician to have it checked out.

The experts at John Hopkins Medicine (https://www.hopkinsmedicine .org) say it is important to do a self-breast exam the same time every month. During the month, your hormone levels fluctuate. This causes changes in your breast tissue. Swelling you may experience during the month decreases when your period starts. When you do the exam at the same time, you will be able to distinguish between something that is normal and something that feels different. They recommend premenopausal women do a self-breast exam toward the end of your period. For postmenopausal women, they suggest you do the exam on the same date every month.

Begin with a baseline self-exam, get naked from the waist up, stand in front of a mirror and look at your breasts. Take each one in from the front and side view. Is one higher or bigger than the other? Do your nipples point forward, to the side or down, or does one or both turn inward? What color are your areolas? Do they have bumps around them, other than when you're cold? Are there any dimples anywhere?

Once you have observed what your breasts look like, the next step is to feel them. Hold them in your hands, and squeeze them. Note if you feel bumps or cysts anywhere. Squeeze your nipple for any discharge, and feel for any lumps. Next, lift your right arm straight over your head, or bend it at the elbow and let your hand hover over the left side of your head, and walk the pad of the fingers on your left hand in small circles over your right breast. Start with light pressure on your skin as you move your fingers over your entire breast. Walk your fingers over it a second time, increasing the pressure. The third time, use stronger pressure, so you can feel deep in your breast. Go all the way over to the hollow area under your arm at the shoulder. Glide the palm of your hand over the skin of your breast and check for areas that may be rough or thick. Do this exam once with your arm over your head and again with your hand on your hip.

Repeat the exercise on your left side, starting with your left arm over your head. When you are done checking your breasts standing up, do it lying on your back. Put a pillow under your right shoulder, lift your right arm above your head and do the exam again. Then move to your left side, and follow the same steps. Doing the exam standing and lying on your back will give you a good standard to go by.

Over the years, there has been a running debate on the value of breast self-examinations (BSE.) Below are two examples of the discussion:

"BSE has been compared with no screening and has been shown to have no benefit in reducing breast cancer mortality."

—*National Cancer Institute*

"Adult women of all ages are encouraged to perform breast self-exams at least once a month. While a mammogram can help you detect cancer before you can feel a lump, 40 percent of diagnosed breast cancers are detected by women who feel a lump, so establishing a regular breast self-exam is very important."

—*Johns Hopkins Medicine*

The decision to perform a monthly breast self-exam is up to you. I wish I were more diligent about doing them. I am still skittish all these years later about finding a lump or another symptom, so I rely on my doctors. I make sure to space my breast surgeon and gynecologist—both do a thorough breast exam for me once a year—six months apart, then I occasionally do a self-exam in between.

Many women have dense breast tissue. That describes the way their tissue appears on a mammogram. It is normal and has nothing to do with the weight, size or firmness of their breasts or how they feel. It means more fibrous connective tissue appears than fatty tissue. It is typically seen in younger women, those with a low body-fat percentage or women on hormone replacement therapy (HRT).

Dense breast tissue shows up white on the images the same way cancer does. This similarity in appearance can make it more difficult to spot something out of the ordinary. Having dense breasts does not mean you will be diagnosed with cancer, but it may make it harder to detect. Discuss your options with your doctor. Talk to him about your and your family's medical history. He may request additional screenings such as a breast MRI—an imaging test that uses powerful magnets and radio waves to create images of the breast and the surrounding tissue—an ultrasound or a 3D mammogram. He also may increase the frequency of your screenings or your physical exams, so he can closely monitor you.

If your doctor has not mentioned dense breast tissue to you, ask him about it after your next mammogram. Not all women have dense breasts, but some doctors do not readily tell their patients when they do. That is changing as more than half the states across the country now legally require a patient be notified of her breast density after a mammogram. Are You Dense? Advocacy Inc. (https://www.areyoudenseadvocacy.org) is an organization working to ensure that women with dense breasts are given information and provided options for early detection.

Tip

Many women have dense breast tissue. That describes the way their tissue appears on a mammogram. It is normal and has nothing to do with the weight, size or firmness of their breasts or how they feel.

Its website provides a state-by-state guide to density reporting laws. Inquire at your next visit if you have dense breasts. Do not assume because your doctor has not discussed it with you that you do not have them.

Breast cancer risks

A risk factor is anything that increases your chances of developing a disease. It does not mean you will get the illness. But you should be aware of them and let your doctor know what might put you at high-risk, so he can more closely monitor your breast health.

Below are risks that increase your chance of a diagnosis:

- Gender: Women are more likely to get breast cancer than men, but 1 percent of all breast cancer patients are men
- Age: Most people diagnosed are over the age of fifty-five, but younger women and men are diagnosed with breast cancer
- Genetics: mutated BRCA1 or BRCA2 gene (breast cancer 1 and breast cancer 2 gene)Women who have inherited these genetic changes are at an increased risk for breast, ovarian and colon cancer. Both men and women carry BRCA1 and BRCA2 genes, and both parents can pass them down to their children
- Having a personal history of breast cancer: Women diagnosed with breast cancer are at higher risk of being diagnosed again
- Radiation therapy to the breast or chest: Women who had radiation therapy to the chest before age thirty for Hodgkin disease, non-Hodgkin lymphoma, or other cancers are at a higher risk for developing breast cancer in the future
- Race or ethnicity: Caucasian women have a slightly higher risk for developing breast cancer than women of color, but women of color are less likely to do as well as white women when they get it
- Long menstrual history: An early period, before twelve years old, and/ or late menopause, after fifty-five years of age, increases a woman's risk
- Using HRT: Hormone replacement medication helps alleviate menopausal symptoms such as hot flashes

- Being overweight or obese: Women who are overweight or obese have a higher chance of being diagnosed than those who are at a normal weight
- Excessive alcohol use: Women who drink more than one drink a day are at higher risk of being diagnosed with breast cancer
- Not being physically active: Lack of exercise or activity puts a woman at higher risk
- Not having children or having children over the age of thirty-five: Late pregnancy or not having children can increase a woman's risk of developing breast cancer
- Not breast-feeding: Breast-feeding reduces the risk of developing breast cancer

How to reduce your risk

The good news is there are some risks you have control over and can reduce.
- Limit your alcohol use: Reduce your intake to one drink a day
- Increase your daily activity: Simple examples—park farther away from the entrance to a store or your office, take the stairs at work instead of the elevator, ride a bike to work
- Avoid the use of HRTs
- Maintain a healthy body weight: Balance your activity with the amount of food you eat
- Breast-feed if you are having children: Breast-feeding for one and a half to two years reduces the chances of developing breast cancer. This includes pumping

Breast cancer symptoms

A symptom is an indicator of something out of the ordinary. Following are symptoms of breast cancer. The symptoms for breast cancer are the same for men as they are for women.
- A lump or mass; most common
- Swelling anywhere on the breast, even if no lump is felt

- Red, hot or swollen breast
- Scaliness or thickening of the nipple or breast skin
- Skin irritation or dimpling of the skin. It sometimes looks like an orange peel
- Breast or nipple pain
- A discharge from the nipple other than breast milk
- Inverted nipple: A nipple that turns inward—if this is not normal for you. Some people are born with an inverted nipple
- Swelling under the arm where your lymph nodes are located.

Breast cancer can spread to the lymph nodes and cause a lump or swelling before the original tumor in the breast is large enough to be felt

Although any of these symptoms can be caused by something other than breast cancer, they need to be investigated quickly—preferably by a breast surgeon; but if one is not available, go to your gynecologist or primary care physician. The doctor will give you a physical examination, review your and your family's medical history, and possibly requests more tests.

Many women do not have any symptoms of breast cancer or a history of the disease among their first-degree relatives (mother, daughter, sister.) Every woman needs to stay on top of her breast health.

How breast cancer is diagnosed

Breast cancer screening starts with a mammogram. It is an X-ray of the breast using a very low dose of radiation. The screening may show something atypical, but a diagnosis cannot be made until a doctor performs a biopsy and takes a tissue sample. A pathologist examines the tissue and determines if it is cancerous and what type, and if positive, recommends the best course of action to address it.

There are two types of mammograms: screening and diagnostic. A screening mammogram is part of a routine health checkup. It is usually two or more images of each breast. A radiologist studies the images for tumors or abnormalities that cannot be felt.

A diagnostic mammogram is done to further study an abnormality that has been found, such as a lump, pain or discharge. It is also what is done for someone with a personal history of breast cancer. The same mammogram machine is used, but more images are taken and from several different angles. The technician can also magnify suspicious areas to produce more-detailed images to help the doctor determine a diagnosis. Check with your insurance carrier for your plan coverage for a diagnostic mammogram. Insurance companies usually do not cover the full cost of the scan. You may have to pay some of the charge.

Digital mammography and traditional mammography both use X-rays to produce an image of the breast. The difference: For traditional mammography, the image is stored on film; for digital mammography, the image is stored as a computer file. The procedure for a digital and a traditional mammogram is the same. The benefit of a digital mammogram is the ability to manipulate the image to enhance or magnify an area for further review. In addition, digital images can be easily shared electronically between breast surgeons and radiologists.

Three-D mammography, also called breast tomosynthesis (tomo, for short), takes multiple X-rays of the breast to create a three-dimensional image on a computer. It is the same exam with the breast compressed between two plates. The only difference a patient may notice is it takes a few more seconds to complete. It is your doctor's preference, traditional or 3D mammogram, that will determine which one you get. Not all insurance companies cover the 3D technology yet. Check with yours before you schedule a screening.

An MRI takes multiple images of the breast that are combined on a computer to create detailed pictures. An MRI supplements a mammogram. Some of the reasons a doctor might recommend an MRI: You have been diagnosed with cancer and need additional screening, have a history of the disease, have a strong family history of breast or ovarian cancer, or have dense breast tissue.

A breast ultrasound uses sound waves to create a black-and-white image of breast tissues and structures. The image produced is called a sonogram. It is helpful when monitoring existing lumps or looking to see if one is filled with fluid or if it is solid. Ultrasounds are also used when performing guided needle biopsies.

As a preventive measure, some women choose to have a bilateral mastectomy to decrease the chances of ever being diagnosed or to reduce their possibility of a recurrence. Although removing both breasts has shown to reduce the chance of a diagnosis by as much as 95 percent, it does not take the chance away completely. Breast cancer can still return to the chest area. If you had a bilateral mastectomy and reconstruction, a mammogram is not necessary, according to the American Cancer Society, (https://www.cancer.org) and CancerCancer.org (https://www.cancercare .org/), but consult with your doctor before making that decision. Some women get an MRI after a single or double mastectomy. Discuss with him what your follow-up care should be.

Have a plan

What to do with all this information? Make an appointment with your doctor, and put together a plan for your breast health. It is simple to do and could save your life.

Find out if there was breast, ovarian or colon cancer on either your mother's or father's side of the family. Any details you can find out are helpful: age when diagnosed; type of cancer; stage diagnosed; if the relative passed, was it the cause of death? It is okay if you do not have a lot of details. Share whatever you know with your doctor. Tell him your health history and what might put you at high risk. Let him know if you have ever felt cysts or abnormalities in your breasts. Discuss with him when you should begin getting mammograms and how often you should have one if you do not had one before.

Together, the two of you can create a plan that makes sense for you. It can always be amended in the future, but you will have a course to follow. If something unusual appears, you will have a timeline and history with helpful information to address it.Make a point to understand the facts about breast health and breast cancer. If you hear something that concerns you or the information sounds questionable, the best place to start is with your doctor. Call his office, or make a note to ask him your questions at your next appointment. A cancer helpline is also a good source for information and to help dispel myths about breast cancer. (See Badass Cancer Resources, Cancer Information, page 244; Patient Support—Helplines, Peer-to-Peer, Live Chats, page 254.)

Your first line of defense against breast cancer starts with you. Education is your best path to taking care of yourself.

Tip

Your first line of defense against breast cancer starts with you. Education is your best path to taking care of yourself.

Recommended Books

Daring Greatly: How the Courage to Be Vulnerable Transforms the Way We Live, Love, Parent and Lead by Berne Brown, Ph.D., LMSW

E2: 9 Do-it-Yourself Energy Experiments That Prove Your Thoughts Create Your Reality by Pam Grant

Full Catastrophe Living: Using the Wisdom of Your Body and Mind to Face Stress, Pain and Illness by Jon Kabat-Zinn

The Last Lecture by Randy Pausch
Achieving your childhood dreams

Little Book of Mindfulness: 10 Minutes a Day to Less Stress, More Peace by Patricia Collard

Mindfulness in Plain English by Bhante Gunaratana

Peace Is Every Step by Thich Nhat Hahn
A guide to mindful living

The Sexy Librarian's Big Book of Erotica by Rose Caraway
Offers twenty-two short stories from dirty fairy tales to sexy dominatrix to inspire your sex life

The Phantom Tollbooth by Jules Feiffer
Stay open to possibilities and never stop learning

The Power of Now by Eckart Tolle
A guide to living in the now

Taking the Leap by Pema Chodron
Lessons in how to work with emotions rather than get rid of them

This Is Water by David Foster Wallace
We have a choice in how we think

When Breath Becomes Air by Paul Kalanithi
Approaching death with grace

Wherever You Go, There You Are: Mindfulness Meditation in Everyday Life
by Jon Kabat-Zinn, Ph.D.

Glossary

A

abscess: A swollen area within body tissue, containing an accumulation of pus. An abscess is a sign of infection.

acupressure: A technique of complementary and alternative medicine that uses the fingers or thumbs on the same pressure points as acupuncture to alleviate pain and other symptoms. Also known as shiatsu.

acupuncture: A technique of complementary and alternative medicine that involves pricking the skin or tissues with needles to alleviate pain and other symptoms.

adenocarcinoma: Cancer that begins in gland-forming tissue. Most cancers of the breast, pancreas, lung, prostate and colon are adenocarcinomas.

adjuvant therapy: Additional cancer treatment given after the primary treatment to reduce the chance of recurrence. Adjuvant therapy may include chemotherapy, radiation or medication.

adrenal gland: Endocrine glands that produce a variety of hormones including adrenaline and the steroids aldosterone and cortisol.

advanced breast cancer: Breast cancer that spreads from the breast to the armpit or other areas of the body. It is also called metastatic, secondary or stage 4 breast cancer.

alopecia: A type of hair loss that occurs when your immune system mistakenly attacks hair follicles, which is where hair growth begins. It is a common side effect of chemotherapy.

anesthesia: A loss of sensation with or without loss of consciousness. Local or regional anesthesia may be used for a specific part of the body, such as the breast, by injection of a drug into that area. This keeps a person from feeling pain during surgery or other medical procedures. General anesthesia numbs the entire body and puts a person to sleep. The drugs are either injected into a vein or inhaled.

areola: The small circular area of dark-colored skin surrounding a nipple.

aromatase inhibitors: Hormone therapy drugs that can slow or stop the production of estrogen in postmenopausal women. Aromatase inhibitors are used to treat hormone receptor-positive early and metastatic breast cancers in postmenopausal women.

aspiration: Removal of fluid or tissue through a needle.

asymmetrical: Not matching.

atypical cell: Mildly to moderately abnormal cell. Also known as dysplasia.

atypical hyperplasia: An accumulation of abnormal cells in the breast.

axilla: The underarm or armpit.

axillary lymph node: A lymph node in the armpit region that drains lymph from the breast and nearby areas.

axillary lymph node dissection: Surgery to remove lymph nodes found in the armpit region.

B

benign: Not harmful in effect. Specifically, with a tumor, means not malignant.

biomarker: A measurable biological property that can be used to identify women at risk. It can also be used to determine how well the body responds to treatment for a disease or condition.

biopsy: Removal of cells or tissue to be tested by a pathologist for cancer cells.

bilateral mastectomy: Surgical operation that removes both breasts.

blood vessel: A tube carrying blood throughout the body.

bone marrow: The soft, spongelike tissue in the center of most bones. It produces blood cells and platelets.

bone scan: A test done to check for cancer in the bones.

BRCA1 and BRCA2 (breast cancer 1 and breast cancer 2): Human genes that produce tumor suppressor proteins. These proteins help repair damaged DNA. A mutation (change) in one of these genes limits

DNA from repairing properly and as a result can lead to additional genetic alterations that increases a person's risk of breast, ovarian and colon cancer.

breast density: A measure used to describe the amount of dense tissue compared with the amount of fatty tissue in the breasts as seen on a mammogram.

breast reconstruction: A surgical procedure that restores the shape, look and feel of the breast after a mastectomy.

C

CA 125 blood test: A blood test that measures the amount of protein CA 125 (cancer antigen 125) in the blood. The test may be used to monitor certain cancers during and after treatment.

calcifications: White spots of calcium deposits in the breast. Calcifications are too small to feel but can be seen on a mammogram. When they show up in tight clusters, irregular shapes or all in a line, it can be a sign of cancer. They are not related to the amount of calcium in a woman's diet.

cancer: A term for diseases in which abnormal cells divide without control or order.

carcinoembryonic antigen (CEA): A type of tumor marker. Carcinoembryonic antigen may help keep track of how well a treatment is working or if a cancer has come back.

carcinogen: Any substance that can cause cancer.

carcinoma: Cancer that begins in the skin or tissue that lines or covers internal organs. Most cancers are carcinomas.

carcinoma in situ (in situ carcinoma): A cancer that remains at the site of its origin and has not spread to deeper tissues or elsewhere in the body. Also called stage 0 cancer.

cell: The basic structural and functional unit of any living thing.

chemotherapy: A systemic drug treatment that uses chemicals to kill cancer cells that remain in the body after surgery. Chemotherapy attacks undetected cancer cells too small to be identified in imaging or other medical tests to prevent them from multiplying.

clear margins (also called negative or clean margins): No cancer cells are seen at the outer edge of the tissue that was removed.

clinical trial: Research study that tests the benefits, the safety and the effectiveness of possible new medical strategies, treatments or devices for humans. These studies also may show which medical approaches work best for certain illnesses or groups of people.

cognitive function: Mental processes related to understanding, such as reasoning, memory, attention, language and problem-solving.

comedo carcinoma: Type of ductal carcinoma in situ in which the cells filling the duct are more aggressive looking.

complementary therapies (integrative therapies): Therapies such as acupuncture, massage, touch therapy and meditation that are used in addition to standard medical treatments. When complementary therapies are combined with standard medical care, they are often called integrative therapies.

contrast material: A dye or other substance that enhances the contrast of structures in the body allowing the radiologist to detect abnormal areas inside the body. Contrast material may be used with X-rays, CT scans and MRIs.

core needle biopsy: A type of biopsy that uses a hollow needle to remove a small core of tissue from an abnormal area in the breast.

cortisol: Hormone that the adrenal gland produces.

cryotherapy: A procedure in which an extremely cold liquid or an instrument called a cryoprobe is used to freeze and destroy abnormal tissue.

CT scan, CAT scan (computerized tomography scan; computerized axial tomography scan): A series of pictures combined from several X-rays to produce a detailed image of structures inside the body.

CT simulation: A procedure in which a patient is placed in a precise and reproducible position for optimum accuracy in radiation therapies.

cyst: Fluid-filled sac.

cystosarcoma phyllodes: A rare, predominantly benign breast tumor.

D

DCIS (ductal carcinoma in situ): A noninvasive condition in which abnormal cells are contained in the inside of the milk ducts. Sometimes referred to as pre-cancer.

diagnosis: The identification of a disease by examining its signs and symptoms.

diagnostic mammogram: X-rays involving two or more views of the breast. Taken after suspicious results on a screening, or after some signs of breast cancer, such as a lump, require further examination.

disease-free survival rate: The length of time after the primary treatment for a cancer ends that the patient survives without any signs or symptoms of that cancer (often five years).

DNA (deoxyribonucleic acid): The nucleic acid that carries hereditary information in cells in humans and almost all other organisms. Almost every cell in a person's body has the same DNA.

duct: A tube or vessel of the body through which fluid passes.

E

early-stage breast cancer: Breast cancer that has not spread beyond the breast or axillary lymph nodes.

edema: Swelling caused by a collection of fluid in the soft tissues.

estrogen: Female sex hormones produced by the ovaries and adrenal glands that promote the development and maintenance of female characteristics of the body.

estrogen receptor (ER): Specific proteins found in cells of the female reproductive tissue, other tissues and some cancer cells. The term "ER positive" (presence of estrogen receptors in the tumor) means a woman's cancer cells may be sensitive to hormone therapy.

excisional biopsy: Surgical procedure that cuts through the skin to remove the entire tumor or suspicious area. This is often done using local or regional anesthesia.

F

false negative: A test result that incorrectly reports a person is disease-free when that person actually has the disease.

false positive: A test result that incorrectly reports a person has a disease when that person does not have the disease.

family history (family medical history): A record of the current and past health conditions of a person's biological (blood-related) family members.

fat necrosis: A benign, noncancerous condition in which fat tissue in the breast or other organs is damaged by injury, surgery or radiation therapy. The damaged fat tissue may be replaced by a cyst or by scar tissue, which may feel like a round, firm lump. This change in fat tissue does not increase the risk of breast cancer.

fibroadenoma: Benign fibrous tumor of the breast.

fine needle aspiration (fine needle biopsy): A biopsy procedure using a fine needle attached to a syringe to take out a small amount of fluid and tissue from the tumor.

first-degree relative (immediate family member): A person's mother, father, sister, brother or child.

G

gene: A linear sequence of DNA that is required to produce a protein.

gene mutation: A permanent change in the DNA of a cell. Gene mutations can be harmful, beneficial or have no effect.

genetic (hereditary): The genetic properties or features of an organism. Heredity is the passing on of its traits from parents to their offspring. The information in a person's genes can be passed on (inherited) from either parent.

genome: All the chromosomes that together form the genetic map.

gland: An organ that makes one or more substances, such as hormones, digestive juices, sweat, tears, saliva or milk.

gynecomastia: Abnormal growth of breast gland tissue in a man or boy.

H

hematoma: A pool of clotted or partially clotted blood in an organ, tissue or body space usually caused by a broken blood vessel. Hematomas may occur in the breast after surgery.

Her-2/neu (human epidermal growth factor receptor 2): An oncogene that appears in the cancer cells of some women with breast cancer and controls cell growth and repair. When overexpressed, leads to more cell growth

heterogeneous: In relation to cancer, refers to the many different types of breast cancer cells that are found within one tumor.

histologic grade: A term used to describe how much the tumor cells resemble normal cells when viewed under the microscope. The higher the histologic grade, the higher the odds of recurrence.

homeopathy (homeopathic medicine): A system based on a belief that the body has the ability to cure itself. Natural substances are specially prepared in small amounts to stimulate the body's own healing processes and restore its good health.

hormone: A chemical substance made by specific glands and tissues in the body that control and regulate the activity of particular cells or organs.

hormone receptors: Specific proteins on cells that hormones attach to. Cancers are called hormone receptor-positive or hormone receptor-negative based on whether they have these receptors.

hormone receptor status: Tells you whether the breast cancer cells have receptors for the hormones estrogen and progesterone. A hormone receptor-positive (estrogen and/or progesterone receptor-positive) cancer needs hormones to grow. A hormone receptor-negative (estrogen and/or progesterone receptor-negative) cancer does not need hormones to grow.

hormone replacement therapy (HRT): Treatment with hormones to effect diminished levels in the body and help alleviate menopausal symptoms and osteoporosis.

hormone therapy (endocrine therapy, endocrine manipulation): Therapy involving drugs or surgery that adds, blocks or removes hormones (estrogen or testosterone) to lower the risk of hormone receptor-positive breast cancer from returning or spreading to a new site.

hyperplasia: Excessive growth of cells in an organ or tissue.

I

immune system: Complex system of cells, tissues, organs and the substances they make by which the body is able to fight infections and diseases.

immunotherapy: A prevention or treatment that uses certain parts of a person's immune system to fight cancer. The therapies stimulate your own immune system to work harder or smarter.

implant (breast implant): Breast-shaped sacks containing silicone, saline or both that is used to restore the breast form after a mastectomy.

incisional biopsy: Surgical biopsy that removes only part of the tumor.

infiltrating cancer: Cancer that grows beyond its site of origin into neighboring tissue. "Infiltrating" has the same meaning as "invasive." It does not imply that the cancer has already spread outside the breast.

inflammatory breast cancer: A rare and aggressive disease in which cancer cells block lymph vessels in the skin of the breast. This type of breast cancer is called "inflammatory" because the breast often looks swollen and red, or inflamed.

informed consent: The process through which a person learns important information about the possible benefits and risks of a treatment plan and then accepts the treatment.

in situ: In its original place. In cancer, "in situ" means the abnormal cells are found only in the place they originally formed.

intensity modulated radiation therapy (IMRT): A type of cancer treatment that uses advanced computer programs to calculate and deliver radiation directly to cancer cells from different angles. It allows people with cancer to receive higher, more effective doses of radiation while limiting the damage to the healthy tissues and organs around it.

internal radiation therapy: A radiation therapy in which low-level radioactive seeds, wires, needles or catheters are placed directly into or near a tumor. The internal radiation therapy allows a higher dose of radiation in a smaller area than might be possible with external radiation treatment.

intraductal: Within the milk duct.

intravenous (IV): The way of giving a drug or other substance through a needle into a vein.

invasive breast cancer: Cancer that has spread from the original location to surrounding normal breast tissue.

invasive ductal carcinoma (IDC): Cancer that forms in the milk duct then breaks through invading nearby tissues.

invasive lobular carcinoma (ILC): Cancer that forms in the milk-producing glands (lobules) then breaks through to the surrounding tissue.

L

lesion: Area of abnormal tissue.

lifetime risk: The chance of developing a disease over the course of a lifetime. Usually defined as birth up to age 85.

liquid biopsy: A test done on a sample of blood to look for cancer cells from a tumor that are circulating in the blood or for pieces of DNA from tumor cells that are in the blood. A liquid biopsy may be used to help find cancer at an early stage.

lobe: A portion of an organ, such as the breast, liver, lung, thyroid or brain.

lobular carcinoma in situ (LCIS): Abnormal cells confined in the lobules that have not spread to surrounding tissue.

lobules: Parts of the breast capable of making milk.

local anesthetic: Anesthesia that affects a certain area of the body.

local recurrence (recurrence): Cancer that has come back to the same breast or near the same place as the original (primary) tumor.

local treatment: Treatment that is directed to a specific organ or limited to an area of the body. Local treatment for breast cancer includes surgery, radiation therapy, cryotherapy, laser therapy or topical therapy (creams or lotion rubbed into the skin).

localized breast cancer: Cancer that is contained in the breast and has not spread to nearby tissue, lymph nodes or other organs.

locally advanced cancer: Cancer that has spread from where it started to nearby tissue or lymph nodes.

lump: Any mass in the breast or elsewhere in the body.

lumpectomy (breast conserving surgery): Surgery that removes only part of the breast containing the tumor and the area closely surrounding the tumor. Also called a partial mastectomy.

lymph: Clear fluid that travels through the lymphatic system and carries cells that help fight infections and diseases. Also called lymphatic fluid.

lymph node (lymph glands): Small bean-shaped structures that act as filters for the lymphatic system. Clusters of lymph nodes are found in the underarms, groin, neck, chest and abdomen.

lymph node status: Tells you if cancer has spread to the lymph nodes. Lymph node-positive means that cancer has spread to the lymph nodes. Lymph node-negative means that cancer has not spread to the lymph nodes.

lymphatic system: The tissues and organs that produce, store and carry white blood cells that fight infections and other diseases.

lymphedema: A condition of localized swelling caused by poor draining of lymph fluid that can occur after removing lymph nodes in surgery or after radiation therapy to the area. It can be temporary or permanent and occur immediately or at a later date.

M

magnetic resonance imaging (MRI): A procedure in which radio waves and a powerful magnet linked to a computer are used to create detailed pictures of areas inside the body. These pictures can show the difference between normal and diseased tissue.

malignant: Cancerous.

mammaprint: A test that is used to help predict whether breast cancer has spread to other parts of the body or come back.

mammogram: An X-ray image of the breast.

mammotome: A device that uses a computer-guided probe to perform breast biopsies.

mastalgia: Breast pain. Can include breast tenderness, sharp burning or tightness in a breast.

mastectomy: Surgical operation that removes the entire breast (or as much of the breast tissue as possible).

mastitis: An inflammation (swelling) of the breast tissue. Usually caused by an infection of the breast. Often seen in nursing mothers.

menopause: The time of life when a woman's ovaries stop producing hormones and menstrual periods stop. A woman is said to be in menopause when she has not had a period for 12 months in a row.

metastasis: A term for cancer that spreads to a different part of the body from where it started, usually through the blood stream (most often the bones, lungs, liver or brain).

metastatic breast cancer: Not a specific type of breast cancer, but rather the most advanced stage (stage IV) of breast cancer.

micrometastasis: A form of metastasis in which the newly formed tumors are too minuscule to be detected, but tumor cells are presumed to have spread to other organs.

modified radical mastectomy: Surgical removal of the breast, the lining of the chest muscles and most, or all, of the lymph nodes under the arm.

mutation: An alteration of the genetic code.

N

needle localization (wire localization): A procedure used to mark a small area of abnormal tissue, so it can be removed by surgery.

neoadjuvant chemotherapy: Chemotherapy treatment used first to shrink tumors before surgery.

neoadjuvant hormone therapy: Hormone therapy used as a first treatment to shrink tumors before surgery.

node-negative (lymph node-negative): Cancer that has not spread to the lymph nodes.

node-positive (lymph node-positive): Cancer that has spread to the lymph nodes.

noninvasive cancer: A cancer that has not spread beyond the ducts or lobules where it began.

noninvasive treatment: A procedure that does not penetrate the skin or body opening with a needle or another instrument.

nonpalpable: Describes a breast lump or abnormal area that cannot be felt but can be seen on an imaging test (such as a mammogram).

nuclear grade: The description of a tumor based on how the cancer cells divide to form more cells. Cancer cells with a high nuclear grade are usually faster growing.

O

oncogene: A gene that is a changed (mutated) form of a gene involved in normal cell growth. In certain circumstances, it can transform a cell into a tumor cell.

oncologist: The physician in charge of planning and overseeing cancer treatment.

oncology: The study of cancer.

oncotype DX: A test for the newly diagnosed that helps identify which women with early-stage estrogen receptor-positive and lymph node-negative breast cancer are more likely to benefit from adding chemotherapy to their hormonal treatment.

P

palliative care: Care given to improve the quality of life of patients who have a serious or life-threatening disease. The goal of palliative care is to prevent or treat as early as possible the symptoms of a disease, side effects caused by treatment of a disease, and psychological, social and spiritual problems related to a disease or its treatment.

partial breast irradiation: Radiation delivered specifically to the part of the breast where the tumor was removed rather than to the whole breast.

partial mastectomy: The removal of cancer and some of the breast tissue around the tumor and the lining over the chest muscles below the cancer. Usually some of the lymph nodes under the arm are also removed. Also called a lumpectomy.

pathologist: The physician who studies the breast tissue and lymph nodes removed during biopsy or surgery and determines whether or not the cells contain cancer.

perimenopause: The time in a woman's life prior to menopause when menstrual periods become irregular and some menopausal symptoms may begin.

PET scan (positron emission tomography): A procedure in which a short-term radioactive sugar is given through an IV so a scanner can show which parts of the body are consuming more sugar. PET is sometimes used as part of a breast cancer diagnosis or treatment, but it is not used for breast cancer screening.

physical therapist: A health professional who administers treatment of disease, injury or deformity through physical methods such as massage, heat treatment and exercise, rather than by drugs or surgery.

plastic surgeon: A surgeon who specializes in reducing scarring or disfigurement that may occur as a result of surgery, accident, birth defects or treatment for diseases.

plastic surgery: A surgery that reconstructs, restores or improves the appearance of the body.

polychemotherapy: Chemotherapy with more than one drug at a time.

progesterone: Hormone produced by the ovary that plays a role in the menstrual cycle and pregnancy.

progesterone receptor (PR): A protein found inside the cells of the female reproductive tissue, some other types of tissue and some cancer cells. The hormone progesterone will bind to the receptors inside the cells and may cause the cells to grow. These cells are generally sensitive to hormone therapy.

prognosis: Expected or probable outcome.

prophylactic mastectomy: Surgery to remove one or both breasts to reduce the risk of developing breast cancer.

prosthesis: A breast prostheses is an artificial breast form that gives women a more natural shape after they have a mastectomy or breast-conserving surgery.

protein: The building block of life, formed from amino acids.

protocol: A detailed plan of a scientific or medical experiment, treatment or procedure.

punch biopsy: A biopsy of skin that punches a small hole into the skin.

Q

quadrantectomy: Removal of a quarter of the breast.

R

radiation oncologist: A physician specializing in the treatment of cancer using targeted, high-energy X-rays.

radiation therapy (radiotherapy): Treatment that uses targeted, high-energy penetrating wave or particle beams to damage or destroy cancerous cells.

radical mastectomy: Surgical removal of the breast, chest muscles and underarm lymph nodes.

radiologist: A physician who reads and interprets X-rays, mammograms and other scans related to diagnosis or follow-up. Radiologists also perform needle biopsy and wire localization procedures.

receptors: Breast cancer cells taken out during biopsy or surgery will be tested to see if they have certain proteins that are estrogen or progesterone receptors. When the hormones estrogen and progesterone attach to these receptors, they fuel the cancer growth.

reconstructive surgeon: A doctor who can surgically reshape or rebuild a part of the body, such as a woman's breast after surgery for breast cancer.

recurrence: A cancer that has come back in the same or opposite breast or chest wall after a period of time when the cancer could not be detected.

reexcision: A surgical procedure to remove the remaining abnormal tissue that was not removed in a previous attempt.

remission: Disappearance of detectable disease.

S

saline-filled breast implants: Silicone shells filled with saline (sterile salt water), used in breast implants.

sarcoma: A type of tumor that develops in connective tissue, such as bone, cartilage or muscle. Sarcomas can be benign (noncancerous) or malignant (cancerous).

sentinel node: The sentinel lymph node is the first node "downstream" from the cancer in the lymph circulatory system. If the cancer were to travel away from the breast tumor and into the lymphatic system, this node would be the first one to show evidence of breast cancer.

sentinel node biopsy: The surgical removal and testing of the sentinel node(s) in the underarm area that is filtering lymph fluid from the tumor. This biopsy is usually done at the time of the initial surgery.

side effect: A problem that occurs when healthy tissues or organs are affected by treatment.

silicone: Synthetic material used in breast implants.

silicone breast implants: Silicone shells filled with silicone gel used in breast implants.

skin-sparing mastectomy: A procedure that surgically removes the breast but keeps intact as much of the skin that surrounds the breast as possible. This skin can then be used in breast reconstruction to cover a tissue flap or an implant instead of having to use skin from other parts of the body.

sonogram: The black-and-white image that an ultrasound creates.

stage of cancer (cancer stage): Describes how much cancer is in the body and where it is. Cancer is always referred to the stage it was given at diagnosis, even if it gets worse.

staging cancer: A classification system (0 to IV) for breast cancers based on the size of the tumor, whether the cancer has spread to the lymph nodes and whether the cancer has spread to other sites in the body. The higher the stage, the more extensive the cancer.

stereotactic mammography: Three-dimensional mammography used to guide a needle biopsy.

stereotactic needle biopsy: Core needle biopsy done with the use of stereotactic (three-dimensional) mammography guidance.

stereotactic radiosurgery: Surgery using radiation, rather than excision with a blade.

subareolar abscess: Infection of the glands under the nipple.

surgeon: Physician who performs any surgery, including surgical biopsies and other procedures related to breast cancer.

surgery (operation): A procedure to remove or repair part of the body or to find out whether disease is present.

surgical oncologist: A physician specializing in the treatment of cancer using surgical procedures.

systematic treatment: Treatment involving the whole body, usually using drugs.

T

tamoxifen: A hormone therapy drug (in pill form) used to treat early- and advanced-stage breast cancers that are hormone receptor-positive. Tamoxifen stops or slows the growth of these tumors by blocking estrogen from attaching to hormone receptors in the cancer cells.

targeted therapy: Drug therapies designed to attach specific molecular agents or pathways involved in the development of cancer.

therapeutic touch: An integrative or complementary therapy in which trained practitioners enter a semi-meditative state and hold their hands just above a person's body to sense energy imbalances brought on by illness. Healing energy is then said to transfer to the person.

3D mammogram: Also called breast tomosynthesis, takes multiple X-rays of the breast to create a three-dimensional image on a computer.

total mastectomy (simple mastectomy): Surgical removal of the whole breast, but axillary tissue is left untouched. Sometimes the sentinel node is removed.

triple negative breast cancer: A breast cancer that is estrogen receptor-negative, progesterone receptor-negative and HER2/neu-negative. These factors limit treatment choice. These breast cancers tend to be aggressive.

tru-cut biopsy: Type of core needle biopsy in which a small core tissue is removed from a lump without surgery.

tumor: An abnormal growth or mass of tissue that may be benign (not cancerous) or malignant (cancerous).

tumor grade: Describes how closely cancer cells look like normal cells and how quickly they are likely to spread. Low-grade cancer cells look more like normal cells and tend to grow and spread more slowly than high-grade cancer cells.

tumor marker: A substance found in tissue, blood or other body fluids that may be a sign of cancer or certain benign (noncancerous) conditions. Most tumor markers are made by both normal cells and cancer cells but are made up in larger amounts by cancer cells.

U

ultrasound: Diagnostic test that uses high-energy sound waves to look at tissues and organs inside the body. Tissues of different densities reflect sound waves differently.

V

vacuum-assisted core biopsy: A biopsy done with a vacuum-assisted device. This method usually removes more tissue than a core biopsy done with a regular needle.

X

X-ray: Radiation used at low levels to make images of the inside of the body. A mammogram is a low-level X-ray image of the breast.

Parts of this glossary were taken or adapted from the National Cancer Institute's *Dictionary of Cancer Terms*, The American Cancer Society *Cancer Glossary*, Susan Love Breast Book *Glossary*, Joint Center for Radiation Therapy *Glossary of Terms*, Susan G. Komen Foundation *Tools & Resources Breast Cancer Glossary*, WebMD. com *Health A-Z*, Breastcancer.org *Treatment*, Radiologyinfo.org *Article Index A-Z*, Merriam-webster.com *Dictionary*, Medicinenet.com *Medical Dictionary A-Z List*, BreastCancer.org *Symptoms & Diagnosis*, Memorial Sloan Kettering Cancer Center *Types of Cancer Treatments*, Cleveland Clinic *Health Library*, BreastCancerFoundation.org *Breast Cancer*, MedlinePlus *Genetics*

Acknowledgments

"Alone we can do so little; together we can do so much."
—*Helen Keller*

This statement describes the writing of *The Upside to Everything, Even Breast Cancer*. I might have been the one who wrote the words on these pages, but it was a collaborative effort. Family, friends and strangers lent their voice, offered advice, shared their knowledge and gave me endless encouragement as I worked toward my goal of writing a book that supports women diagnosed with breast cancer. I am so thankful.

I am grateful beyond measure for the following people: my husband, **Michael Cleeff**; his unwavering support when I got my breast cancer diagnosis barely three years into our marriage and again when I was writing this book confirms that I have won the lottery in this lifetime. My sister, **Bonnie Drescher West**, for her unyielding belief in me always and for understanding me in a way only a sister can. **Wendy Marcus**, a better friend, or more talented copy editor, a person could not ask for; she was the key to my confidence and courage as a writer. I will never be able to adequately express my appreciation. **Gay Walley** and her Wednesday night reading group; their feedback, questions and surprised reaction to a day in the life of a cancer patient reminded me of the rude shock of the experience and further validated the need for this book. It is more insightful because of them. **Arlene Matlick** for involving me in SHARE Cancer Support Pink and Teal Seminars to educate women about the signs of breast cancer. Answering questions and teaching hundreds of women how to care for their breasts remind me to never take my knowledge about the disease for granted. **Kerri Conan, Robert Schoenlank** and **David Stoner**, respectively, for the idea, title and confirmation of the last chapter, "Prelude to a Postscript." I did not know how important a chapter it was until I completed the book. **Rhonda Johnson** for her intuitive direction on the book's concept and her clarity about how I should approach the book. **Christine Baczewska** for her keen eye, creativity and hand-holding on all things visual regarding *The Upside to Everything*. **Margie Bauml** for putting me in the right place at the right time to make my book a reality. **John Alexander**, my friend and champion in all my endeavors.

Dr. Deborah Axelrod for inviting me to partake in a study on the diagnosis of breast cancer when she was at Beth Israel Medical Center; it saved my life. Her empathy for the cancer patient is unparalleled and the profession a safer and healthier place because of her. Cancer specialist **Dr. Eugene Thiessen**, who founded SHARE Cancer Support 45 years ago so no one would have to experience breast cancer alone. Millions of women have benefited from his generous and compassionate heart, me included. My most heartfelt thank-you goes to the women who trusted me with their fears, expectations and darkest thoughts. The opportunity to support them as they grappled with their disease has been one of the most rewarding experiences of my life.

Having *The Upside to Everything, Even Breast Cancer* published feels like the culmination of a cancer saga that started when I was a child. When Dr. Axelrod told me I had breast cancer, the first person I thought of was my mother and when she got her diagnosis. Dr. Axelrod wrote down two things: SHARE Cancer Support and *Dr. Susan Love's Breast Book*. She told me to call the first and buy the second. Both had a huge impact on how I coped with my diagnosis. To be able to share my knowledge from the SHARE helpline, dedicate this book to my mother, and have Dr. Axelrod and Dr. Love endorse it are upsides to the experience of breast cancer I did not see coming twenty-plus years ago.

Bibliography

Chapter 1—I Have What?!

Mandal, Ananya, Dr. "Lymph Node Removal," News Medical, http://www.news-medical.net, 5 June 2019, http://www.news-medical.net/health/Lymph-node-Removal.aspx

"Every 2 Minutes, A Woman in the United States Is Diagnosed With Breast Cancer," Breast Cancer Research Foundation, www.bcrf.org, 14 Aug. 2014, https://www.bcrf.org/blog/every-2-minutes-woman-us-diagnosed-breast-cancer

"Reading a Pathology Report," Cancer.Net, www.cancer.net, January 2016, https://www.cancer.net/navigating-cancer-care/diagnosing-cancer/reports-and-results/reading-pathology-report

"Treatment for LCIS," Breastcancer.org, www.breastcancer.org, 9 Sept. 2016, http://www.breastcancer.org/symptoms/types/lcis/treatment

"What Can You Tell Me About Sentinel Node Biopsy?" Breastcancer.org, www.breastcancer.org, 19 Aug. 2014, http://www.breastcancer.org/questions/sentinel_node

Chapter 2—Doctors, Doctors and More Doctors

Pantilat, Steve, M.D. "What is a Hospitalist?" The Hospitalist, https://www.the-hospitalist.org, February 2006, https://www.the-hospitalist.org/hospitalist/article/123072/what-hospitalist

Singal, Jessie, "A Lot of Cancer Patients Aren't on the Same Page as Their Doctors," The Cut, www.thecut.com, 12 July 2016, https://

www.thecut.com/2016/07/a-lot-of-cancer-patients-arent-on-the-same-page-as-their-doctors.html

"Choosing a Doctor and a Hospital," American Cancer Society, www. cancer.org, 26 Feb. 2016, https://www.cancer.org/treatment/finding-and-paying-for-treatment/choosing-your-treatment-team/choosing-a-doctor-and-a-hospital.html

"Choosing a Doctor: Quick Tips," U.S. Department of Health and Human Services, https://healthfinder.gov, 22 Feb. 2018, https://healthfinder .gov/HealthTopics/Category/doctor-visits/regular-check-ups/choosing-a-doctor-quick-tips

"Choosing Your Doctor," National Breast Cancer Foundation Inc., www.nationalbreastcancer.org, 21 Mar. 2018, http://www.national breastcancer.org/breast-cancer-doctors

Communication, Lincoln Medical and Mental Health Center, Morrisania Diagnostic and Treatment Center, June 2014, *New Employee Orientation Self Study Manual*, page 42, July 2015

Customer Service, Lincoln Medical and Mental Health Center, Morrisania Diagnostic and Treatment Center, June 2014, *New Employee Orientation Self-Study Manual*, page 41, July 2015

"RN vs Nurse Practitioner (NP) What Is the Difference?" Herzing University, https://www.herzing.edu/, https://www.herzing.edu/difference/rn-vs-np

"The Oncology Team," Cancer.Net, https://www.cancer.net, August 2020, https://www.cancer.net/navigating-cancer-care/cancer-basics/cancer-care-team/oncology-team

"Questions to Ask Your Surgeon About Breast Reconstruction," American Cancer Society, www.cancer.org, 12 Sept. 2017, https://www.cancer .org/cancer/breast-cancer/reconstruction-surgery/questions-to-ask-your-surgeon-about-breast-reconstruction.html

"Questions to Ask Your Surgeon About Breast Reconstruction," Breastcancer.org, www.breastcancer.org, 20 July 2016, http://www. breastcancer.org/treatment/surgery/reconstruction/questions-to-ask

"What Doctors Wished Their Patients Knew," Consumer Reports Health, www.consumerreports.org, February 2011, https://www.consumerreports. org/cro/2012/04/what-doctors-wish-their-patients-knew/index.htm

"What Is the Difference Between a Nurse and a Nurse Practitioner?" The College of St. Scholastica, https://www.css.edu/, 19 June 2018, https://www.css.edu/about/blog/what-is-the-difference-between-a-nurse-a-nurse-practitioner/

Chapter 3—Next Steps

Kim, Ben, Dr. "How Fast Does Cancer Grow," Experience Your Best Health, http://drbenkim.com, 8 Sept. 2015, http://drbenkim.com/how-fast-does-cancer-grow-spread

"After a Breast Cancer Diagnosis: Questions to Ask Your Doctor," CancerCare, https://www.cancercare.org, 30 Nov. 2016, https://www.cancercare.org/publications/46-after_a_breast_cancer_diagnosis_questions_to_ask_your_doctor

"Breast Cancer: Questions to Ask the Health Care Team," Cancer.Net, https://www.cancer.net/, July 2020, https://www.cancer.net/ cancer-types/breast-cancer/questions-ask-health-care-team

"Inpatient, Outpatient or Observation," NYU Langone Medical Center, Apr. 2016, *Patient Information & Education*, Page 1, January 2010

"Questions to Ask Your Doctor About Breast Cancer," American Cancer Society, https://www.cancer.org, 25 Sept. 2017, https://www.cancer .org/cancer/breast-cancer/understanding-a-breast-cancer-diagnosis/questions-to-ask-your-doctor-about-breast-cancer.html

"Questions to Ask Your Surgeon About Breast Reconstruction," Breastcancer. org, http://www.breastcancer.org, 20 July 2016, http://www.breastcancer. org/treatment/surgery/reconstruction/questions-to-ask

"What You Need to Know About Breast Cancer," National Cancer Institute, U.S. Department of Health and Human Services, https://www.nih.gov/ NIH Publication No. 12-1556, April 2012, https://tawam.seha.ae/assets/uploads/2021/03/Breast-Cancer-English-122.pdf

Chapter 4—Now What?

MoSCoW Method, Wikipedia, https://www.wikipedia.org/, 4 Feb. 2018, https://en.wikipedia.org/wiki/MoSCoW_method

Chapter 5—Appointments, Tests and Procedures

Gillikin, Jason, "What is the Difference Between Pre-authorizations & Pre-certification Insurance?" PocketSense, www.pocketsense.com, 25 Oct. 2017, https://pocketsense.com/what-is-the-difference-between-preauthorization-pre-certification-insurance-12314906.html

Houseman, Kaitlyn, "The Importance of Preauthorization," Revele, https://www.revelemd.com/, 16 Nov. 2015, https://www.revelemd.com/blog/bid/74087/the-importance-of-preauthorization

Umansky, Diane, "If the Doctor Asks for Your Social Security Number, Do This," Consumer Reports, https://www.consumerreports.org, 11 Oct. 2019, https://www.consumerreports.org/cro/news/2015/03/what-to-do-if-your-doctor-asks-for-your-social-security-number/index.htm

Medical Portal, MyChart at NYU Langone Health, NYU Langone Health, 2018

"Tests and Visits Before Surgery," MedlinePlus Medical Dictionary, https://medlineplus.gov, 27 Feb. 2016, https://medlineplus.gov/ency/patientinstructions/000479.htm

Chapter 6—Surgery

Grannell, Rachael, "7 Things You Should Absolutely Know Before Going to the Hospital," HuffPost.com, https://www.huffingtonpost.com, 12 June 2014, Updated, 6 Dec. 2017, https://www.huffingtonpost.com/2014/06/12/hospital-facts_n_4856009.html

"Breast Cancer: Questions to Ask the Health Care Team," Cancer.Net, www.cancer.net, April 2017, https://www.cancer.net/cancer-types/breast-cancer/questions-ask-health-care-team

About Your Breast Surgery, Memorial Sloan Kettering Cancer Center, *Patient & Caregiver Education*, pages 3-4, 2013

Health Care Proxy, NYU Langone Medical Center, May 2016, *Patient Information & Education, Advance Directives*, page 1, Jan. 2010

Patient Visitors, NYU Langone Medical Center, Apr. 2016, *Patient Information & Education*, Jan. 2010

Preparing for Your Surgery, Memorial Sloan Kettering Cancer Center, 2013, *Patient & Caregiver Education*, pages 7-8

Surgical Margins, Breastcancer.org, https://www.breastcancer.org/, 19 Sept. 2018, Surgical Margins | Breastcancer.org

Chapter 7—Treatment

"A Guide to Clinical Trials for Cancer," U.S. National Library of Medicine, Medical Encyclopedia, https://medlineplus.gov, January 2021, https://medlineplus.gov/ency/patientinstructions/000823.htm

"The Basics of Clinical Trials," American Cancer Society, https://www.cancer.org, 3 Mar. 2016, https://www.cancer.org/treatment/treatments-and-side-effects/clinical-trials/what-you-need-to-know/clinical-trial-basics.html

"Breast Cancer: Questions to Ask the Health Care Team," Cancer.Net, https://www.cancer.net/ , April 2017, https://www.cancer.net/cancer-types/breast-cancer/questions-ask-health-care-team

"Medical Definition of Clinical Trials," MedicineNet.com, https://www.medicinenet.com, 13 May 2016, https://www.medicinenet.com/script/main/art.asp?articlekey=2752

"Phases of Clinical Trials," Cancer.Net, https://www.cancer.net, 20 Sept. 2017, https://www.cancer.net/research-and-advocacy/clinical-trials/phases-clinical-trials

"Questions to Ask Your Doctor About Breast Cancer," American Cancer Society, https://www.cancer.org, 20 Sept. 2019, https://www.cancer.org/cancer/breast-cancer/understanding-a-breast-cancer-diagnosis/questions-to-ask-your-doctor-about-breast-cancer.html

Chapter 8—Rights, Responsibilities and Privacy

"Consumer Rights and Protections," Medline Plus, www.medlineplus .gov, 5 Mar. 2018, https://medlineplus.gov/ency/article/001947.htm

"HIPPA, Health Insurance Portability & Accountability Act," Lincoln Medical and Mental Health Center, Morrisania Diagnostic and Treatment Center, New Employee Orientation Self-Study Manual, *Patient Rights and Responsibilities*, page 72, June 2014

"Patient's Bill of Rights," Lincoln Medical and Mental Health Center, Morrisania Diagnostic and Treatment Center, New Employee Orientation Self-Study Manual, *Patient Rights and Responsibilities*, Page 79, June 2014

"Summary of the HIPPA Privacy Rule," U.S. Department of Health and Human Services, www.hhs.gov, 26 July 2013, https://www.hhs.gov/ hipaa/for-professionals/privacy/laws-regulations/index.html

Chapter 9—Dealing With the Bureaucracy of Cancer

Dagher, Veronica, "How to Handle a Large, Unexpected Medical Bill," *The Wall Street Journal Markets*, www.wsj.com, 15 Aug. 2017, https:// www.wsj.com/articles/how-to-handle-a-large-unexpected-medical- bill-1502811927

Fitch, Andrew, "Tips for Appealing a Denied Health Insurance Claim," NerdWallet, https://www.nerdwallet.com, 2 Sept. 2014, https:// www.nerdwallet.com/blog/health/managing-health-insurance/tips- appealing-denied-health-insurance-claim/

Grant, Kelli B., "Avoid the Pain of a Surprise Medical Bill," CNBC, https:// www.cnbc.com, 28 Aug. 2015, https://www.cnbc.com/2015/08/28/ avoid-the-pain-of-a-surprise-medical-bill.html

Snider, Susannah, "How to Get Help Paying Medical Bills," *U.S. News*, https:// www.usnews.com/, 9 Sept. 2020, https://money.usnews.com/money/ personal-finance/debt/articles/how-to-get-help-paying-medical-bills

Woodruff-Santos, Mandi, "How to See Through Opaque Health Care Costs," Yahoo, https://finance.yahoo.com, 16 Sept. 2014, https://finance.yahoo.com/news/5-ways-to-save-at-the-doctor-s-office-180221261.html

"Appealing Health Plan Decisions," U.S. Department of Health and Human Services, www.hhs.gov, 31 Jan. 2017, https://www.hhs.gov/healthcare/about-the-law/cancellations-and-appeals/appealing-health-plan-decisions/index.html

"Explaining Our Time of Service Collection Policy," NYU Langone Medical Center, 23 May 2013

"Hints for Good Note Taking," Chapman University, https://www.chapman.edu, April 2018, https://www.chapman.edu/students/academic-resources/tutoring-center/resources-success/study-strategies/note-taking/index.aspx

"Insurance Coverage Denials and the Appeals Process," The Cancer Advocacy Project, The City Bar Justice Center, Oct. 2014, pages 1-4

"Quick Guide to Cobra," Triage Cancer, http://triagecancer.org, 24 Aug. 2017, http://triagecancer.org/wp-content/uploads/2017/01/2017-COBRA-Quick-Guide.pdf

Chapter 10—Family, Friends and Illness

Clear, James, "Handling Criticism: How to Deal With People Judging You and Your Work," Buffer, https://buffer.com/ 9 Oct. 2013, https://blog.bufferapp.com/haters-and-critics-how-to-deal-with-people-judging-you-and-your-work

Manson, Mark, "How We Judge Others, Is How We Judge Ourselves," Mark Manson, www.markmanson.net, 30 Mar. 2018, https://markmanson.net/how-we-judge-others

"Helping Children When a Family Member Has Cancer: Dealing With Diagnosis," American Cancer Society, https://www.cancer.org, 20 July 2012, https://www.cancer.org/treatment/children-and-cancer/when-a-family-member-has-cancer/dealing-with-diagnosis.html

"Talking to Your Spouse or Life Partner," Breastcancer.org, www.
breastcancer.org, 10 May 2016, http://www.breastcancer.org/tips/
telling_family/spouse

"Telling Others About Your Cancer," American Cancer Society, https://
www.cancer.org, April 2016, https://www.cancer.org/treatment/
understanding-your-diagnosis/talking-about-cancer/telling-others-
about-your-cancer.html

Chapter 11—Telling Children About Cancer

Fayed, Lisa, "Telling Friends and Family That You've Been Diagnosed With
Cancer: What to Say to Your Spouse, Kids, and Employer," VerywellHealth,
https://www.verywellhealth.com, 7 Feb. 2018, https://www.verywellhealth.
com/how-to-tell-your-children-that-you-have-cancer-514230

Jacobs, Hollye, RN, MS, MSW, 2014, "The Silver Lining; A Supportive
& Insightful Guide to Breast Cancer," Children Always Know, pages
40-63, Atria Books, 17 July 2018

Love, Susan M., M.D. 2010 *Dr. Susan Love's Breast Book*, Fifth Edition,
"Coping: What to Tell Your Children," pages 268-271, Da Capo
Press, 17 July 2018

"For Parents: Talking With Children About Cancer," Dana-Farber Cancer
Institute, http://www.dana-farber.org, 2018, http://www.dana-farber.
org/for-patients-and-families/care-and-treatment/support-services-
and-amenities/family-connections/for-the-patient/talking-with-
children-about-cancer/

"Talking to Children When a Loved One Has Cancer," CancerCare,
https://www.cancercare.org), 29 Mar. 2017, https://www.cancercare
.org/publications/22-helping_children_when_a_family_member_
has_cancer#!explaining-the-diagnosis

"How to Tell a Child That a Parent Has Cancer," American Cancer
Society, https://www.cancer.org, 20 Dec. 2016, https://www.cancer
.org/treatment/children-and-cancer/when-a-family-member-has-
cancer/dealing-with-diagnosis/how-to-tell-children.html

"Talking to Kids About Cancer," Cancer Council, https://www.cancervic
.org.au/, December 2015, https://www.cancervic.org.au/downloads/
resources/booklets/talking-to-kids-about-cancer/Talking-to-Kids-
About-Cancer.pdf

"Talking With Children About Cancer," Cancer.Net, https://www.cancer
.net/, August 2017, https://www.cancer.net/coping-with-cancer/
talking-with-family-and-friends/talking-about-cancer/talking-with-
your-children-about-cancer

"Talking to Children About Cancer," Canadian Cancer Society, http://
www.cancer.ca/en/?region=on, 2018, http://www.cancer.ca/en/
cancer-information/cancer-journey/talking-about-cancer/telling-
children/?region=on

"Telling Kids About Cancer: Age Appropriate Advice," Telling Kids About
Cancer, http://www.tellingkidsaboutcancer.com, 2012, http://www.
tellingkidsaboutcancer.com/AgeAppropriateAdvice

Chapter 12—Cancer and Work

Borstelmann, Nancy, LICSW, MPH, "How Do I Tell My Boss I Have
Cancer? Step-by-Step Approach," Dana-Farber Cancer Institute,
https://blog.dana-farber.org, 6 July 2016, https://blog.dana-farber.
org/insight/2012/01/how-to-tell-your-boss-you-have-cancer/

"The ADA: Your Employment Rights as an Individual With a Disability,"
U.S. Equal Employment Opportunity Commission, https://www.eeoc.
gov, 1 Jan. 2009, https://www.eeoc.gov/eeoc/publications/ada18.cfm

"How the ADA Law Protects Patients at Work," Patient Advocate Foundation,
https://www.patientadvocate.org, 2018, https://www.patientadvocate.
org/explore-our-resources/maintaining-employment-employment-
benefits/how-the-ada-law-protects-patients-at-work/How the ADA
Law Protects Patients at Work – Patient Advocate Foundation

"Whom to Tell," Cancer + Careers, https://www.cancerandcareers.org/en,
2 Feb. 2018, https://www.cancerandcareers.org/en/at-work/where-
to-start/sharing-the-news/who-to-tell

Chapter 13—Identity Crisis

Granger, Kari, "How to Deal With the 'Victim Mentality' in Others," Medium Corporation, Personal Growth, www.medium.com, 12 Dec. 2016, https://medium.com/personal-growth/dealing-with-the-victim-mentality-in-others-a9d6f2270f72

Guthrie, Catherine, "Why More Breast Cancer Survivors Are Going Flat," Oprah.com, Oprah.com, 20 Sept. 2017, http://www.oprah .com/inspiration/going-flat-why-some-women-reject-breast-reconstruction-surgery

Michaelson, Peter, "When You Feel Bad About Yourself," WhyWeSuffer .com, www.whywesuffer.com, 29 Oct. 2012, http://www.whywesuffer .com/when-you-feel-bad-about-yourself/

Norris, Dawn R., Ph.D. "Keeping Your Job, Losing Your Identity," *Psychology Today*, www.psychologytoday.com, 29 Aug. 2017, https:// www.psychologytoday.com/us/blog/the-next-step/201708/keeping-your-job-losing-your-identity

Parks-Ramage, Jonathan, "Cancer Was My Identity, Until I Created a New One," Refinery 29, www.refinery29.com, Aug. 2015, https://www. refinery29.com/how-to-deal-with-cancer-diagnosis

"Breast Reconstruction," Breastcancer.org, www.breastcancer.org, 31 Oct. 2017, http://www.breastcancer.org/treatment/surgery/reconstruction

"Positive Thinking: Reduce Stress by Eliminating Negative Self-Talk," Mayo Clinic, www.mayoclinic.com, 18 Feb. 2017, https://www. mayoclinic.org/healthy-lifestyle/stress-management/in-depth/positive-thinking/art-20043950?pg=2

"The Struggle for Personal Identity in Cancer Patient," MedicalxPress. com, https://medicalxpress.com, 20 May 2011, https://medicalxpress. com/news/2011-05-struggle-personal-identity-cancer-patient.html

"What Is the Difference Between a Victim and a Survivor? And Who Will You Choose to Be?" Dating a Sociopath, https://datingasociopath .com, 30 Oct. 2013, https://datingasociopath.com/2013/10/30/what-is-the-difference-between-a-victim-and-a-survivor-and-who-will-you-choose-to-be/

Chapter 14—Emotional Rescue

Chaplin, Diana, "5 Awesome Ways to Nourish Your Spirit," Mind Body Green, MindBodyGreen.com, 30 Oct. 2016, http://www.mindbodygreen.com/0-6834/5-Awesome-Ways-to-Nourish-Your-Spirit.html

Cherry, Kendra, "Overview of the 6 Major Theories of Emotion," VerywellMind, Verywellmind.com, 25 Feb. 2018, https://www.verywellmind.com/theories-of-emotion-2795717

Courtley, Cade, "SEAL Training Tips: Mental Preparation," Military, Military.com 2012, http://www.military.com/special-operations/seal-training-mental-preparation.html

Durnell, Linda, "Train Your Brain Using the Navy SEAL Mental Toughness Program," HuffPost, https://www.huffpost.com/, 25 Aug. 2014, https://www.huffpost.com/entry/train-your-brain-using-th_b_5527152

Goodhart, Frances, M.D., and Lucy Atkins, "The Downside of Beating Cancer," DailyMail.com, http://www.dailymail.co.uk, 14 June 2011, http://www.dailymail.co.uk/health/article-2003214/Cancer-survivors-Depression-exhaustion-anger-downside-beating-disease.html

Gregoire, Carolyn, "Depression Might Literally Color the Way We See the World," Huffingtonpost.com, 16 Oct. 2017, https://www.huffingtonpost.com/entry/depression-color-perception-research_us_55e86ba0e4b0aec9f35657f6

Higuera, Valencia, "Situational Depression or Clinical Depression," Medical News Today, https://www.medicalnewstoday.com/, 28 Sept. 2018, https://www.medicalnewstoday.com/articles/314698

Nappi, Allison, "5 Lies You Were Told About Grief," Rebelle Society, Rebellesociety.com, 18 Dec. 2013, http://www.rebellesociety.com/2013/12/18/5-lies-you-were-told-about-grief/

Seltzer, Leon F., Ph.D. "A Powerful Two-Step Process to Getting Rid of Unwanted Anger," *Psychology Today*, Psychologytoday.com, 16 Aug. 2012, https://www.psychologytoday.com/blog/evolution-the-self/201208/powerful-two-step-process-get-rid-unwanted-anger

Singal, Jessie, "Stop Telling Your Depressed Friends to Cheer Up," The Cut, https://www.thecut.com, 12 June 2014, https://www.thecut.com/2014/06/stop-telling-your-depressed-friends-to-cheer-up.html

Smith, Melinda, M.A., Robinson, Lawrence, and Segal, Jeanne, Ph.D. "Depression Symptoms and Warning Signs," HelpGuide, https://www.helpguide.org, Jan. 2018, https://www.helpguide.org/articles/depression/depression-symptoms-and-warning-signs.htm

Tong, Laura, "40 Ways to Let Go of Anger Right Now," Tiny Buddha, www.tinybuddha.com/blog, 8 Apr. 2018, https://tinybuddha.com/blog/40-ways-to-let-go-of-anger-right-now/

Tsaousides, Theo, Ph.D. "7 Things You Need to Know About Fear," *Psychology Today*, PsychologyToday.com, 19 Nov. 2015, https://www.psychologytoday.com/blog/smashing-the-brainblocks/201511/7-things-you-need-know-about-fear

Van Epps, Heather, Ph.D. "Seeing Red: Coping With Anger During Cancer," CURE, https://www.curetoday.com, 10 June 2012, https://www.curetoday.com/publications/cure/2012/summer2012/seeing-red-coping-with-anger-during-cancer

Wilson, Robert Evans, Jr. "The Most Powerful Motivator—How Fear Is Etched Into our Brains," *Psychology Today*, www.psychologytoday.com, 23 Sept. 2009, https://www.psychologytoday.com/us/blog/the-main-ingredient/200909/the-most-powerful-motivator

"Coping With Anger," ASCO Cancer.Net, Managing Emotions, http://www.cancer.net, January 2016, http://www.cancer.net/coping-with-cancer/managing-emotions/coping-with-anger

"Living as a Breast Cancer Survivor," American Cancer Society, Living as a Breast Cancer Survivor, Cancer.org, 22 Aug. 2017, https://www.cancer.org/cancer/breast-cancer/living-as-a-breast-cancer-survivor/emotions-and-breast-cancer.html

"Emotional, Mental Health, and Mood Changes," American Cancer Society, Cancer.org, 24 May 2016, https://www.cancer.org/treatment/treatments-and-side-effects/physical-side-effects/emotional-mood-changes.html

Chapter 15—Cancer and Sex

Lenbuck, Jonathan, "How Does Sex Differ From Intimacy?" PsychCentral, www.psychcentral.com, 26 Apr. 2013, https://psychcentral.com/ blog/ how-does-sex-differ-from-intimacy/

Mapes, Diane, "Your Body, After Cancer," Fred Hutch, https://www. fredhutch.org/en.html , 6 Mar. 2015, https://www.fredhutch.org/ en/news/center-news/2015/03/your-body-after-cancer.html

Mapes, Diane, "The Sexual Aftermath of Cancer," Fred Hutch, https://www. fredhutch.org/en.html, 28 July 2016, https://www.fredhutch.org/en/ news/center-news/2016/07/the-sexual-aftermath-of-cancer.html

Mapes, Diane, "Your Post-Cancer Treatment Sex Rx," Fred Hutch, https:// www.fredhutch.org/en.html, 29 July 2016, http://www.fredhutch .org/en/news/center-news/2016/07/your-post-cancer-treatment- sex-advice.html

"Female Sexual Health After Cancer," Livestrong, https://www.livestrong .org, 12 Feb. 2018, https://www.livestrong.org/we-can-help/ finishing-treatment/female-sexual-health-after-cancer

"How Surgery Can Affect the Sex Life of Females With Cancer," American Cancer Society, http://www.cancer.org, 12 Jan. 2017, http://www. cancer.org/treatment/treatmentsandsideeffects/physicalsideeffects/ sexualsideeffectsinwomen/sexualityforthewoman/sexuality-for- women-with-cancer-breast-surgery

"Self-Image and Sexuality," National Cancer Institute, https://www.cancer. gov/, 12 Feb. 2021, https://www.cancer.gov/about-cancer/coping/ self-image#dating

"Single Women: Finding Your Way," Breastcancer.org, www.breast cancer. org, 1 Mar. 2017, http://www.breastcancer.org/tips/intimacy/single

"Managing Female Sexual Problems Related to Cancer," American Cancer Society, Sex and the Woman With Cancer, http://www.cancer.org, 12 Jan. 2012, https://www.cancer.org/treatment/treatments-and- side-effects/physical-side-effects/fertility-and-sexual-side-effects/ sexuality-for-women-with-cancer/problems.html

"The Use of Vaginal Estrogen in Women With a History of Estrogen-Dependent Breast Cancer," The American College of Obstetricians and Gynecologists, Obstetrics & Gynecology (*The Green Journal*), https://www.acog.org, March 2016, https://www.acog.org/Clinical-Guidance-and-Publications/Committee-Opinions/Committee-on-Gynecologic-Practice/The-Use-of-Vaginal-Estrogen-in-Women-With-a-History-of-Estrogen-Dependent-Breast-Cancer

Chapter 16—Getting Support

Bianchi, Jane, "Things You Should Never Say to Someone Who Has Cancer," YahooLife, https://www.yahoo.com, 8 Aug. 2014, https://www.yahoo.com/lifestyle/things-you-should-never-say-to-someone-who-has-cancer-93414490137.html

Miller, Elana, M.D. "44 Ways to Make the Day of Someone With Cancer," HuffPost, www.huffingtonpost.com, 12 Aug. 2014, https://www.huffpost.com/entry/living-with-cancer_b_5660514

"Support After a Breast Cancer Diagnosis," Susan G. Komen, https://ww5.komen.org. 2017, https://ww5.komen.org/uploadedFiles/_Komen/Content/About_Breast_Cancer/Tools_and_Resources/Fact_Sheets_and_Breast_Self_Awareness_Cards/Getting%20the%20Support%20you%20Need.pdf

"Cancer Support Groups," National Cancer Institute, www.cancer.gov, 2 Dec. 2014, https://www.cancer.gov/about-cancer/coping/adjusting-to-cancer/support-groups

Chapter 17—Caregivers and Supporters

Levine, Carol, "Top 10 Things Caregivers Don't Want to Hear," Well Spouse Association, http://www.wellspouse.org, 2006, http://www.wellspouse.org/spousal-caregiving/top-10-things-caregivers- don-t-want-to-hear.html

Span, Paula, "The Reluctant Caregiver," *The New York Times*, https://newoldage.blogs.nytimes.com, 20 Feb. 2013, https://newoldage.blogs.nytimes.com/2013/02/20/the-reluctant-caregiver/

Stalter, Michael, "Keeping It Together When Your Wife Has Cancer," The Good Men Project, https://goodmenproject.com, 8 Sept. 2018, https://goodmenproject.com/featured-content/keeping-it-together-when-your-wife-has-cancer-dg/

"Caregiver Burnout and Stress," Help for Cancer Caregivers, https://www.helpforcancercaregivers.org, 2018, https://www.helpforcancercaregivers.org/content/caregiver-burnout

"How to Be a Friend to Someone With Cancer," American Cancer Society, www.cancer.org, 25 Jan. 2016, https://www.cancer.org/treatment/understanding-your-diagnosis/talking-about-cancer/how-to-be-a-friend-to-someone-with-cancer.html

"Support for Caregivers of Cancer Patients," National Cancer Institute, https://www.cancer.gov, 6 Nov. 2017, https://www.cancer.gov/about-cancer/coping/caregiver-support

Chapter 18—Remission, Recurrence, Survivor

Carr, Kris, "Living With Cancer: Eight Things You Need to Know," *Scientific American*, www.scientificamerican.com, 16 July 2008, https://www.scientificamerican.com/article/living-with-cancer-8-things/

Gubar, Susan, "Living With Cancer: Chronic, Not Cured," *The New York Times*, www.nytimes.com, 5 June 2014, https://well.blogs.nytimes.com/2014/06/05/living-with-cancer-chronic-not-cured/

Hendriksen, Ellen, Ph.D. "Six Tips for Handling Survivor Guilt," *Psychology Today*, www.psychologtoday.com, 22 Nov. 2017, https://www.psychologytoday.com/us/blog/how-be-yourself/201711/six-tips-handling-survivor-guilt

Kneier, Andrew, Ph.D., Rosenbaum, Ernest, M.D., Rosenbaum, Isadora R., M.A., "Coping With Cancer: Ten Steps Toward Emotional Well-Being," Stanford Medicine, Ernest and Isadora Rosenbaum Library, http://med.stanford.edu, 2018, http://med.stanford.edu/survivingcancer/coping-with-cancer/coping-with-cancer.html

Roland, James, "Stage 4 Breast Cancer Recurrence and Remission," Healthline, https://www.healthline.com/, 26 Aug. 2020, https://www.healthline.com/health/stage-4-breast-cancer-recurrence- and-remission

Weiss, Marisa, M.D., Wojciechowski, Brian, M.D., Gupta, Sameer, M.D., M.P.H. "Recurrent Breast Cancer," Breastcancer.org, http://www.breastcancer.org, 14 Feb. 2018, https://www.breastcancer.org/symptoms/diagnosis/recurrent

"13 Facts About Metastatic Breast Cancer," Metastatic Breast Cancer Network, http://www.mbcn.org, 2018, http://www.mbcn.org/13-facts-about-metastatic-breast-cancer/

"Breast Cancer Recurrence," Susan G. Komen, https://ww5.komen .org, 9 May 2017, https://ww5.komen.org/BreastCancer/ReturnofCancerafterTreatment.html

"Managing Cancer as a Chronic Illness," American Cancer Society, https://www.cancer.org, 16 Feb. 2016, https://www.cancer.org/treatment/survivorship-during-and-after-treatment/when-cancer-doesnt-go-away.html

"Metastatic Breast Cancer Symptoms & Diagnosis," Breastcancer.org, http://www.breastcancer.org, 6 Feb. 2018, http://www.breastcancer.org/symptoms/types/recur_metast/metastic

"Second Cancers After Breast Cancer," American Cancer Society, https://www.cancer.org, 21 Aug. 2017, https://www.cancer.org/cancer/breast-cancer/living-as-a-breast-cancer-survivor/second-cancers-after-breast-cancer.html

"Treatment of Stage IV (Metastatic) Breast Cancer," American Cancer Society, https://www.cancer.org, 1 Feb. 2018, https://www.cancer.org/cancer/breast-cancer/treatment/treatment-of-breast-cancer-by-stage/treatment-of-stage-iv-advanced-breast-cancer.html

"What is 'Cure'?" Memorial Sloan Kettering Cancer Center, https://www.mskcc.org, 2018, https://www.mskcc.org/experience/living-beyond-cancer/resources-survivors/what-cure

Chapter 19—The New Normal

Annis, Bonnie, "Treatment Is Over, Now What? Transitioning Back Into Life Before Cancer," Cure, https://www.curetoday.com, 2 Mar. 2016, https://www.curetoday.com/community/bonnie-annis/2016/03/treatment-is-over-now-what-transitioning-back-into-life- before-cancer

Florida, Richard, "It's Not the Food Deserts: It's the Inequality," City Lab Equity, https://www.citylab.com, 18 Jan. 2018, https://www.citylab.com/equity/2018/01/its-not-the-food-deserts-its-the-inequality/550793/

Jaquad, Suleika, "Lost in Transition After Cancer," *The New York Times*, https://well.blogs.nytimes.com, 16 Mar. 2015, https://well.blogs.nytimes.com/2015/03/16/lost-in-transition-after-cancer/

"Stress Diaries Identifying Causes of Short-Term Stress," Mindtools, https://www.mindtools.comhttps://, 2018, www.mindtools.com/pages/article/newTCS_01.htm

"The Importance of Follow-Up Care," Cancer.Net, https://www.cancer.net, April 2018, https://www.cancer.net/survivorship/follow-care-after-cancer-treatment/importance-follow-care

"Transitioning Your Breast Cancer Care From MSK to a Primary Care Doctor," Memorial Sloan Kettering Cancer Center, Memorial Sloan Kettering Cancer Center (mskcc.org), 28 Oct. 2016, https://www.mskcc.org/cancer-care/patient-education/transitioning-your-breast-care-mskcc-primary-care-doctor

Chapter 20—Prelude to a Postscript

Beaumont, Atalanta, "We Need to Talk About Death," Psychology.com, Psychologytoday.com, 9 Mar. 2018,https://www.psychologytoday.com/us/blog/handy-hintshumans/201703/we-need-talk about-death

Block, Sandra, "4 Key End-of-Life Documents to Get in Order," Kiplinger's, https://www.kiplinger.com, 2014, https://www.kiplinger.com/article/retirement/T021-C000-S002-4-key-end-of-life-documents-to-get-in-order.html

Curtis, Glenn, "6 Estate Planning Must-Haves," Investopedia, https://www.investopedia.com, 13 Dec. 2017, https://www.investopedia.com/articles/pf/07/estate_plan_checklist.asp

Dokoupil, Tony, "Grave Gardening: Tending More Than Just Flowers," CBS News, www.cbsnews.com, 22 Apr. 2018, https://www.cbsnews.com/news/grave-gardening-tending-more-than-just-flowers/

Klosowski, Thorin, "One Day, You're Going to Die. Here's How to Prepare for It," Lifehacker, https://lifehacker.com/, 28 Mar. 2013, https://lifehacker.com/5992722/one-day-youre-going-to-die-heres-how-to-prepare-for-it?commerce_insets_disclosure=on&utm_expid=66866090-48.Ej9760cOTJCPS_Bq4mjoww.2&utm_referrer=https%3A%2F%2Fwww.google.com%252

Pennington, Jackie, "Morbid History: The Victorian Art of Mourning," The Pennington Edition, Tiny Comical History, www.thepenningtonedition wordpress.com, 22 Feb. 2012, https://thepenningtonedition.wordpress .com/2012/02/22/the-victorian-art-of-mourning/

Sayward, Suzanne, "Five Ways in Which a Trust Is Better Than a Will," Samuel, Sayward & Baler, https://ssbllc.com/, 8 May 2018, https://ssbllc.com/articles/five-ways-in-which-a-trust-is-better-than-a-will/

Sabitino, Charles, JD, "Advance Directives," Merck Manual, https://www.merckmanuals.com/home , 2016, https://www.merckmanuals.com/home/fundamentals/legal-and-ethical-issues/advance-directives

Villet-Lagomarsino, Ann, "Hospice vs Palliative Care," National Caregivers Library, http://www.caregiverslibrary.org/, 31 Aug. 2017, http://www.caregiverslibrary.org/caregivers-resources/grp-end-of-life-issues/hsgrp-hospice/hospice-vs-palliative-care-article.aspx

Wood, Ruth, "We Need to Talk About Death: Why We Should All Make End-of-Life Preparations," The Telegraph Lifestyle, https://www.telegraph.co.uk/, 26 July 2015, We http://www.telegraph.co.uk/lifestyle/11756068/We-need-to-talk-about-death.html

"Coping With Impending Death," WebMD, https://www.webmd.com/, 26 Aug. 2015, https://www.webmd.com/mental-health/features/coping-with-impending-death#4

"Deciding About Health Care," New York Department of Health, *A Guide for Patients and Families*, pages 1-6, May 2010

"End of Life: Caring for a Dying Loved One," Mayo Clinic, https://www.mayoclinic.org/, 5 Apr. 2017, https://www.mayoclinic.org/healthy-lifestyle/end-of-life/in-depth/cancer/art-20047600

"Estate Planning—Keeping Track of Passwords, Access Keys and PINs," FindLaw, Estate Planning, https://www.findlaw.com/, 19 Mar. 2018, http://estate.findlaw.com/planning-an-estate/estate-planning-keep-track-of-passwords-access-keys-and-pins.html

"Estate planning: Types of trusts," CNN Business, https://money.cnn.com, 24 Mar. 2017, https://money.cnn.com/pf/money-essentials-trusts/index.html

"Hospice Care," Medline Plus, MedlinePlus.gov 13 Oct. 2016, MedlinePlus .gov, 19 Mar. 2018 https://medlineplus.gov/hospicecare.html

"How to Prepare for the Death of a Loved One," wikiHow, https://www.wikihow.com, Sept. 2017, https://www.wikihow.com/Prepare-for-the-Death-of-a-Loved-One

"Palliative Care in Cancer," National Cancer Institute, Cancer.gov, 20 Oct. 2017, https://www.cancer.gov/about-cancer/advanced-cancer/care-choices/palliative-care-fact-sheet#q1

"Palliative Care," Medline Plus, MedlinePlus.gov 26 Mar. 2015, https://medlineplus.gov/palliativecare.html

"What Is Estate Planning?" Estate Planning, https://www.estate planning.com, 2018, https://www.estateplanning.com/What-is-Estate-Planning/

Afterword: Breast Health

Bramlet, Kellie, "3D Mammograms: What You Should Know," MD Anderson Cancer Center, www.mdanderson.org, Oct. 2015, https://www.mdanderson.org/publications/focused-on-health/october-2015/FOH-3D-mammography.html

Foy, Kenya, "8 Completely Natural Ways Your Breasts Change as You Grow Older," Hello Giggles, www.hellogiggles.com, 1 June 2017, https://hellogiggles.com/lifestyle/health-fitness/ways-breasts-change-get-older/

Matlick, Arlene, "How to Become an Empowered Patient," SHARE Cancer Support, https://www.sharecancersupport.org/, 2018, https://www.sharecancersupport.org/educational-programs/pink-and-teal-seminars/

Miller, Redonda, M.D. "Breast Cancer Screening," National Center for Biotechnology Information, www.ncbi.nih.gov, 16 Mar. 2001, https://www.ncbi.nlm.nih.gov/pmc/articles/PMC1495188/

"Breast Cancer Risk Factors You Cannot Change," American Cancer Society, www.cancer.org, 6 Sept. 2017, https://www.cancer.org/cancer/breast-cancer/risk-and-prevention/breast-cancer-risk-factors-you-cannot-change.html

"Breast Cancer Signs and Symptoms" American Cancer Society, www.cancer.org, 22 Sept. 2017, https://www.cancer.org/cancer/breast-cancer/about/breast-cancer-signs-and-symptoms.html

"Breast Exams," Johns Hopkins Medicine, https://www.hopkinsmedicine.org, 2018, Breast https://www.hopkinsmedicine.org/kimmel_cancer_center/centers/breast_cancer_program/treatment_and_services/risk_and_prevention/breast_exam.html

"Breast Health," Jean Hailes for Women's Health, https://jeanhailes.org.au, 2018, https://jeanhailes.org.au/health-a-z/breast-health

"Breast Self-Exam for Breast Awareness," MayoClinic, https://www.mayoclinic.org, 2018, https://www.mayoclinic.org/tests-procedures/breast-exam/about/pac-20393237

"Breast Ultrasound" American Cancer Society, www.cancer.org, 2018, https://www.cancer.org/cancer/breast-cancer/screening-tests-and-early-detection/breast-ultrasound.html

"Dense Breast Tissue: What It Means to Have Dense Breasts," Mayo Clinic, Mammograms, www.mayoclinic.org, 23 Mar. 2018, https://

www.mayoclinic.org/tests-procedures/mammogram/in-depth/dense-breast-tissue/art-20123968

"Eat Healthy, Active Living Videos," American Cancer Society, Healthy Living, Active Living Videos, https://www.cancer.org, 2015, https://www.cancer.org/healthy/eat-healthy-get-active/healthy-eating-active-living-videos.html

"Mammograms," National Cancer Institute, https://www.cancer.gov/, 7 Dec. 2016, https://www.cancer.gov/types/breast/mammograms-fact-sheet

"Digital vs. Film Screening Mammography," Susan G. Komen, https://ww5.komen.org, 7 May 2018, https://ww5.komen.org/Breast Cancer Table31Digitalmammographyversusstandardmammography forbreastcancerscreening.html

"What Are the Risk Factors for Breast Cancer?" Centers for Disease Control and Prevention, www.cdc.gov, 27 Sept. 2017, https://www.cdc.gov/cancer/breast/basic_info/risk_factors.htm

Index

About the Author

Theresa Drescher is a life and career coach, an entrepreneur, the director of a nonprofit and a twenty-two-year breast cancer survivor. She is the author of *The Upside to Everything, Even Breast Cancer.*

Ms. Drescher moved to New York City in 1982 and spent the next twenty-five years traveling the world as a buyer and product development manager, eventually becoming a director of marketing and product development for Avon Products, Inc. In 1999, two months after she left her corporate job and started her own design company, she was diagnosed with breast cancer. After she survived her ordeal, she knew she had to share her valuable knowledge to help others manage their cancer experience.

In 2000, she started volunteering for a breast cancer helpline in New York City to share with other women what she had learned about being diagnosed. For more than twenty years she answered questions, gave advice, explained documents, laid out action plans, lent an ear and supported women through tough times and triumphs, all of which she shares in this book. Since 2014 she has spoken publicly about the signs of breast cancer and how to become an empowered patient.

In 2001, she founded City Santa Inc., an all-volunteer nonprofit she runs with her husband, Michael, that benefits children in cancer hospice, at-risk youth, women and children in domestic violence shelters, adults in homeless shelters, and families in crisis. Theresa and Michael live in the East Village of New York City.